A LEARNING SYSTEM IN HISTOLOGY

CD-ROM

DEBORAH W. VAUGHAN, PH.D.
LARS HANSEN

AND GUIDE

DEBORAH W. VAUGHAN, PH.D.

OXFORD
UNIVERSITY PRESS

2002

Oxford   New York

Auckland   Bangkok   Buenos Aires   Cape Town   Chennai
Dar es Salaam   Delhi   Hong Kong   Istanbul   Karachi   Kolkata
Kuala Lumpur   Madrid   Melbourne   Mexico City   Mumbai   Nairobi
São Paulo   Shanghai   Singapore   Taipei   Tokyo   Toronto

and associated companies in
Berlin   Ibadan

Published by Oxford University Press Inc.,
198 Madison Avenue, New York, New York 10016
http://www.oup-usa.org

Oxford is a registered trademark of Oxford University Press.

Library of Congress Cataloging-in-Publication Data
Vaughan, Deborah W.
A learning system in histology : CD-ROM and guide/
Deborah W. Vaughan.
p. cm.   ISBN 0-19-515173-9
I. Histology—Laboratory manuals.
I. Title
QM555 . V38 2002   611'.018—dc21   2001050006

For technical support *only* :
Email: techsupport@oup-usa.org
Fax: 1-914-747-3590
Toll Free Tel: 1-877-773-4325
Direct Tel: 1-914-773-4325

For all other customer service requests, call: 1-800-445-9714

2 4 6 8 9 7 5 3 1

Printed in the United States of America
on acid-free paper.

A Learning System in Histology

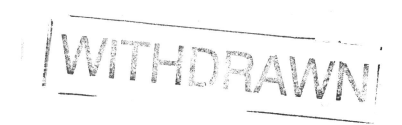

An accompanying

CD is enclosed

inside this book

PREFACE

The printed Guide and multiplatform CD-ROM provide a virtual histology laboratory experience for the user. The CD-ROM database contains over 2000 page files. Most of the CD-ROM images are grouped in nested series of images that progress from low-power views useful for orientation to higher-power views, following the standard approach to studying histology microscope slides in the laboratory. Over 75 ultrastructural images are included on the CD-ROM reflecting the increasing importance of electron microscopy in understanding cell structure and function.

The CD-ROM and the Guide are designed to be used together, but they can also be used separately. The CD-ROM might be used alone for self-study, for reference, or to review for licensing board examinations. The Guide offers a highly organized approach to the laboratory study of microscopic anatomy, and provides concise text emphasizing key concepts. The Guide and CD-ROM together are designed to supplement a comprehensive histology textbook or course.

PEDAGOGIC DESIGN

This two-part set is uniquely designed as a learning system. The printed Guide not only provides a structured laboratory experience but also promotes a means to learn microscopic anatomy in a manner that makes it understandable and intuitive. In recognition of the importance of context for successful recall of the vocabulary and images of histology, the Guide emphasizes three contexts:

- the context of a morphological continuum from gross anatomy to the light microscopic and sometimes ultrastructural level,
- the context of structure–function relationships within and between cells, tissues, and organs, and
- the context of vocabulary word roots, many of which provide clues to functional or morphological features.

The main section of the CD-ROM provides a virtual microscope experience with the advantages of speed, volume, flexibility, and interactivity possible with this medium. It is organized into the same laboratory topics as the Guide. Within each topic, the user selects the desired microscope slide from the list and, by clicking on its name, loads a full color low-power image similar to what is visible with an unaided or 10x examination of such a slide. All images to which sequentially higher magnification images are linked are marked with a simple box representing hotspot(s) linked to those images. The location of the box(es) corresponds to the location of the linked images. To promote understanding of relationships and structural variability, most linked higher magnification images are similar to the tissue section to which they are linked, but not necessarily derived from the same tissue section. Multiple examples are provided to illustrate certain organs or parts of organs.

Every light microscope image in the CD-ROM laboratory exercise is a full color image from which the user can toggle to a grey-scale, comprehensively labeled identical image. No text accompanies the images in the main database other than an occasional annotation of function or categorization within the confines of the image.

GUIDE

The printed Guide is designed like a Histology Laboratory Guide. The first two chapters, however, set the philosophy for successful cognitive processing of the terms and images. The following 20 chapters cover the standard histology topics of cells, tissues, organs, and systems. Each chapter begins with an overview of the topic: its general purpose and basic structural patterns. Each chapter lists its topic-specific vocabulary with word roots to aid in understanding and recall of the names. In most chapters the subject matter is diagrammatically organized in a flowchart format, progressing from general structures to more specific structures, to illustrate relationships among the component parts. To establish the macroscopic end of the morphological continuum, most system chapters include a simple anatomical diagram indicating the location of the organs represented in the chapter's tissue images. Summary tables are included in several of the chapters. The virtual laboratory exercise itself proceeds sequentially through a series of microscope slides, just as in an actual laboratory exercise, using images on the CD-ROM. In the printed Guide, each microscope slide image series is introduced with a small grey-scale reproduction of the lead-in image on the CD-ROM, with a list of the higher magnification images that are linked to the lead-in image. Each of these printed images in the Guide is accompanied by a description of the histological stain, embedding medium and section thickness, and source.

CD-ROM

The CD-ROM is the truly unique component of this learning package. Its program is designed to be user-friendly and efficient. The interface is standard and consistent throughout the program and the toolbar is intuitive: the user can toggle between labeled and unlabeled images, move back one image, move to the main topic page, and activate a help page.

The CD-ROM offers multiple routes into the database of images:

- BY TOPIC (the main index). The user can select from 21 standard topics of histology. These topics correspond to the chapters of the Guide. Within each of these standard topics, a list of the relevant microscope slides (identified by label and stain) provides links to low-power images that are in turn linked to higher-power images. In addition, on each topic page a comprehensive list of the identifiable cells and structures is included for that topic; each item in the list of cells and structures is linked to at least one labeled image page.
- BY ANATOMICAL FIGURE. A simple diagram of an anatomical figure illustrates the system of interest. The location and orientation of the slides (images) in the database are indicated on this anatomical figure, and the user can click on the slide number and load that image page. Links are made to both light and electron microscope images.
- BY SCHEMATIC, TABLE, OR CHART. Summary information, such as tables describing the comparative features of blood vessels or schematics of the terminal differentiation of hemopoietic cells are provided. Illustrating images are linked to items in the charts, tables and schematics.
- BY THUMBNAIL. Thumbnail low-power images of each lead-in tissue section (the 2–15X views) are provided with slide and item's name and histological stain, organized by topic. Each thumbnail image is linked to the unlabeled image page.
- BY SLIDE NUMBER. A sequential list of all of the microscope slides in the collection is provided. Slides that are used to illustrate more than one feature are repeated for each feature. Each is linked to the low-power image pages in the database.
- BY KEYWORD. This is a comprehensive list of structures illustrated in the database and it serves as a valuable entry point for the user who seeks specific information. All of the items listed have at least one link to a labeled image page.
- COMMON CONFUSIONS. Certain organelles, cells, tissues, and organs are commonly confused by students of histology. In this section, images are used in conjunction with text to enable the student to differentiate among

two to four similar structures. The explanations are based on functionally relevant distinguishing morphological features.

- APPENDICES. There are three appendices:

    A. Histological Stains. This appendix includes descriptions of commonly used histological stains with linked examples of those stains.

    B. Taxonomic Key. This is a comprehensive guide to differentiating among organs and subdivisions of organs.

    C. Glossary. This section includes definitions of common terms. An extensive list of common Latin and Greek prefixes, suffixes, and word roots is provided to help the user understand the vocabulary of histology.

TECHNICAL NOTES

The images of the CD–ROM are derived from the collection of microscope slides and electron micrographs used in the Boston University School of Medicine medical histology course. Most of the microscope slides used for the images have been prepared by our own histology technicians over several decades, using human and nonhuman primate material.

With regard to the technical design of the CD-ROM program, image resolution was selected to have the ideal balance between high quality imaging and small file size so the images are quick loading and illustrate what needs to be seen. Images of different magnification are individual files, all of approximately the same file size. All images are designed to fit the screen of a standard laptop computer, so there is no need for scrollbars or resizing windows. The images are scientifically and aesthetically consistent.

Boston, Massachusetts   D.W.V

Contents

A LEARNING SYSTEM IN HISTOLOGY

1. INTRODUCTION: BASIC SKILLS

This chapter provides an introduction to both the art and the science of histology. It presents the following basic topics to facilitate the successful mastery of histology:

- the vocabulary of histology
- standard planes of section encountered in histology
- the appearance of solid objects in tissue sections
- standard preparative procedures used to produce tissue sections
- a systematic thinking strategy to facilitate the identification of cells and organs

There is no shortcut to learning how to recognize and identify the microscopic features of tissues and organs accurately. Like any discipline, there is a vast amount to absorb and understand and apply. Yes, it is necessary to memorize hundreds of new names and terms as part of mastering this discipline, but developing a context for all those cells and structures will facilitate successful recall. The skills required to interpret microscope images involve the application of acquired knowledge about the microscopic structure of the body. This chapter explains how to organize and approach microscopic anatomy in an intelligent manner so that what is learned remains retrievable and easily integrated into other areas of study.

A comprehensive textbook provides more details about the functional significance of the morphological features illustrated in this Guide and CD-ROM. It is important to recognize the inseparability of structure and function, as this connection is key to the ability to interpret and understand a microscope image. In this Guide, simple structure–function relationships are described to encourage that thoughtful approach and to make the images more meaningful, interesting, and easier to remember.

THE VOCABULARY OF HISTOLOGY

Many of the terms in histology, like the vocabulary of most sciences, have Latin or Greek word roots that reveal details about the cell or structure, usually details of its function or morphology. If you translate the name, you have a valuable clue as to what that cell or structure looks like or what it does. Many of these word roots are included in this Guide, and a compiled list of common word roots, prefixes, and suffixes, is included in Appendix C of the CD-ROM.

Histology is a visual discipline that uses standardized descriptions of its microscopic entities. Chapter 2 introduces some of the general terms that are used to describe cells and their morphological characteristics — the basic working tools of descriptive histology. The exercises that follow present terms that are used to describe cells and tissues in specific organs and systems. As with all biomedical sciences, precise terms describe specific entities, and in order to communicate effectively, it is necessary to learn the vocabulary of histology.

STANDARD PLANES OF SECTION
ENCOUNTERED IN HISTOLOGY

Relating two-dimensional images to the three-dimensional structures from which they come is one of the more challenging aspects of histology and it is a skill that comes more easily to some people than to others. The standard planes of section into which a solid object may be cut are always expressed with respect to the long axis of that object, whether that object be an organelle, a part of a cell, a tissue, an organ, or a part of an organ. Thus in the diagram in Figure 1-1, the drawn object can represent any one of

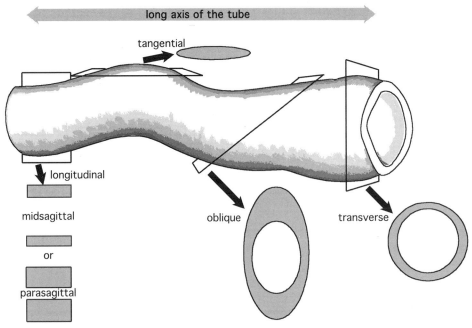

Figure 1-1. Diagrammatic representation of a tubular structure penetrated by plates in four standard planes of section. The arrows point to profiles of sections typical of those produced by sectioning in each of these planes.

these structures. The standard planes are as follows:

- Longitudinal or sagittal: a tissue section that is oriented parallel to the long axis of the object. Parasagittal refers to a longitudinal section that is located to the side of the center of the object. A section that is located in the center plane is termed a midsagittal section.
- Tangential: a glazing section through the edge of the object.
- Oblique: a section oriented at an angle to the long axis of the object.
- Transverse: a section oriented perpendicular to the long axis of the object.

The appearance of histological structures can vary considerably with the plane of section: a tangential section through a sheet of epithelial cells may appear to be an abnormal multicellular tumor to the unprepared student, or a section through an intestinal villus may appear to be a cluster of cells floating free in the lumen of the gut. It is possible to interpret successfully all planes of section by examining histological material thoughtfully first at low magnification and searching for clues that reveal the shape of the solid object from which the tissue section is derived. With time, the ability to "see" a solid object in a single representative tissue section will develop.

THE APPEARANCE OF SOLID OBJECTS IN TISSUE SECTIONS

A single whole cell in an unsectioned preparation, such as in a smear of peripheral blood that has been spread on a glass microscope slide and stained, can appear quite different from that same cell cut into 2 μm–thick sections. Most histological material is examined in tissue sections that have been prepared by cutting a solid block of tissue into sections that can range in thickness from less than a micrometer to several micrometers. A histological tissue section is therefore only a thin slice through a whole cell or organ and since the section is only a part of the whole it may not have all the mophological characteristics of the whole. As your experience increases, you will develop a sense of which morphological features of a cell, structure, or organ are critically important to enable your correct identification and which features do not have to be present in order to identify the cell or structure. An understanding of the effects of sectioning, in addition to an understanding of the functional significance of various morphological characteristics, will aid in the correct interpretation of microscopic images.

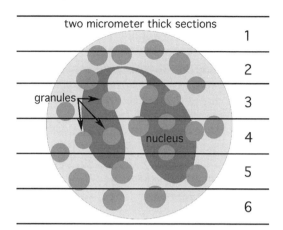

Figure 1-2. Diagrammatic representation of an eosinophil sectioned into a series of six sections, each 2 μm–thick.

Consider the eosinophil, one of the cells present in peripheral blood that is examined in a blood smear preparation in Chapter 2. The name of this cell reflects the presence of pink-stained eosinophilic (*eosin,* a standard histological stain + *-philic,* liking) granules in its cytoplasm. Such a cell is schematically diagrammed in Figure 1-2. In a blood smear preparation the cells of blood are spread thinly on a glass microscope slide and dried onto the surface; the cells are viewed in their entirety and all their morphological features are present. The eosinophil is seen to have a circular cell profile with a diameter of approximately 12 μm, a segmented nucleus (meaning nuclear lobes connected by a thin nuclear strand), and cytoplasm filled with uniform bright pink-stained granules. When that eosinophil is sectioned as part of a tissue block, all these morphological features may not be present, but that should not prevent its correct identification.

Consider the consequences of sectioning a cell like the eosinophil into a series of six 2 μm–thick sections. To help visualize this phenomenon in three dimensions, consider the analogy of a hard-boiled egg cut into slices. As with that egg, all sections passing through the cell do not pass through its largest dimension, so all the profiles (pieces) are not equal in diameter. As illustrated in the diagram (Figure 1-2), the diameters of the tangential 2–μm sections, numbers 1 and 6, are less than the diameters of the sections passing through the cell's center, numbered 3 and 4. Also, observe that of the six sections, only four (numbered 2–5) contain enough of the lobed nucleus to be recognizable in section. Furthermore, in this cell with its segmented nucleus, the nucleus appears as one piece in section number 2 and as two separate pieces in sections numbered 3, 4, and 5. Finally, sections 1 and 6 consist of cytoplasm containing only the cell-specific granules.

With this concept of a sectioned cell in mind, it is understandable why it is possible to correctly identify a given cell when only part of it is visible in a tissue section. Many cells, like this eosinophil, have very characteristic cytoplasmic or other morphological features. In the case of this eosinophil, you will learn that this is the only cell with eosinophilic granules that is normally present in peripheral blood and in connective tissue. Therefore, a cellular fragment containing eosinophilic granules (in standard histological preparations) can only be part of an eosinophil.

This kind of logical reasoning, based on learned expectations regarding the tissue section, can be applied to every cell, structure, tissue, and organ examined in histological slides or images. It is key to the skills that lead to mastery in histology.

STANDARD PREPARATIVE PROCEDURES USED TO PRODUCE TISSUE SECTIONS

Section thickness, plane of section, and tissue preparation all affect the visual image of solid cells and tissues and their parts. To this end, part of the learned expectations brought to the material examined in histology is a set of expectations regarding the effects of various standard preparative procedures on the tissue section. Attempt to relate the static image of a tissue section to the dynamic, functioning organ from which it came.

To produce most of the microscope slides like those depicted in the CD-ROM, a tissue block of an organ is fixed, processed, and embedded in plastic (a methyl methacrylate) or paraffin, sectioned with a microtome, and stained with hematoxylin and eosin (commonly abbreviated as H&E). The plastic embedding medium is typically a harder substance than paraffin and the increased hardness enables the production of relatively thinner tissue sections. Thinner sections can provide improved visualization of microscopic details because there is less superimposition of section components when you look through the section mounted on a slide. As an example of this visual phenomenon, imagine looking at a row of people standing on a theater stage in front of you: it is easier to see details of individual people if they are standing in a single row rather than standing in rows three or more people deep.

Hematoxylin and eosin are the standard and most frequently used histological stains, and they are usually used in combination with one another. With H&E, materials that exist with a net negative charge in tissue sections, such as nucleic acids and glycosaminoglycans, stain blue with hematoxylin, and materials that exist with a net positive charge in tissue sections, such as myofibrils and collagen, stain pink with the eosin. Materials with no net charge do not bind the charged stain molecules. This simple differentiation can provide the histologist with a great deal of information about the structure, function, and activity of the cells and tissues. Most of the images on the CD-ROM are stained with H&E, but the image database also includes material that has been stained with other common histological stains, stains that are used to demonstrate specific cellular or extracellular materials in the tissue sections. A summary of the staining characteristics of commonly used histological stains is included in Appendix A of the CD-ROM.

A SYSTEMATIC THINKING STRATEGY TO FACILITATE CORRECT IDENTIFICATION OF CELLS AND ORGANS

The exercises in this Guide will enable you to identify several hundred cells and structures that comprise the microscopic anatomy of organs. To simplify this activity, it is useful to develop a systematic thinking process (not unique to this discipline) that can lead to the successful identification of cells, tissues and organs in histology. Without such a strategy, you would have to memorize thousands of morphological images and sort thorough hundreds of possibilities in your mind each time you seek to identify a cell, part of a cell, an organ, or part of an organ. Clearly, such a cumbersome process is not only inefficient but also unreliable. With an organized strategy, you use your learned expectations and systematically progress from the unknown to the known.

The key to identifying any histological material is to begin with broad categorizations, and systematically rule out possibilities as you examine the slide material. From the broad beginning you progress to a narrower set of expectations, and on to the next narrower set until finally you ask the final question to correctly identify what you are examining. The art of histology lies in developing an intuition for the series of the expectations you bring to your slide, and anticipating the questions that will narrow those expectations. This cognitive strategy will enable you to identify nearly everything you encounter in a microscope slide, both the normal and the abnormal.

This methodical strategy is illustrated here using the peripheral blood smear examined in the following (Chapter 2)as an example. To begin, at the first level of discovery you identify the material as a smear of peripheral blood cells. It is not difficult to recognize such a preparation of peripheral blood because nearly 99% of the cells spread out on the slide are uniform cells containing no nucleus. You know it is a smear because entire cells are dispersed on the slide and not cut into sections. Because it is a smear, you can expect to see all the appropriate morphological characteristics for each of the cells. All these expectations are to be learned from histology laboratory exercises and from a comprehensive histology course. From this point in your systematic analysis, you can further expect that if this is a normal peripheral blood smear, there are only seven cell types present — not the 200+ in the body. Furthermore, those seven cell types fall into two distinct groups: those with a nucleus and those without a nucleus. Your expectations will progress through a series of decision-trees, followed by elimination. For example, those cells without a nucleus subdivide into two distinctly different populations: a population that is very uniform in size (approximately 7 μm in diameter), round in profile, comprising the vast majority of blood cells, and a population of small (2–4 μm) cellular fragments, approximately one–tenth as numerous as the former. The former are red blood cells, and the latter, platelets. The nucleated cells also subdivide into two distinct groups: those whose nucleus is segmented (nuclear lobes connected by a thin nuclear strand), and those whose nucleus is not segmented. Your expectations tell you that within the former group of nucleated cells there are only three types of cells, and each type is uniquely characterized by the presence of cell–specific granules in its cytoplasm in this typical blood smear: one with blue-stained granules, one with pink-stained granules, and one with unstained (neutral) granules. This deductive reasoning process can be applied in both a forward and backward direction. For example, with regard to the cell with unstained granules (that is, you do not see stained granules in its cytoplasm) you can identify the cell correctly because you know (expect) that all the cells in peripheral blood that have a segmented nucleus also have granules, and if you cannot see pink or blue ones, the granules must be the neutral ones.

This diagnostic decision–making process is summarized diagrammatically above. The Guide includes several such diagrammatic flow charts to provide relevant organizational overviews. This decision–tree approach to the material can also be organized in the form of a taxonomic key, as illustrated in Chapter 2, for this same material. A comprehensive taxonomic key covering all the organs illustrated in the CD-ROM is included in Appendix B of the CD-ROM. With either approach — the diagram or the taxonomic key — the basic strategy is to begin broadly and progressively narrow your choices to a final indentification. The order you establish for this process is based on your learned expectations.

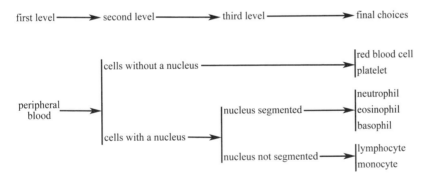

In summary, the key to the successful identification of histological images is to progress systematically to a conclusion based on the expectations you bring to the material. The expectations you bring are acquired in laboratory exercises like the ones simulated in this Guide, supplemented by a comprehensive histology course. These learned expectations include those based on understanding the preparative procedures employed in histology, as well as both the appropriate functional and broad morphological contexts.

2. PERIPHERAL BLOOD CELLS

This chapter examines peripheral blood and introduces the concept of a cell. The cell is the basic structural and functional unit of histology. Cells of the body come in a vast array of shapes and sizes, which typically relate to the variety of functions they perform. In the body, tissues and organs are composed of cells assembled together to perform functions that cannot be performed adequately by single cells alone. It is often difficult to discern individual cells in the microscope but it is very important to establish the concept of individual cells early in the study of histology. Normal and pathological events occur at the cellular level, and so the individual cell and its place in the hierarchy of progressively more complex structural units of histology cannot be underestimated.

This exercise examines the cells of peripheral blood in a smear preparation for which the cells have been dispersed on a microscope slide and stained. This chapter introduces some of the general terms used to describe cells and their morphological characteristics.

The following cells are illustrated in this section. Know the definition, morphology, and function of each. Many cells and structures in histology have more than one name, and you should be familiar with all of them. The Latin or Greek word roots of each of these names are also provided to aid in the recall of the names. Because there is a simple pattern to the construction of most histological names, understanding the source of the name or term will often facilitate remembering the cell and/or its function.

>red blood cell (RBC), erythrocyte (*erythro-*, red + -*cyte*, cell)
>white blood cell (WBC), leukocyte (*leuko-*, white + -*cyte*, cell)
>granulocyte (*granulo-*, granule + -*cyte*, cell)
>agranulocyte (*a-*, no + *granulo-*, granule + -*cyte*, cell)
>neutrophil, polymorphonuclear neutrophil (PMN, poly) (*poly-*, many + *morpho-*, form + -*nucleus*, a little nut or kernel; *neuter*, neither + -*phil*, liking)
>eosinophil, polymorphonuclear eosinophil (PME) (*eosin-*, referring to the stain eosin + -*philic*, liking)
>basophil, polymorphonuclear basophil (PMB) (*bas-*, referring to basic stains + *philic*, liking)
>lymphocyte (*lympha*, spring water + -*cyte*, cell)
>monocyte (*mono-*, one, referring to its unsegmented nucleus + -*cyte*, cell)
>platelet, thrombocyte (-*let*, a diminutive ending of *plat*, a flat object; *thrombos*, clot + -*cyte*, cell)

The formed elements of blood are studied by spreading a drop of fresh peripheral blood on a slide to produce a single layer of dispersed cells. A Romanovsky–type dye mixture (Wright's or Giemsa stain, described in Appendix A: Staining and Commonly Used Stains in the CD-ROM) is used to stain the nuclei, cytoplasm, and cytoplasmic granules of the cells that then can be identified and differentiated by type. The analysis of the morphology and relative numbers of white blood cells is a common and useful clinical test because variation in morphology and relative numbers of cells can reflect the presence of disease. The clinical test that provides the relative numbers of white blood cells in blood is known as the differential blood count.

COMMON DESCRIPTIVE FEATURES OF CELLS

Some of the characteristics used to identify cells in histology are described below. Understand the functional significance of each of these features and their variations.

- nuclear morphology. Is the cell's nucleus round? Oval? Indented? How many segments or lobes, if any? Is the nucleus dark and condensed? Pale? Absent? Is a nucleolus present? If so, how many?
- relative cell size and shape. Is the cell larger or smaller than the rather uniform red blood cells? By how much? Are the cells within the population uniform in diameter? What is the cell's shape?
- staining characteristics of cytoplasm. What stains were used in the preparation of the slide and what color is the cell's cytoplasm? What does the intensity and the hue of the coloration of the red blood cells reveal in this and any microscope preparation?
- morphology of cytoplasmic inclusions. Are there any inclusions? What size and color are they? Are they uniform in size and color?
- relative number of cells. In normal tissue (what we study in histology) information regarding the relative numbers of each cell type can be as much a key to identification as cellular morphology. However, it is necessary to scan a real peripheral blood smear to ascertain relative numbers of cells. In the series of images on the CD-ROM, you are able to surmise only that there are typically more red blood cells than white blood cells. You can learn nothing about the relative numbers of each type of white blood cell without systematically scanning a large sample area of the blood smear and recording each cell type you encounter.

CD-ROM Notice: The images examined in this chapter are identified numerically in this Guide and on the CD-ROM by their microscope slide number as they might be listed in a standard histology laboratory. There are four initial images on the CD-ROM for this exercise. One of those images, termed a lead-in image, has higher magnification images linked to hotspots. The images linked to the lead-in image on the CD-ROM are listed as higher magnification images in the notation below.

THE CELLS OF PERIPHERAL BLOOD

CELLS WITHOUT A NUCLEUS

RED BLOOD CELL. The red blood cells (erythrocytes) are the cells that contain the respiratory pigment hemoglobin that transports oxygen in the blood. Mature red blood cells have no nucleus, and because of their biconcave shape, their centers may appear pale due to the relative thinness at the center of the cell. They are uniform in shape and diameter, and measure approximately 7 µm in a dried smear preparation. They normally account for nearly 99% of the total cells in peripheral blood.

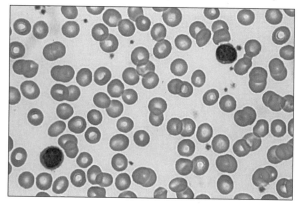

PERIPHERAL BLOOD
Slide #17: Peripheral Blood Smear; Wright's stain; smear preparation; human.

Blood smear images:
- lymphocytes and platelets
- neutrophils
- monocyte
- granulocytes
- (higher) neutrophil and eosinophil
- (higher) basophil

In all histological material, including the smear, red blood cells are invariably present and provide two valuable pieces of reference that are useful in the interpretation of histological material: (*1*) an indication of the expected coloration of acidophilic material in the preparation, and (*2*) an internal unit of measure. Among the learned expectations to be brought to this slide is that the hemoglobin of the red blood cells is acidophilic (*acid*, referring to acid stains + -*philic*, liking). How the red blood cells stain will provide a sense of how other acidophilic material will stain in a preparation. If the erythrocytes of the slide appear grayish, then the coloration of all cells will be shifted to the blue end of the spectrum, and if they appear red, the shift will be to the red end. With regard to the size of red blood cells, they are normally uniform in size, approximately 7 µm in the dried smear and approximately 8 µm in diameter in well-fixed tissue preparations.

BLOOD PLATELETS. These are small (2–4 µm) ovoid bodies that are responsible for the clotting function of blood. This function accounts for the alternative name, thrombocytes. Platelets usually stain pale blue and contain a few azurophilic (*azure*, a purplish oxidation product in the Wright's stain + -*philic*, liking) granules. The central zone (called the granulomere; *granulo-*, granule; -*mere*, a part) of the platelet appears darker than the almost clear periphery (called the hyalomere; *hyalos*, glass). Platelets are highly organized fragments pinched off of the cytoplasm of megakaryocytes (large cells located in bone marrow) and contain biologically active substances that are either synthesized by the parent cells or absorbed from the blood. The number of platelets in the blood is approximately 5%- 10% the number of red blood cells.

BLOOD CELLS WITH A NUCLEUS
The remaining cells of peripheral blood are collectively termed white blood cells (or leukocytes). There are five types of leukocytes, three of them contain cell–specific granules in their cytoplasm, and two do not. The former are classified as granulocytes and the latter are agranulocytes. The relative numbers of these leukocytes maintain a predictable range in the peripheral blood of a normal healthy individual, but that range can be exceeded in disease states.

GRANULOCYTES. These cells notably contain specific granules in their cytoplasm. This group of cells is also characterized by having a segmented nucleus, each of the several nuclear segments or lobes being connected by a thin strand of nuclear material. Because of this nuclear characteristic the cells are also known as polymorphonuclear cells. The polymorphonuclear designation is followed typically by an indication of the staining characteristics of the cell–specific granules present in the cytoplasm.

NEUTROPHIL. (polymorphonuclear neutrophil [PMN or poly]) These are typically the most numerous of the granulocytes, and also the most numerous of all the leukocytes. Neutrophils measure 12—15 µm in diameter, approximately 1.5 times the diameter of a red blood cell. Their most obvious characteristic is the highly segmented nucleus, which usually has three to five connected segments or lobes. The number of PMNs in peripheral blood with just two, or more than five, nuclear segments is a clinically relevant feature of blood. The nuclear chromatin is condensed, which for these cells is a visible sign that the cell is terminally differentiated and no longer capable of mitotic division. The cytoplasm is finely granular, owing to the presence of three classes of granules, none of which are easy to see in standard light microscope sections: small (< 0.5 µm) pale staining neutrophilic granules predominate (80%–85% of the total number of granules), accompanied by an equal number of purplish azurophilic granules and pale tertiary granules (15%–20%). The neutrophilic granules contain antibacterial proteins and enzymes; the azurophilic granules are typical lysosomes, and the tertiary granules facilitate the movement of neutrophils through connective tissue where they carry out their principal function after leaving the blood stream. Together with macrophages (*macro-*, large; *phage*, eat), the neutrophils are the principal phagocytes (*phag-*, eat; -*cyte*, cell) of the body.

EOSINOPHIL. (polymorphonuclear eosinophil; [PME]) These cells are comparatively rare in peripheral blood, typically occurring in a ratio of about one for every 50 circulating neutrophils. The nucleus is segmented, but normally has fewer lobes (2–3 lobes) than the nucleus of neutrophils. The cytoplasm is filled with uniform, relatively large, refractile, eosinophilic granules, making it easy to identify this cell type. The refractile nature of the granules is difficult to capture in photomicrographs. Eosinophils are active in immunological reactions, ingesting antigen-antibody complexes and inactivating the pharmacologically active agents formed during host responses to allergens. They are also responsive to parasitic worm infections.

BASOPHIL. (polymorphonuclear basophils; [PMB]) Basophils are the rarest of the white blood cells, often absent from normal differential white blood cell counts. The nucleus is usually bilobed, but may be obscured by the dense blue–black, basophilic cytoplasmic granules. The specific granules are not uniform in size or shape, but may be as large as those of eosinophils. The staining is largely attributable to the granules' content of the anticoagulant heparin. Basophils function in certain types of allergic reactions.

AGRANULOCYTES

These white blood cells do not have distinct cell–specific granules in their cytoplasm, and the nucleus is not segmented.

LYMPHOCYTE. The three classes of cells, B lymphocytes, T lymphocytes, and null lymphocytes, are similar in appearance in routinely stained light microscope preparations. Together these lymphocytes are the most numerous of the agranulocytes. In peripheral blood they are predominantly small cells, approximately the diameter of erythrocytes (5–8 µm); larger ones may measure 10–12 µm in diameter. In the smaller lymphocytes the nucleus occupies most of the cell, leaving a narrow rim of clear basophilic cytoplasm. Some of the medium– and large–sized lymphocytes have more cytoplasm and it may contain small azurophilic granules. The nucleus is round and its chromatin condensed. Such a nucleus is typically termed a heterochromatic nucleus (*hetero-*, other + *chroma*, color), referring to the condensed, transcriptionally inactive chromatin (*chroma*, color). Special histochemical methods or immunocytochemical stains are required to distinguish among major functional subdivisions of lymphocytes, or among their subgroups.

MONOCYTE. These are the largest of the leukocytes, ranging 14–20 µm in diameter. The nucleus is eccentrically (*ec-*, out of + *kentron*, center) located and may be indented, sometimes so as to appear kidney–shaped or folded. The finely clumped chromatin of the nucleus is more dispersed, and less condensed, than that of the lymphocyte. The cytoplasm tends to stain gray rather than the clear blue of lymphocytes because this cell usually contains a variety of small, irregular inclusions in addition to azurophilic granules.

Monocytes are cells that have been generated in the bone marrow and are passing through the blood stream en route to the tissues and organs where they contribute to the resident macrophage populations. These macrophage populations are collectively referred to as the mononuclear phagocyte system. Macrophages are discussed in Chapter 5: Connective Tissue.

TAXONOMIC KEY TO PERIPHERAL BLOOD CELLS

In Chapter 1 a diagrammatic flow chart illustrates a logical cognitive strategy that can be used to systematically identify the cells in normal peripheral blood. You can alternatively use a decision–tree strategy in the form of a taxonomic key, as illustrated here. Either way, the basic strategy is to begin broadly and progressively narrow the choices down to a final few. It is not necessary to memorize these tables, but to recognize them as a means to organize the facts in a systematic way so that all the terms and details of histology can be easily remembered and retrieved.

A comprehensive taxonomic key encompassing all the organs and subdivisions of organs described in this guide are compiled in Appendix B of the CD-ROM.

GENERAL CAVEAT

Observe that the percentage composition of blood provided in texts and atlases characterizing the relative percentage composition of formed elements in peripheral blood are not in exact agreement. Minor discrepancies such as these are not uncommon among references.

THE TAXONOMIC KEY

To use this key, first select between the choice #1's, then under the appropriate #1, select between the #2's, and for leukocytes select the appropriate #3 to reach the correct identification.

1) nucleus absent

    2) uniform cell size; approximately 7.5 µm; pink to gray cytoplasmic staining; most numerous cell type in smear...   *...red blood cell*

    2) smallest elements; irregular shapes; pale basophilic cytoplasm with centrally clumped azurophilic (violet–pink) granules; tend to be in clumps...   *...platelet*

1) nucleus present (leukocytes)

    2) distinct cytoplasmic granules

        3) highly segmented nucleus (typically 3–5 lobes); a few fine azurophilic (violet–pink) granules in cytoplasm; cell 12–15 µm; constitute 50%–77% of total leukocytes...   *...neutrophil*

        3) nucleus typically bilobed; large, uniform, refractile, eosinophilic (pink) granules; constitute 1%–5% of total leukocytes...   *...eosinophil*

        3) nucleus typically obscured by relatively large basophilic (blue–black) granules; least numerous of the leukocytes (0%–2% of total leukocytes)...   *...basophil*

    2) few or no cytoplasmic granules

        3) spherical to ovoid nucleus; range in size from diameter of RBC (small) to diameter of neutrophil (large), 6–18 µm; basophilic cytoplasm forms rim around nucleus; the larger cells with more cytoplasm may have fine azurophilic granules; constitute 15%–50% of total leukocytes...   *...lymphocyte*

        3) eccentrically located and indented nucleus; nucleus less dense than lymphocyte nucleus; largest leukocyte; 14–20 µm in diameter; finely clumped pale basophilic cytoplasm; may have azurophilic granules; comprise 3%–10% of total leukocytes...   *...monocyte*

3. Tissues, Layers, and Organs

This chapter provides an introduction to the concept of how cells, the fundamental building blocks of the body, are assembled into tissues and how tissues assemble into organs in order to perform complex functions necessary for the operation of the body. There are four basic tissue types in the body — epithelial tissue, connective tissue, muscle tissue, and nervous tissue — and they are represented in most organs. Usually one tissue type predominates, reflecting the principal function of that organ.

Just as there are standardized terms for describing morphological characteristics of cells, there are general terms commonly used in histology to describe the layers in the wall of a hollow organ. These are used like shorthand terms for tissues, or combinations of tissues, in specific locations. The following items are illustrated in this chapter.

> lumen (inside cavity; *lumen*, light, window)
> mucous membrane or mucosa (*mucosa*, referring to the clear, viscous secretion
>   often associated with the surface of these moist membranes)
> lamina propria or lamina propria mucosae (*lamina*, layer; *propria*, one's own;
>   *mucosae*, of the mucosa)
> muscularis mucosae (*muscularis*, muscle; *mucosae*, of the mucosa)
> submucosa (*sub-*, beneath + *mucosa*, the mucosa)
> muscularis externa (*muscularis*, muscle; *externa*, external)
> serous membrane or serosa (*serosa*, referring to the watery substance covering
>   these surfaces)
> adventitia (*adventitia*, coming from abroad, referring to the fact that the
>   adventitia does not form a functionally integral part of the organ)

This chapter also examines the morphological continuum that exists between the macroscopic image of an organ, through light microscope images, to electron microscope images. The electron microscope view is referred to as ultrastructure (*ultra-*, beyond + structure) or fine structure. Successful interpretation of a light microscope image is influenced by understanding the fine structure of cells and tissues. Ultrastructural details fall beyond the resolution of the light microscope, so it is important to appreciate how ultrastructural characteristics appear in standard light microscopic preparations. Much of what is understood of the structure–function relationship is based on knowledge of a cell's ultrastructure. Chapter 22 (Ultrastructure of the Cell) in this Guide summarizes cellular ultrastructure and the functional significance of ultrastructural details.

It is valuable in the study of microscopic structure to progress through images of increasingly greater magnification and then reverse the steps and return to the lower magnification so as to reinforce the perspective of organization that is often lost with higher magnifications. Remember that the cells of the body operate within the context of their surroundings and to understand the normal and abnormal functions of these cells, tissues, and organs, it is important to think of them as they really exist.

CD-ROM Notice: The images examined in this chapter are listed numerically on the CD-ROM by microscope slide number and electron micrograph plate number as they might be listed in a standard histology laboratory exercise. All the lead–in images on the CD-ROM are labeled with the numbers indicated in this chapter. The images linked to the lead–in image on the CD-ROM are indicated is this Guide as the higher magnification images.

LIGHT MICROSCOPE IMAGES

This low magnification view represents how this section appears without the aid of a microscope. The tissue section has a fairly uniform circular profile; it is a transverse section of the tube-shaped intestine. Examine its wall at an intermediate level of magnification. Higher magnification will provide additional detail of the wall. Go back to the low magnification image and note how, having seen an increased level of detail, you now can actually discern more detail in the lower magnification image. After examining all of the tissues that make up the wall of this organ up to the ultrastructural level, examine the section in the reversed order of magnifications. You will find that your observations at higher magnifications have greatly enhanced your perception of what you see at lower powers.

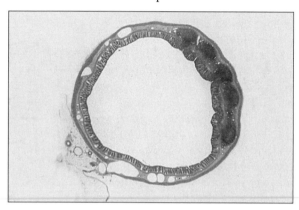

TISSUES AND LAYERS: TRANSVERSE SECTION OF GUT
Slide #1: Exercise A; H&E; 2 µm-thick methacrylate plastic section; rat large intestine.

Higher magnification images:
- (medium) complete thickness of organ wall
- (high) luminal epithelium
- (high) outer region of the wall
- (higher) muscularis externa and ganglion

AN INTRODUCTION TO TISSUES

Each of the four basic tissues of histology is represented in the wall of this organ. Epithelial tissues, which cover most of the free surfaces of the body, line the central lumen as well as the outside surface of this tube. Because of different functional requirements, these two epithelial tissues lining the inside and the outside of the tube are morphologically different from each other. However, they share one common characteristic of all epithelia: each forms a surface-parallel sheet of cells. Muscle tissue is present in two distinct layers in the wall of this tube: an inner one that can independently modify the shape of the lumen and an outer one that facilitates the propulsion of intestinal contents in a process termed peristalsis (*peri-*, around + *stalsis*, constriction). Nervous tissue is present in the wall to direct and coordinate the activity of the muscle layers. Connective tissue, which generally serves to maintain the other tissues in their proper three–dimensional relationships as well as to provide the means of metabolic support to these other tissues, is present in layers located between the other tissues. In subsequent chapters of this guide each of these basic tissue types is examined in more complete detail.

TERMINOLOGY

Specific terms are used for the tissue layers comprising the wall of this tube. The tube is lined by a three–part membrane that consists of (*1*) an epithelium (in this case, a simple columnar epithelium), (*2*) a layer of loose connective tissue upon which the epithelium rests, and (*3*) a layer of smooth muscle. These layers constitute what is termed the mucosa, or mucous membrane. A mucous membrane lines the moist interior cavities of the various hollow organs in the body; its composition is modified according to the functional needs of its location.

   This organ is suspended in the abdominal cavity of the body and its outer surface is covered by another membrane, which consists of (*1*) an epithelium on the free surface and (*2*) an underlying layer of connective tissue. This underlying connective tissue may be of substantial thickness, or barely noticeable, depending on location and the organ. These two tissues comprise the serous membrane, or serosa. Organs that are embedded in the body wall do not have a serosa. For these organs, the connective tissue that lies deep to the muscularis externa becomes continuous with that of the body wall and it is called the adventitia.

All organs that have an outer surface that faces a body cavity — the peritoneal cavity, pericardial cavity, or pleural cavity — are covered by a serous membrane that enables the organ to move with minimal friction within the confines of its cavity. In fact, each of the aforementioned body cavities is lined with a serous membrane that is continuous with that covering the organ. Thus, part of a serosa lines the cavity's containing wall and the other part is reflected over the outside of the organ suspended within that cavity. These two parts of the serosa are specifically designated the parietal portion (*paries*, pl. *parietes*, wall) of the serosa, which lines the cavity wall, and the visceral portion (*viscus*, pl. *viscera*, the internal organs) of the serosa, which covers the organs. The serosa lining each of the three body cavities has a specific name. The serous membrane is known as the peritoneum in the peritoneal cavity (*periteino*, to stretch over); it is known as the pericardium, in the pericardial cavity (*peri-*, around + *cardia*, heart); and it is known as the pleura, in the pleural cavity (*pleura*, a rib). Thus, the serosa covering the outside of this tissue section of the large intestine is specifically termed the visceral peritoneum, because it covers the gut and the gut is contained within the peritoneal cavity.

To simplify reference to the two layers of connective tissue and the two layers of smooth muscle in the wall of this general tube structure, each of these has a specific name. Thus, the loose connective tissue underlying the epithelium that lines the lumen is referred to as the lamina propria a designation that is more precise than referring to it as the layer of connective tissue underlying the epithelium that lines the lumen. The deeper connective tissue, located between the two muscle layers, is the submucosa referring succinctly to its location deep to the mucosa. The two layers of smooth muscle are designated the muscularis mucosae, which is part of the mucosa, and the muscularis externa, which is outermost in this organ's wall.

These general histological terms are adapted to describe tissues in the walls of organs in several organ systems, including the respiratory, reproductive, urinary, and digestive systems. The tissue layers forming the walls of the tubes comprising the circulatory system are known by their own special names.

Consider the wall of the gut again. It provides another source of confusion, especially for students who have difficulty visualizing three–dimensional relationships in histology. In the gut, both the muscularis mucosae and the muscularis externa are composed typically of two contiguous orthogonally–orientated layers of smooth muscle fibers. By convention, the muscle cells within each of these contiguous layers are designated by their general orientation with respect to the long axis of the tube, in this case the large intestine. Thus, in both the muscularis mucosae and the muscularis externa, the innermost muscle fibers form the circular layer, in which the muscle fibers encircle the tube, and the outermost fibers form the longitudinal layer, in which the muscle fibers are oriented parallel to the tube's long axis. Although this designation is not difficult to understand, interpretation can be tremendously confusing because in a transverse section of the tube the individual elongate muscle cells of the inner circular muscle layer are sectioned longitudinally and the muscle cells of the outer longitudinal layer are sectioned in their transverse plane. Remember that the plane of section is expressed with respect to the long axis of that object, be it a tube, a solid body, a cell, or an organelle. So in this tube's longitudinal plane of section (oriented at right angles to the transverse plane of this light microscope tissue section), the muscle fibers of the outer longitudinal layers are sectioned longitudinally whereas the fibers of the inner circular layers are sectioned transversely. It helps to visualize a solid model of this tube and its orthogonally arrayed muscle fibers.

ULTRASTRUCTURAL IMAGES

Knowing the ultrastructure of cells and tissues provides additional understanding necessary for complete interpretation of light microscope images and appreciation of structure–function relationships.

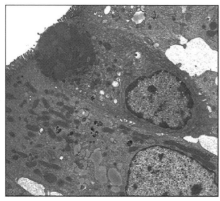

LUMINAL EPITHELIUM
Electron Micrograph #4: Simple Columnar Epithelium; goblet cell and absorptive cell; rat intestine.

Higher magnification images:
- intercellular interdigitation
- mucinogen inclusions

The luminal epithelium of the intestine is a simple columnar epithelium. It is composed of mucus–secreting goblet cells, named because of the goblet shape the apical (*apex*, summit, tip) accumulation of mucinogen granules gives the cell, and absorptive cells, called enterocytes (*entero-*, intestines + *-cyte*, cell)). In this micrograph one goblet cell is situated between two absorptive cells. The lumen of the organ is the empty appearing area in the upper left of the plate. Although the electron microscope image is quite similar to what is seen at high magnification in the light microscope, it provides details of functionally important features of this epithelium. For example, the set of intercellular junctions, which serves to attach the epithelial cells firmly together, isolates the luminal space from the lamina propria below. Material that passes from the lumen into the subjacent lamina propria must pass through the selective barrier provided by the epithelial cells themselves before entering the basal or lateral spaces. Intercellular interdigitation physically reinforces this sheet of cells. The electron micrographs also provide increased detail of the elaborate absorptive surface specialization that characterizes the enterocytes.

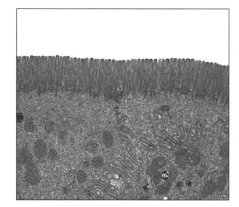

MICROVILLOUS BORDER
Electron Micrograph #5: Microvillous Border; intestine of rat.

Higher magnification views:
- junctional complex
- microvilli

The luminal surface of the absorptive cells is characterized by microvilli (*micro-*, small + *villus*, shaggy hair) that serve to increase the surface area of the enterocytes. Proteins associated with the enterocyte plasma membrane facilitate the movement of material across that membrane and into the cell. Increased plasma membrane surface area provides increased means to absorb material from the lumen. In the light microscope this microvillous border of the absorptive epithelium appears as a solid narrow band on the luminal surface of the enterocytes; electron microscopy is required to reveal the true functional significance of this surface modification. The paired serpentine lines in the lower half of the plate represent the interdigitating plasma membranes of the contiguous cells. A set of three specific intercellular junctions make up the composite structure termed the *junctional complex* that characterizes the absorptive epithelium of the gut. This junctional complex will be examined in detail in Chapter 4 (Epithelial Tissues).

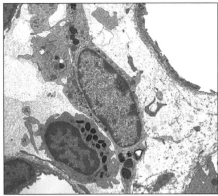

LAMINA PROPRIA
Electron Micrograph #9: Macrophage and Eosinophil; rat connective tissue.

Higher magnification views:
- macrophage cytoplasm
- granules and residual bodies
- fenestrated capillary

The lamina propria is a loose connective tissue and in both the light and the electron microscope it is seen to contain a variety of cell types dispersed in an extracellular (*extra-*, outside, beyond + *cella*, a storeroom, a chamber) matrix of fibrillar material and nonfibrillar ground substance. Although neither the standard light nor the electron microscope image reveals the biochemical nature of the many different molecules that make up the ground substance, it is important to recognize that the ground substance plays a very important role in the control and maintenance of the microenvironment of the cells that reside within and around it. In this image, portions of the thin curved walls of two capillaries are visible in the upper and lower corners of the plate. Although capillaries are visible in the light microscope, this level of morphological detail of their walls is not visible light microscopically. The distinction among different categories of capillaries is based on such functionally important morphological features (covered in Chapter 11: Circulatory system). The specific organelles and inclusions in the two cells depicted in this plate reflect their different functions. These cells are identified and discussed subsequently in Chapter 5: Connective Tissue. These two cells also are easily distinguishable in the light microscope.

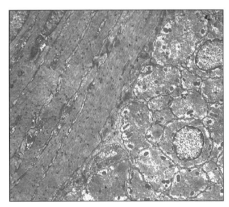

MUSCULARIS EXTERNA
Electron Micrograph #17: Smooth Muscle; intestine of rat.

Higher magnification views:
- smooth muscle and gap junctions
- Auerbach's plexus and caveolae

In both the light and electron microscope preparation, the elongate smooth muscle cells appear to be two different cell types when sectioned in planes oriented transverse to and longitudinal to their long axis. To clarify this confusing image, consider an analogy with a commercial package of wieners: imagine how the collected profiles of the wieners appear if you section a whole plastic–wrapped package in a plane oriented parallel to, rather than perpendicular to, the wiener's long axis. Like the elongate smooth muscle cells, in transverse plane the wiener profiles are circular, but the profiles are long and narrow when viewed in the longitudinal plane of section. One of the major challenges in histology is to be able to recognize solid cells, parts of cells, organs, and parts of organs in a variety of planes of section. It is a basic skill that is absolutely central not only to histological work but also to radiological imaging work as well.

Special intercellular junctions located between the smooth muscle cells are visible only in the electron microscope. These junctions, called gap (or nexus) junctions, permit the electrical coupling of smooth muscle cells, thus enabling the sheet of smooth muscle cells to contract in a coordinated manner. The junctions are called gap junctions because a very narrow gap of approximately 2 μm exists between the two membranes. The small pale profiles of axons, which influence the behavior of the smooth muscle of the muscularis externa, are visible between the two layers of smooth muscle and can be identified in both light and electron microscope preparations.

4. Epithelial Tissue

Epithelial tissues (also epithelium, pl. epithelia) are collections of contiguous cells that form surface parallel sheets. Epithelia line most free surfaces in and on the body, form ducts, and comprise the parenchyma (the specific cells of a gland or organ) of glands. Because of their location, epithelia are among the easiest tissues to recognize and identify and functionally they are among the most important tissues of the body. Clinically, epithelia are the most common source of cancerous tumors in adults, so it is important to appreciate the normal structure of various classes of the epithelia, as well as their normal function and location.

Understanding the structure and function of epithelia is the key to the successful identification of most organs. Ideally the structure–function relationship will become intuitive, such that you can look at an epithelium and automatically know its function. An everyday analogy for such a learned structure–function relationship is a door. Think about it: you rarely look at a standard door without knowing its function, and no matter whether the door is open or closed (a structural detail), you know its intended use. Furthermore, doors come in a variety of forms — elevator doors, revolving doors, sliding doors — and you cannot look at any one of these varieties without associating its specific name with its use, function, and typical location. Your goal in histology is to recognize histological features in that same way: for each cell, tissue, and organ, learn its name along with its morphology, function, typical location and the inseparability of these three features. A comprehensive histology text elaborates on the functions that are referenced only superficially in the context of these exercises.

This chapter examines the following categories of epithelial tissues. Learn to relate the name and morphology with the function and location of each.

> simple squamous epithelium (*squama*, a scale; *epi-*, upon + *thele*, nipple, from a term originally applied to the thin skin covering the nipples)
> endothelium (*endo-*, within + epithelium)
> mesothelium (*mesos*, middle + epithelium)
> simple cuboidal epithelium (refers to the cell shape and number of cell layers)
> simple columnar epithelium (refers to cell shape and number of layers)
> transitional epithelium (refers to an epithelium with an appearance that differs depending on its state of stretch)
> pseudostratified ciliated epithelium (*pseudo-*, false + *stratum*, a layer; *cilium*, an eyelid)
> pseudostratified epithelium with stereocilia (*stereo*, solid + cilia)
> stratified squamous, keratinized epithelium (*keras*, horn)
> stratified squamous, nonkeratinized epithelium

A variety of surface specializations, located on the apical, lateral, and basal surfaces of the epithelial cells, facilitates the function of epithelia. Learn to recognize and identify these specializations in light microscope preparations (LM) as well as in electron microscope preparations (EM). In the electron microscope the structures often have identifiable component parts, and in the list below, the component parts are listed offset below the main structure. Associate the morphology and location of each of these specializations with a specific function.

> terminal bar(LM) = junctional complex (EM)
> > tight junction or zonula occludens (*zonula*, a small band; *occludens*, occluding)
> > zonula adherens (*zonula*, a small band; *adherens*, adhesive)

desmosome or macula adherens (*desmo-*, a band + *some*, a body; *macula*, spot)

basement membrane(LM) = basal lamina plus lamina reticularis (EM)
> basal lamina (*basal*, base; *lamina*, thin plate)
> lamina densa (*lamina*, a thin plate; *densus*, thick)
> lamina lucida or lamina rara (*lamina*, a thin plate; *lucidus*, clear; *rarus*, thin)
> lamina reticularis (*lamina*, a thin plate; *reticulum*, a small net)

brush or striated border (LM) = microvillous border (EM)
microvillus, pl. microvilli (*micro-*, small + *villus*, shaggy hair)
stereocilium, pl. -cilia (*stereo-*, solid + *cilium*, eyelid)
cilium, pl. cilia (*clium*, eyelid)
axoneme (*axo-*, axis + *nema*, a thread)
basal striations (LM) = basal enfoldings (EM)

This chapter on epithelial tissues includes an introduction to some of the standard terminology related to glands. Glands are derived from epithelial tissue. Specific glands are covered in subsequent sections of this Guide. such as Chapter 14: Oral Cavity and Chapter 16: Liver, Gall bladder and Pancreas. The structure, function and location of the following items are described in this chapter.

endocrine gland (*endo-*, within + *-crine*, to separate)
exocrine gland (*exo-*, outside + *-crine*, to separate)
goblet cell (name refers to its goblet-like shape)
serous acinus, pl. acini (*acinus*, grape or berry)
mucous acinus, pl. acini (*acinus*, grape or berry)
serous demilune (*demi-*, half + *-lune*, moon)
myoepithelial cell (*myo-*, muscle + epithelium)

CD-ROM Notice: The images examined in this chapter are listed numerically on the CD-ROM by microscope slide number as they might be listed in a standard histology laboratory. Some microscope slides appear more than once because, as in a real laboratory exercise, a single tissue section is used to demonstrate more than one structure. All the lead–in images on the CD-ROM are labeled, and have links, that are appropriate for the tissue or structure being illustrated, and each is so designated in the CD-ROM list. To avoid confusion resulting from selecting the wrong nested series of images, read the label on the CD-ROM list carefully.

EPITHELIA

Epithelia are located on free surfaces of the body. They cover the external body surface; they form the internal linings of hollow organs such as the stomach, trachea, heart, blood vessels, and urethra; and they line the body cavities such as the thoracic and abdominal cavity. Therefore, when you look for epithelium, this tissue is usually immediately adjacent to a space.

Consider the following diagrammatic overview of the hierarchical organization of the epithelial tissues examined in this exercise. You are not expected to memorize this flow chart, but simply to recognize it as one means to organize the tissue categories in a systematic way so that all of them can be easily and accurately remembered. Most epithelia are classified according to two features: the shape of the cells and the number of cellular layers. Some epithelia in specific locations have special names, like the endothelium that lines blood vessels. Special epithelia, such as the germinal epithelium lining the seminiferous tubules and the neuroepithelium of the retina, are examined in Chapters 18 and 21 (the Male Reproductive System and the Eye, respectively).

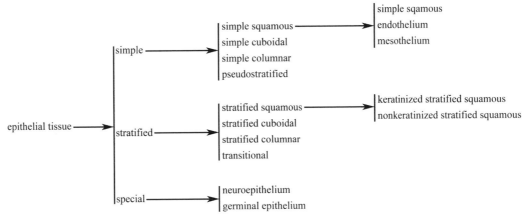

SIMPLE EPITHELIA

A simple epithelium is a sheet of cells that is only one cell thick. This cellular monolayer always rests on an extracellular (*extra-*, outside + *cella*, a storeroom, a chamber) basement membrane, which is examined subsequently in this Chapter.

SIMPLE SQUAMOUS EPITHELIUM. An example of this epithelial type is seen in the kidney tissue section. The structure of the kidney is discussed in Chapter 13; at this point simply learn to recognize a simple squamous epithelium.

Look in the cortical region of the kidney and find the renal corpuscles. These are

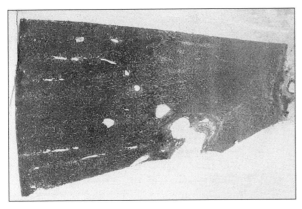

SIMPLE SQUAMOUS EPITHELIUM
Slide #160: Kidney; radial section; H&E stain; 4 μm thick methacrylate section; nonhuman primate.

Higher magnification image:
• (high) simple squamous epithelium

spherical structures within which are tufts of blood capillaries. The outer lining of this sphere is a simple squamous epithelium (called the parietal layer of Bowman's capsule). The lumen it encircles is normally filled with the filtrate of blood that has passed out of the capillaries as the first step in the production of urine.

ENDOTHELIUM. A special variety of simple squamous epithelium lines the blood vessels.

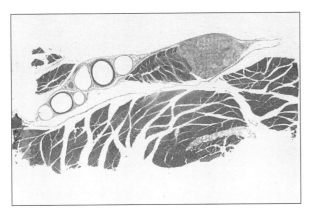

ENDOTHELIUM
Slide #52: Neurovascular Bundle (radial artery, vein and nerve fascicles, transversely sectioned); H&E stain; 4 μm thick methacrylate section; nonhuman primate.

Higher magnification image:
• (high) endothelium

In this location this epithelium is specifically known as endothelium. Locate endothelial cells lining the lumen (central space) of the vessels in this tissue section. This tissue was fixed by vascular perfusion and so these blood vessels are relatively distended and free of blood. The endothelial cells are extremely flattened and elongated along an axis that is parallel to the long axis of the vessel. Because of their orientation, the small dark nuclei of the endothelial cells may be located close together in a transversely sectioned vessel. The wall of a very small diameter vessel, like a capillary, may be formed from a single endothelial cell.

At this point, you can safely assume that if a structure is a blood vessel, it is lined with an endothelium. The rest of the blood vessel wall is described in the Circulatory System Chapter (Chapter 11) of this Guide.

MESOTHELIUM. Observe the mesothelium (another specific kind of simple squamous epithelium) lining the outside surface of the distended urinary bladder. This tissue section has two sides, an inner concave side adjacent to the bladder's lumen (to the left side of this image) and the outer convex side that faces the peritoneal cavity. The epithelia that line serous body cavities and cover the free surfaces of organs that project into these serous cavities are specifically referred to as mesothelia. Mesothelia provide smooth surfaces moistened with serous fluid that facilitate the movement of these organs in a relatively frictionless environment.

The mesothelium is part of a layer termed the serosa, or serous membrane, in association with underlying connective tissue. For many organs, such as the heart and lungs, the serosa has an organ-specific name, such as visceral pericardium and visceral pleura, respectively. Organs that project into the peritoneal cavity, such as the urinary bladder and most of the organs of the alimentary canal, are covered by a serous membrane specifically termed the peritoneum.

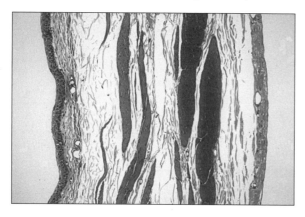

MESOTHELIUM
Slide #166: Urinary Bladder; Lee's stain; 4 μm thick methacrylate section; nonhuman primate.

Higher magnification image:
• (high) mesothelium

SIMPLE CUBOIDAL EPITHELIUM. The testis is an egg-shaped solid organ, and this tissue section is from a block that has been prepared by trimming off the curved faces from two sides of the organ, leaving the central region of the testis. Observe the network of anastomosing canals identified as the rete testis (*rete*, a net; *testis*, in the testis) embedded in the core of this organ. There are a variety of ducts and tubules in this block of tissue and the manner in which the morphology of each one reflects its special function is discussed in Chapter 19 (Male Reproductive System).

In the area of the rete testis, the predominant canals are lined with cells that are shaped like cubes in which the length, width, and height of the cells are all about equal. Note the size, shape, and position of the nucleus within these cells: it is typically spheroid and located in the middle of the cell. The boundaries between the cells are not evident because the thickness of the plasma membrane is beyond the resolution of the light microscope. However, you can envision the shape of the cells because each of these cells has one nucleus and you can assume that the cellular interfaces occur

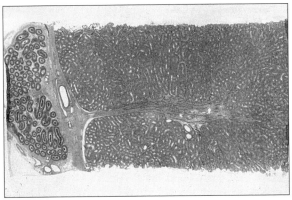

SIMPLE CUBOIDAL EPITHELIUM
Slide #171: Rete Testis in Testis; H&E stain: 4 μm thick methacrylate section; nonhuman primate.

Higher magnification image:
* (high) simple cuboidal epithelium

approximately halfway between adjacent nuclei. In this tissue section, the numerous irregular channels among the rete testis that are lined with endothelium are lymphatic vessels.

SIMPLE COLUMNAR EPITHELIUM. The organ in this tissue section has obvious inside and outside surfaces. The outside surface is covered by a mesothelium because this region of intestine is normally suspended within the peritoneal cavity of the body. A simple columnar epithelium lines the lumen where it functions to absorb selectively intestinal contents for the body's use. Observe the size and shape of these epithelial cells and the position and shape of their nuclei. The columnar cells of the epithelium are tall and narrow, and their nuclei are also elongated and typically located in the base of the cell. The columnar shape of the cells is best seen in regions of epithelium that are sectioned in a plane that is oriented perpendicular to the sheet of cells. Although the intestine has been cut in transverse section in this tissue section, many of the cells comprising the simple columnar epithelium have been sectioned obliquely. When you look at the geometry of the mucosa in the low magnification image, you should not be surprised that most of the lining epithelial cells are sectioned obliquely and therefore do not show a perfectly columnar profile.

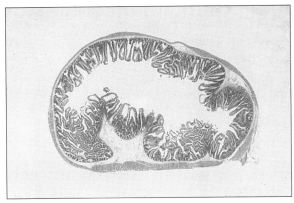

SIMPLE COLUMNAR EPITHELIUM
Slide #117: Jejunum (small intestine); eosin & toluidine blue stain; 4 μm thick methacrylate section; nonhuman primate.

Higher magnification image:
* (high) simple columnar epithelium

It is important to be able to interpret the image of a sheet of columnar cells that has been sectioned in planes other than the perfect perpendicular one. When the plane of section through the epithelial sheet is oriented tangentially, or parallel to the epithelial free surface, the outlines of the individual columnar cells appear as polygons and the nuclear profiles are circular. Furthermore, it should not be surprising that the distance from the base of the epithelium to the luminal surface increases with increasing the angle the section varies from the perfect perpendicular plane. Conversely, if you are searching for a region where an epithelium is sectioned most perfectly perpendicular to its horizontal plane, you should seek the region where the epithelium appears thinnest. You can safely assume that in most normal material the epithelium that lines the lumen of an organ, lines the entire lumen.

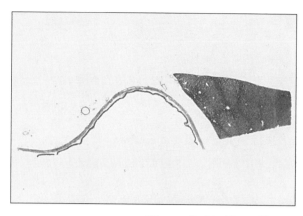

SIMPLE COLUMNAR EPITHELIUM (OBLIQUE SECTION)
Slide #155: Liver and Gall Bladder; Lee's stain; 4 μm thick methacrylate section; nonhuman primate.

Higher magnification image:
- (medium) adventitial and serosal wall
- (high) simple columnar epithelium

The gall bladder, illustrated in Slide #155, is lined with a simple columnar epithelium that facilitates the absorption of water and ions from the bile stored within its lumen. The gall bladder shares part of its wall with the liver, and so it has both an adventitia and a serosa.

These columnar epithelial cells are functionally and morphologically polarized. The side facing the lumen is referred to as the luminal or apical side, and the side facing the lamina propria is referred to as the basal or abluminal side (*ab-*, away from + lumen).

PSEUDOSTRATIFIED EPITHELIUM. A pseudostratified epithelium lines the lumen of the extrapulmonary bronchus in this next tissue section. Principally this epithelium contains columnar ciliated cells with single mucus–secreting cells dispersed among them. The mucinogen granules in the mucus–secreting cells are preserved and stained magenta by the PAS stain. Additional populations of cells are present in this epithelium and are described in Chapter 18 (Respiratory System) of this Guide. The distinguishing feature of a pseudostratified epithelium is that the nuclei of the cells appear at different levels in the epithelium as if the epithelium were stratified, yet all of the cells in this epithelium are in contact with the basement membrane. Thus, a pseudostratified epithelium may be considered in a topological sense as a variant of simple epithelium. It is necessary to learn which epithelia in the body are pseudostratified because in tissue sections typically they appear to be stratified. Another example of a pseudostratified epithelium is examined in this chapter in the context of its specific surface special-ization, stereocilia.

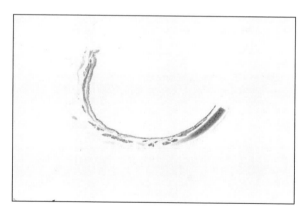

PSEUDOSTRATIFIED EPITHELIUM: UNICELLULAR GLANDS
Slide #131: Extrapulmonary Bronchus; Periodic Acid Schiff (PAS) stain and lead hematoxylin; 4 μm thick methacrylate section; nonhuman primate.

Higher magnification image:
- (medium) wall
- (high) pseudostratified epithelium and single-cell gland

Because the ciliated pseudostratified epithelium with mucus–secreting cells is so characteristic of the trachea, bronchi, and nasopharynx it is often termed respiratory epithelium.

STRATIFIED EPITHELIA

These epithelia have two or more layers of cells, with the cells of the deeper layers usually differing in appearance from those at the surface. These epithelia are named according to the shape of the cells comprising the free surface layer of the epithelium.

STRATIFIED SQUAMOUS KERATINIZED EPITHELIUM. This tissue section appears to have two rough surfaces: the deep surface is rough because it has been cut from the body and the outer surface is irregular because of the response of the thick outer layer of cells to the preparative histological procedures. The epidermis (*epi-*, upon + *dermis*, skin) of this tissue section is a stratified squamous epithelium in which the superficial cells have become modified (filled with keratin filaments) to provide protection for the under–lying tissue from mechanical abrasion. The cells of the epithelium are generated in its basal layer and they differentiate as they are pushed toward the surface by newly forming cells. Learn to look at an epithelium like this and think of the process that produces it: as each new cell progresses from the basal layer to the free surface it loses its nucleus and becomes filled with filamentous keratin. Examine the cells comprising this epithelium and note the differences in the size and shape of the cells and the nuclear condition — present or absent, pyknotic (*pykno-*, thick, dense) or not. The cells of the basal layer are cuboidal or low columnar. Cells at more superficial levels are irregular in shape and larger. In the outermost keratinized layer, the cells are flattened, lack a nucleus, and the cytoplasm is largely replaced by keratin. Not surprisingly, the layer of keratinized cells is thicker in the skin that covers the palm of the hand and the sole of the feet like this one, compared to the skin of the rest of the body. In Chapter 10 (Integument), the names of the morphologically distinct layers of this epithelium are provided.

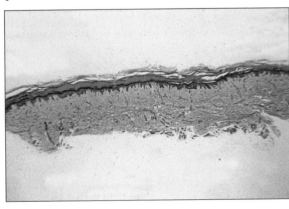

STRATIFIED SQUAMOUS KERATINIZED EPITHELIUM
Slide #84: Plantar Skin; H&E stain; 10 μm thick paraffin section; human.

Higher magnification image:
- (high) stratified squamous keratinized epithelium

STRATIFIED SQUAMOUS NONKERATINIZED EPITHELIUM. Although in most tissue sections the organ's lumen corresponds to the concave surface, you should recognize that this is not always true. Think about a block of tissue that has been removed as a biopsy (*bio-*, life + *-ops*, vision) sample: as the block is immersed in a fixative, the more solidly packed underlying tissues contract and stretch the weaker tissues of the luminal surface into a convex surface. Learn to examine all edges of a tissue section to gain a sense of orientation to the solid object from which it came.

A stratified squamous nonkeratinized epithelium occurs where surfaces inside the body require special protection from abrasive forces, although not against dehydration since these surfaces are normally moist. Examples of stratified squamous nonkeratinized epithelia are found in the esophagus, mouth, epiglottis, and vagina. In the tissue section of the vagina note the variation in the size and shape of the epithelial cells and the character of the nuclei throughout the full depth of this epithelium. New cells are generated only at the basal surface and they are pushed toward the free surface from which they are sloughed off. Unlike the keratinized epithelium, the squamous surface cells of this epithelium are nucleated and not packed with keratin.

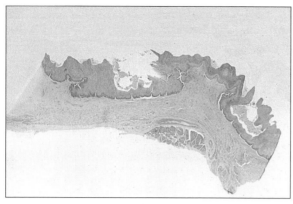

STRATIFIED SQUAMOUS NONKERATINIZED EPITHELIUM
Slide #196: Vagina; H&E stain; 10 μm thick paraffin section; human.

Higher magnification images:
- (high) stratified squamous epithelium
- (higher) superficial layers

Variation in the apparent thickness of this epithelium occurs because of undulations in the sheet of cells with respect to the plane of section. Just looking at this low power image suggests that the wall of the vagina is uneven and, in fact, is characterized by large folds called rugae (*ruga*, a wrinkle).

TRANSITIONAL EPITHELIUM. The chief characteristic of this stratified epithelium that lines the lumen of the urinary bladder is that its appearance varies with its degree of stretch, hence the name transitional epithelium. As the urinary bladder becomes filled, the epithelium stretches and becomes thinner. Observe the epithelium lining the lumen of the relaxed urinary bladder. There are several cell layers. Note that the basal cells of this

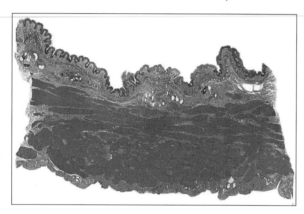

TRANSITIONAL EPITHELIUM: CONTRACTED
Slide #165: Urinary Bladder, relaxed; hematoxylin & toluidine blue/phloxinate stain; 4 μm thick methacrylate section; nonhuman primate.

Higher magnification image:
- (high) transitional epithelium

epithelium are small and irregular in shape. In the middle layers the cells are larger and often pear-shaped. On the free surface some cells are quite large, often swollen, and have bulging convex apices (*apex*, pl. *apices*, summit, tip). Luminal cells that have two nuclei are believed to result from the fusion of two cells. Surface cells that resemble parasols with a broad rounded top and extended narrow stem may be termed umbrella cells. Do not confuse this epithelium with stratified cuboidal epithelium, which

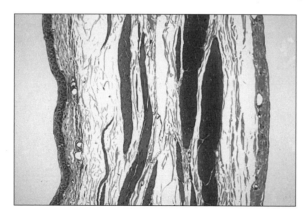

TRANSITIONAL EPITHELIUM: DISTENDED
Slide #166: Urinary Bladder, Distended; Lee's stain; 4 μm thick methacrylate section; nonhuman primate.

Higher magnification images:
- (medium) bladder wall
- (high) transitional epithelium

generally has no more than two layers and whose surface cells have a comparatively flat luminal surface.

The stretched, or distended, transitional epithelium has as few as two layers, and the interface with the underlying lamina propria is stretched and no longer undulating, The cells in the superficial layer are large and relatively squamous. This epithelium should not be confused with a stratified squamous epithelium, because the latter has many more layers of cells.

Because this epithelium lines the passageways and bladder of the urinary system, it is also termed a urothelium.

STRATIFIED CUBOIDAL AND STRATIFIED COLUMNAR EPITHELIUM. Examples of stratified cuboidal epithelium and stratified columnar epithelium are illustrated in subsequent sections of this Laboratory Guide, in Chapter 10 (Integument) and Chapter 19 (Male Reproductive System), respectively. A stratified cuboidal epithelium lines the ducts of sweat glands, and a stratified columnar epithelium lines the distal end of the penile urethra.

CELL SURFACE SPECIALIZATIONS

In this diagrammatic overview the various surface specializations are first categorized by the surface of the cell on which they occur. Microvilli are subcategorized by light microscope (LM) terms commonly used for light microscopically distinct microvillous borders. The intercellular junctions of the cell's lateral surface are initially subcategorized by function. The basement membrane of light microscopy (LM) has two ultrastructural (EM) components.

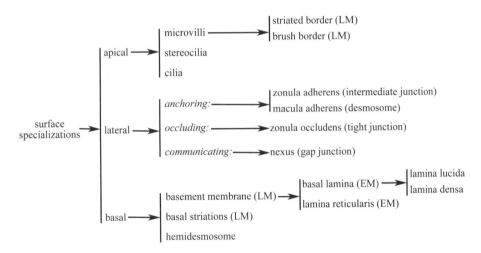

LATERAL SPECIALIZATIONS

TERMINAL BAR AND INTERCELLULAR JUNCTIONS. Locate the simple columnar epithelium lining the lumen of the duodenum. In a region of the tissue section where the columnar cells are cut vertically (i.e., in a plane parallel to the columnar cell's long axis), observe that just beneath, and parallel to, the free surface of the cells, there are a series of small, dark spots connected with a thin dark line stained the same pink color. This structure is termed the terminal bar apparatus and it is a belt-like structure that encircles the apical region of the cell. You can detect the geometry of this belt by examining a region of epithelium that is sectioned in a tangential plane (or sectioned parallel to the free surface) through the apical region of the columnar cells. Look in such an area for the pink–stained structure that has the same staining characteristics as the terminal bar apparatus you identified in the vertical section of the epithelium. Observe how in the tangential section the fine pink lines of the terminal bar apparatus form circumferential

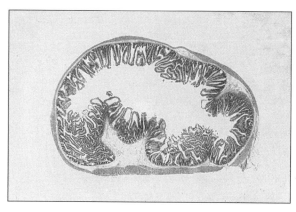

TERMINAL BAR
Slide #117: Jejunum; (small intestine); eosin & toluidine blue stain; 4 μm thick methacrylate section; nonhuman primate.

Higher magnification image:
- (high) terminal bar and striated border

hexagonal arrays. The technique of looking around a tissue section is a valuable means to develop a sense of the three-dimensional geometry of objects depicted in these two-dimensional tissue sections.

When viewed in the electron microscope the terminal bar apparatus is shown to be a set of three intercellular junctions termed the *junctional complex*. This specific complex of junctions is situated in the apical region of the epithelial cells in a location that corresponds to the location of the terminal bar apparatus identified in light microscope preparations of this tissue. The intercellular junctions — the zonula occludes, the zonula adherens, and the macula adherens — each have their own specific transmembrane and extracellular protein components. It is the extracellular components of these junctions that are principally responsible for the pink-stained belts seen in the light microscope. The intercellular interdigitation of the lateral surfaces of the cells in this micrograph provides an additional means to interlock the cells of this absorptive epithelium; this interdigitation is not apparent in light microscope preparations.

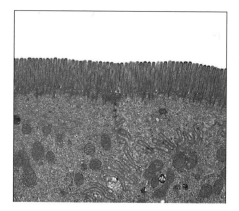

JUNCTIONAL COMPLEX
Electron Micrograph #5: Microvillous Border; rat intestine.

Higher magnification images:
- junctional complex of absorptive epithelium and terminal web.
- microvilli

Do not confuse the terminal bar apparatus with the terminal web of the cell. Terminal web refers to the dense intracellular concentration of actin microfilaments and intermediate filaments that occurs within the apical portion of the epithelial cell. Filaments within this apical meshwork insert into the intercellular junctions to secure the cytoskeletal interior of one cell to the cytoskeletal interior of the adjacent cells.

Electron Micrograph #6 is an oblique section through the luminal surface of an epithelium like the one in Electron Micrograph #5. The multiple circular profiles at the top of this image are the transversely sectioned microvilli that project into the lumen. The junctional complex consists of three individual intercellular junctions whose roles are collectively critically important to the function of this epithelium. Of the three intercellular junctions, the one located closest to the lumen is a tight junction, or zonula occludens. Its two-fold purpose is (*1*) to seal off the intercellular space so that luminal materials cannot flow between adjacent cells into the underlying lamina propria but must pass through the cells themselves, and (*2*) to limit the membrane domains of free-

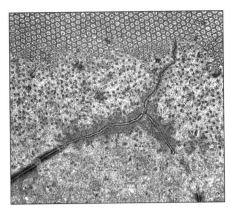

MICROVILLOUS BORDER AND JUNCTIONAL COMPLEX
Electron Micrograph #6: Junctional Complex, oblique section;
rat intestine.

Higher magnification images:
* tight junction (zonula occludens)
* desmosome and zonula adherens
* microvilli

floating integral membrane proteins such that those of the apical domain are restricted to that part of the cell and those of the basolateral domain remain in their region.

The second of the three intercellular junctions in this complex is the intermediate junction (zonula adherens) and the third junction is the desmosome (macula adherens). Both of these latter two junctions serve to bind the cells together so that the epithelium can withstand stresses and other tensile forces without losing its physical integrity. Cytoskeletal actin filaments in the terminal web are linked to transmembrane proteins of the zonula adherens and tonofilaments (bundles of cytokeratin intermediate filaments) are linked to transmembrane proteins of the desmosome. Thus the cytoskeletons of these cells are bound by these intercellular junctions; if only the membranes were attached, the cells could be easily separated from each other.

Both the zonula adherens and the zonula occludens completely encircle the apical region of each epithelial cell, whereas the desmosome is in the form of a patch or spot. Desmosomes occur randomly on the lateral surface of the columnar cell and are not restricted to the region of the junctional complex. A modified desmosome, called the hemidesmosome (hemi-, one half + desmosome), serves to attach an epithelium to its underlying connective tissue.

These three intercellular junctions occur separately or together between cells in other locations of the body. For example, tight junctions may occur between endothelial cells in capillaries (Chapter 11), a form of the intermediate junction occurs between cardiac muscle cells (Chapter 9), and desmosomes link the cells of the epidermis (Chapter 10).

A fourth class of intercellular junction, termed the gap (also nexus, or communicating) junction, occurs among cells in a variety of tissues where it permits electrical coupling and the intercellular passage of small molecules between cells. The gap junction is not part of the junctional complex of an absorptive epithelium like this one, although it may be part of other complexes of junctions in other tissues. You will examine gap junctions in smooth and cardiac muscle cells (Chapter 9).

Two opposing faces of a plasma membrane forming a zonula occludens are illustrated in Electron Micrograph #7. The freeze-fracture technique in which a small block of tissue is rapidly frozen and split, preferentially splits the plasma membrane between its two lipid leaflets. This preparation reveals the intramembranous arrangement of the transmembrane linker proteins that comprise the tight junction. Depending on the functional requirements of the tissue in which they occur, tight junctions may be very tight and completely isolate the luminal compartment from the basolateral compartment of an epithelium, or they may have varying degrees of leakiness. The

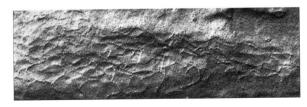

TIGHT JUNCTION
Electron Micrograph# 7: Tight Junction; freeze-fracture preparation; nonhuman primate.

tightness of the tight junction is determined by the physical complexity of the inter-connected strands of transmembrane particles that form the belt encircling the cell. If the interlocking strands are loosely arranged, material can pass between the cells by following an indirect path around the strands.

APICAL SPECIALIZATIONS

MICROVILLI AND GLYCOCALYX. Microvilli are tiny, finger-like projections of the cell's surface membrane, each supported by a central bundle of actin filaments. A single microvillus is approximately 1–2 μm high and approximately 80 nm wide. Microvilli are typically too small and too tightly packed together to be seen individually in a light microscope preparation.

In tissue sections of H&E stained small intestine examined earlier in this chapter, a distinct faintly eosinophilic strip appears on the apical surface of the columnar absorptive cells. In the intestine this strip is called the striated border and it corresponds to many hundreds of small microvilli massed together on the apical surface of each absorptive epithelial cell. Observe the striated border on the luminal surface of the PAS–stained tissue section illustrated below. The striated border stains magenta because of the PAS–positive glycocalyx. The glycocalyx (*glyco-*, sweet + *-calyx*, shell) is a well–developed surface coat composed principally of oligosaccharide extensions of phospholipids and integral membrane proteins. In some areas on this section the individual microvilli are slightly shrunken and separated from each other, providing an indication of their numbers and sizes.

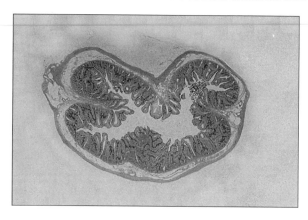

MICROVILLI AND GLYCOCALYX
Slide #122: Jejunum, PAS-lead hematoxylin stain; 4 μm thick methacrylate section; nonhuman primate.

Higher magnification image:
• (high) striated border and glycocalyx

The fine structure of microvilli is illustrated in Electron Micrographs #5 and #6 of the CD-ROM, which were examined previously in this chapter in the context of the intercellular junctions. The image of the longitudinally sectioned microvilli in Electron Micrograph #5 illustrates clearly how microvilli can substantially increase the luminal surface area of the absorptive cell. The greater the surface area of the plasma membrane, with its complement of absorption–facilitating integral proteins, the greater is the capacity of the enterocytes to absorb material from the lumen. The core of the microvillus is a bundle of 25 to 30 actin filaments that provides skeletal support for these fingerlike extensions and inserts into the matted terminal web in the apex of the cell. The fuzzy coat of glycocalyx is also evident in this micrograph. In Electron Micrograph #6 the orientation of the tissue section illustrates the close packing of the microvilli. This obliquely sectioned preparation also illustrates the uniform bundles of actin filaments that form the cores of the microvilli and insert into the terminal web of the absorptive cell.

Microvilli vary in numerical density and length, depending of the function of the cell. In the kidney, the microvillous border of the proximal tubules is referred to as the brush border, and the individual microvilli are longer than those of the gut and often tangled together in the lumen of the tubules in which they occur. You can observe the brush border in the kidney tissue section used to illustrate the basement membrane later in this chapter. Compare the fine structure of the microvilli in the kidney tubules with those of the gut in the electron micrograph (Electron Micrograph #19) used to illustrate basal striations later in this chapter.

STEREOCILIA. Very long microvilli are associated with the cells that line the ductus epididymis. These ducts are part of a structure, the epididymis, that caps the posterior surface of the testis. These long microvilli are specifically termed stereocilia. In this tissue section the stereocilia form tufts of slender processes arising from the apical surfaces of the pseudostratified columnar epithelium. The stereocilia resemble microvilli more than cilia in that the stereocilia have a supporting central core of actin and they are nonmotile. Sometimes they are branched. Like the shorter microvilli, their role is believed to be absorptive given that this epithelium plays a role in concentrating the seminal fluid produced by the seminiferous tubules of the testis. Stereocilia occur only in the epididymis and on the hair cells of the inner ear. In the inner ear the stereocilia serve as mechanical transducers of sound waves.

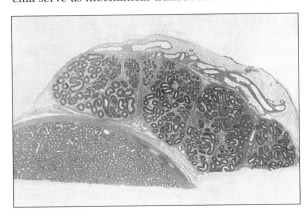

STEREOCILIA
Slide #169: Epididymis and Tubuli Recti; H&E stain; 4 mm thick methacrylate section; nonhuman primate.

Higher magnification image:
- (high) pseudostratified epithelium with stereocilia

CILIA. Cilia project from the surface of the pseudostratified epithelium of the conducting airways of the respiratory system. They are longer (5–10 μm) than microvilli, and thicker with a diameter of 0.2–0.3 μm. Cilia can be individually visualized in tissue sections principally because there are fewer of them per cell than there are microvilli on a typical absorptive cell. The dark staining line at the apical end of the ciliated cells corresponds to the row of basal bodies in the apical cytoplasm into which each cilium inserts. The cilia are motile and, in the bronchus and trachea, beat toward the pharynx to transport mucus over the surface of the epithelium for the purpose of clearing the airway of inhaled debris.

Ciliated epithelia occur in several areas of the body where they serve to move material in a surface-parallel unidirectional direction. Examples include the oviduct, the efferent ductules of the male reproductive system, and the ventricles of the brain. In normal living tissue they beat rapidly and in one direction.

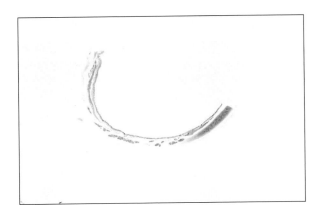

PSEUDOSTRATIFIED: CILIA
Slide #131: Extrapulmonary Bronchus; PAS stain and lead hematoxylin; 4 μm thick methacrylate section; nonhuman primate.

Higher magnification image:
- (high) ciliated pseudostratified epithelium

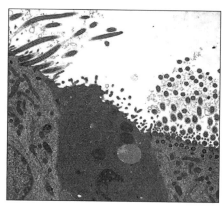

CILIATED EPITHELIUM
Electron Micrograph, #18: Cilia in Rat Trachea.

Higher magnification images:
* transversely sectioned cilia and the axoneme
* cilia and basal bodies
* longitudinally sectioned cilia

The low packing density of the individual cilia is evident in Electron Micrograph #8. Because of their long and narrow shape, and the thinness of the EM tissue section, the cilia in this micrograph appear as profiles of obliquely and transversely sectioned pieces floating freely in the lumen. The special core complex of longitudinal microtubules in the interior of each cilium is termed the axoneme. Observe that the axoneme is an arrangement of two single microtubules surrounded by nine doublet microtubules that are uniformly spaced around the central ones. At the base of each cilium, the axoneme is continuous with a basal body. Each basal body has nine triplet microtubules that are continuous with the doublets of the axoneme but has no central microtubules, as the central ones of the axoneme do not continue past the base of the cilium.

The scanning Electron Micrograph #20 illustrates both cilia and microvilli on the apical surfaces of cells lining the ventricles of the brain. Compare the size and packing density of these surface specializations. The ciliated cells are ependymal cells that line the ventricles and move cerebrospinal fluid through the ventricular system. The choroid plexus, which produces the cerebrospinal fluid in the ventricles, is a system of looped capillaries covered by modified ependymal cells with microvilli instead of cilia. These microvilli of the choroid plexus cells are not so long or organized as those on the apical surface of an absorptive cell.

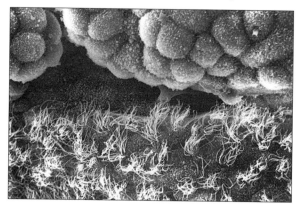

CILIA AND MICROVILLI
Electron Micrograph, #20: Cilia and Microvilli; rat brain ventricle; scanning electron micrograph.

BASAL SPECIALIZATIONS

BASEMENT MEMBRANE AND BASAL LAMINA. All epithelia rest on an extracellular basement membrane. This kidney tissue section (Slide #161) has been processed with the PAS stain to demonstrate the basement membrane, which is PAS–positive because of the proteoglycans that are present within it. The basement membrane appears as the thin magenta line upon which all the epithelia rest. Observe the PAS stain on the luminal side of some of tubules in the cortex. These tubules have a brush border of microvilli which, like the striated border of the intestine, is accentuated by the PAS–stained glyco-calyx. This brush border is illustrated with the basal striations of these kidney cells in Electron Micrograph #19.

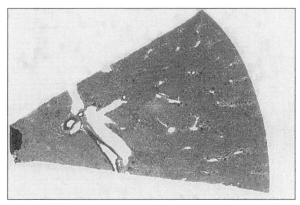

BASEMENT MEMBRANE
Slide #161: Kidney, radial section; PAS stain; 3 μm thick methacrylate section; nonhuman primate.

Higher magnification images:
• (middle) kidney cortex
• (high) proximal and distal tubules

The basement membrane seen in the light microscope corresponds in part to a two–layered extracellular structure located on the basal surface of an epithelium, termed the basal lamina. This is illustrated in Electron Micrograph #22. The two parts of the basal lamina are (*1*) an electron lucent layer immediately subjacent to the basal plasmalemma of the epithelial cell called the lamina lucida or lamina rara, and (*2*) an electron dense felt-like layer called the lamina densa. The lamina reticularis is an additional fine structural component of this region of attachment between the epithelium and the underlying connective tissue; it contains coarser fibers and anchoring proteins that bind the basal lamina (which is firmly attached to the epithelium) to the underlying connective tissue.

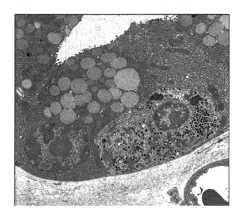

BASAL LAMINA
Electron Micrograph #22: Chief Cells and Enteroendocrine Cell; epithelium of the stomach; rat.

Higher magnification images:
• basal surface of the cells

A two–layered structure like the basal lamina surrounds peripheral nerves and muscle fibers. In such a location this extracellular structure is preferably termed the external lamina, rather than the basal lamina, because it surrounds a cell's entire circumference. Like the basal lamina of epithelia, the external lamina also functions to attach cells to the connective tissue with which they are associated. The external lamina of peripheral nerves is illustrated in Electron Micrographs #12, #13, and #28 on the CD-ROM.

BASAL STRIATIONS AND BASAL ENFOLDINGS. Examine the submandibular gland and observe the intralobular duct system (*intra-*, within + lobule, a diminutive of *lobos*, lobe). Some of these ducts have walls whose cells are low cuboidal, but the walls of other ducts are composed of columnar cells whose spheroid nuclei are located near the center of the cell. The greatly enfolded basal membrane accounts for the unexpected position and shape of the nucleus (for a columnar cell). The striations in the basal portion of these cells are difficult to discern in the light microscope.

In the electron microscope the basal striations correspond to an elaboration and folding of the basal plasma membrane. Basal striations represent the means by which a cell increases its basal surface area just as microvilli represent a means for a cell to

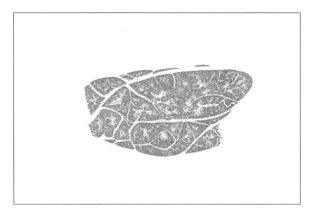

Basal Striations
Slide #102: Submandibular Gland; H&E stain, 4 μm thick methacrylate section; nonhuman primate.

Higher magnification images:
- (middle) ducts and secretory elements
- (high) striated duct

increase the surface area of its luminal membrane. The basal membrane contains transmembrane proteins that facilitate the pumping of ions from the cell into the underlying connective tissue; the more membrane there is, the greater the number of ions that the cell can pump across its membrane. The presence of so many mitochondria associated with the enfolded basal membrane reflects the high energy requirement for this pumping process.

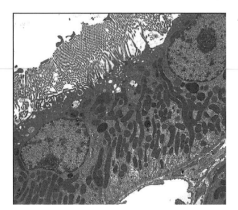

Basal Enfoldings
Electron Micrograph #19: Microvilli and Basal Enfoldings; proximal tubule; the rat kidney.

Higher magnification images:
- basal enfoldings
- microvillous border

GLANDS

Some epithelia are organized into glands, such as the sweat glands, salivary glands, and the liver. Glands can be classified using a variety of different criteria, including the mechanisms of secretion, the geometric arrangement of the secretory cells, the branching patterns of ducts, and the chemical nature of the secretions.

Glands can be broadly divided into exocrine glands, which usually secrete via a duct onto surfaces continuous with the body's exterior (e.g., alimentary tract, respiratory passage, etc.) and endocrine glands, which are ductless glands that secrete locally or directly into the circulatory system. Endocrine glands will be examined in Chapter 17 (Endocrine System) and so they are not included in the following classifications.

Classification based on numbers of cell

Unicellular glands. Unicellular (*uni-*, one + *cella*, chamber) glands represent the simplest form of a gland. An example is the single cell that is incorporated into an epithelium. Both the mucus–secreting goblet cell occurring among enterocytes in the intestine and the mucus–secreting cell located within the pseudostratified epithelium of the respiratory system have been observed previously in light microscope tissue sections. In both of these examples, observe the shape of the entire cell, the shape and position of the nucleus, and the shape and size of the secretion reservoir storing the mucinogen inclusions. The secretory product is stored in the part of the cell adjacent to the lumen into which it will be released.

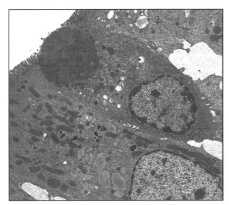

UNICELLULAR GLAND
Electron Micrograph #4: Goblet Cell and Enterocytes; intestinal epithelium of rat.
Higher magnification images:
  • goblet cell cytoplasm
  • mucigen inclusions

The electron micrograph reveals more detail of the goblet cell than a light microscope view does: the cytoplasmic cup portion of the cell that surrounds the secretory product is termed the theca (*theca*, box) whereas the base is termed the stem or base of the goblet cell. The characteristic shape of these cells observed in standard light microscope preparations is not reflected in electron microscope preparations because the preparative procedures for light microscopy cause an artifactual swelling of the mucinogen droplets in the apex of the cell.

MULTICELLULAR GLANDS. The cells of multicellular glands form simple, coiled, or branched tubular structures, or they assemble as terminal sacs called acini (*acinus*, grape or berry) or alveoli (*alveolus*, small hollow sac or cavity). The cells of multicellular glands discharge their product into a duct such as the striated duct observed previously, or directly onto an epithelial surface. Multicellular glands are illustrated in the following tissue sections of the parotid gland and the submandibular gland.

CLASSIFICATION BASED ON TYPE OF SECRETION

In addition to the classification of glands based on their geometric characteristics, glands can be classified on the basis of the chemical nature of their secretion. Histochemical and immunocytochemical techniques are necessary for demonstrating differences in the chemical nature of secretions. Morphological differences in the secretory cells can be used to distinguish between two broad classes of secretion: mucous and serous. Many glands associated with the respiratory, digestive, and urogenital system are classified according to these secretions. Mucous glands secrete mucinogen, which is a mixture of large glycosylated proteins that form a thick viscous protective lubricant upon hydration, termed mucin, that is a major component of mucus. Serous glands secrete an enzyme-rich watery fluid.

SEROUS SECRETION. The parotid gland, one of the major salivary glands, is a purely serous gland. Observe that the secretory cells are arranged in acini or alveoli around a small lumen into which they secrete their product. The nucleus is relatively spherical and

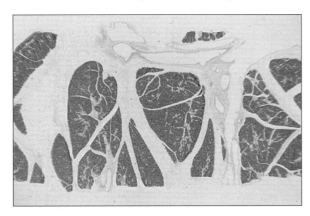

SEROUS GLAND
Slide #101: Parotid Gland; H&E stain; 4 mm thick methacrylate section; nonhuman primate.

Higher magnification image:
  • (middle) secretory acini

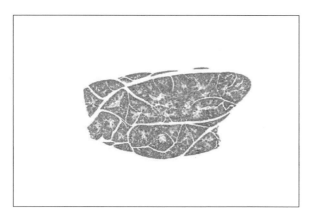

MIXED SEROMUCOUS GLAND
Slide #102: Submandibular Gland; H&E stain, 4 μm
thick methacrylate section; nonhuman primate.

Higher magnification images:
* (middle) mucous and serous cells
* (high) mucous and serous acini
* (high) mucous acinus and serous demilune

situated basally in the cell. The cytoplasm of the secretory cells is somewhat granular
and basophilic. The secretory granules are stored in the apical portion of the cells where
they remain until a signal causes them to be released. The watery secretions of these
cells contain mainly glycoproteins; in the oral cavity, the secretions include a bactericide
along with some digestive enzymes.

MIXED SEROMUCOUS SECRETION. The submandibular gland is a mostly serous gland but
also contains mucous acini, and so is classified as a mixed seromucous gland. Observe
that the mucous cells, which form the multicellular mucous acini, have pale frothy
cytoplasm. A flattened or crescent–shaped nuclei situated in the base of the cells. The
cells appear frothy or empty because the mucinogen product has been dissolved and
washed out during tissue processing. Serous cells, in contrast, have a less flattened
nucleus and a granular basophilic cytoplasm that is consistent with a protein-producing
cell.

Some of the mucous acini are capped by a crescent–shaped cluster of serous cells.
This cap-like group of cells is termed a serous demilune and their enzyme–rich product
reaches the lumen via small canals between the mucous cells.

An epithelial cell modified for its ability to contract, and termed a myoepithelial
cell, is applied to the basal surface of the secretory acinus. This cell contains myofila-
ments in its cytoplasm and has cellular processes that extend around the perimeter of
the acinus, like fingers of a hand holding a ball. When stimulated, these myoepithelial
cells contract and force secretory product into the lumen of the acinus.

5. CONNECTIVE TISSUE

Connective tissue is one of the four basic tissue types in histology. It is unique in comparison to the other types because its cells are dispersed in an extracellular matrix (*matrix*, womb) of fibers and interfibrillar ground substance. Connective tissues are present throughout the body where they serve to hold other tissues in their proper three–dimensional relationships. There is considerable morphological variability among connective tissues, not only in the relative proportions of cells to matrix, but also in the types of cells and in the amounts and organization of the extracellular fibrillar and nonfibrillar material. Learn to relate the morphology of the cells and matrix to the functions of the connective tissue.

In some connective tissues, components of the extracellular matrix predominate. The principal functions of these connective tissues are structural and their physical properties are related to the composition and organization of the extracellular matrix. In other connective tissues, one or more of the resident cell types predominate and the roles of these connective tissues rest principally in the functions of the cells. Knowing the normal behavior and interactions of the resident cells and the mechanical properties of the matrix, enables you to examine a tissue section of connective tissue and understand its function. The ability to interpret a light microscope image of connective tissue is actually an ability you already have, except that you presently apply a different set of learned expectations. Think about looking at a news photograph and how you get a sense of who, what, where, and even sometimes how just by examining the static images of the people, their expressions, clothing or uniforms, and the setting. In pathology, the abnormal presence or absence of any of the elements of connective tissue provides insight into suspected pathological events and, often how to deal therapeutically with them.

Fewer than ten different connective tissue cell types typically reside in connective tissue proper. The characteristic morphology of each cell is distinctly different from that of the others. Do not simply memorize each cell's morphological features, but attempt to relate its unique morphology to its function. For example, the cell whose principal role involves secreting protein usually has blue–staining cytoplasm because of its numerous protein–producing basophilic ribosomes; the phagocytic (*phag-*, eat; *-cyte*, cell) macrophage shows morphological evidence of intracellular digestion; and the cell responsible for storing the body's energy reserves contains a large droplet of lipid, the body's stored source of chemical energy.

This chapter examines the following cells. Some of these cells also appear in peripheral blood because they use the blood for transport to the connective tissue from the bone marrow where they were born.

> fibroblast (*fibro-*, a slender filament + *-blast*, germ, indicating an immature cell)
> lymphocyte (*lympho-*, combining form relating to lymph + *-cyte*, cell)
> plasma cell (*plasma*, something formed)
> macrophage (*macro*, large + *-phage*, to eat)
> mast cell (*Mast*, German word for food)
> neutrophil (polymorphonuclear neutrophil; *neutro-*, neither + *-phil*, liking)
> eosinophil (polymorphonuclear eosinophil; *eosin-*, the histological stain + *-phil*, liking)
> adipocyte or fat cell (*adipo-*, fat + *-cyte*, cell)
> unilocular adipocyte or white fat cell (*uni-*, one + *-loculus*, a small compartment)
> multilocular adipocyte or brown fat cell (*multi-*, multiple + *-loculus*, a small compartment)

Recognize the appearance, arrangement and physical properties of the following fibers in connective tissues.

collagen fiber; collagen fibrils (*col-*, glue + *-gen*, producing)
elastin fibers (*elastreo*, drive or push)
reticular fibers (*reticulum*, a small net)

Connective tissues are classified according to the relative density of fibers and cells, or by the predominant fiber or cell type. Bone and cartilage are special connective tissues that will be examined in a subsequent exercise. The following connective tissues are examined in this exercise.

loose (areolar) connective tissue (*area*, a courtyard + *-olar*, suffix denoting diminutive)
dense irregular connective tissue
dense regular connective tissue
reticular tissue (*reticulum*, a small net)
white adipose tissue
brown adipose tissue

CD-ROM Notice: The images examined in this chapter are listed numerically on the CD-ROM by microscope slide number as they might be in a standard histology laboratory. Observe that some microscope slides are listed more than once because, as in a real laboratory exercise, a single tissue section is used to demonstrate more than one feature. The appropriate lead-in images on the CD-ROM are labeled, and have the appropriate links, for the tissue or structure being illustrated. To avoid confusion resulting from selecting the wrong nested series of images, read the label on the CD-ROM list carefully.

In several of the image series in this exercise, the usual linked hotspot format is substituted for, or supplemented by, listing additional linked images either below the standard lead-in image or with a box-like graphic in a corner of the image.

CONNECTIVE TISSUE PROPER

This exercise begins with an examination of the variety of cells observed in general connective tissue, termed connective tissue proper. After examining the cells, examine the fibers of connective tissue, and conclude this chapter by considering examples of different classes of connective tissues. Consider the following diagrammatic overview of the composition of generalized connective tissue.

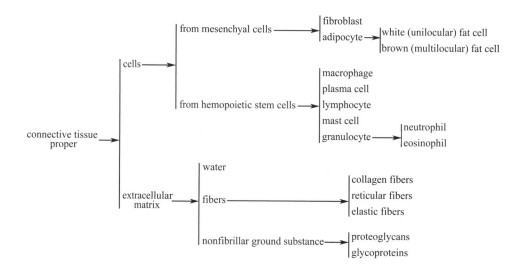

THE CELLS OF CONNECTIVE TISSUE PROPER

A variety of cells typical of loose connective tissue are present in the trachea. Identify the following cells in this 2-µm thick plastic section.

FIBROBLAST. Fibroblasts are thin and elongated cells that contain a relatively long and narrow, dark nucleus. Their attenuated (*attenuatus*, to make thin), branching, eosinophilic cellular processes are often too fine to be seen in the light microscope, or they blend into the wisps of collagen fibers, which also stain with eosin. Fibroblasts are distributed throughout the lamina propria and are usually the most numerous cells in a loose connective tissue. They are responsible for the synthesis and turnover of the principal components of the extracellular matrix: both the fibers and the nonfibrillar ground substance.

It is possible to interpret the level of activity of these cells by their morphology: when the rate of matrix turnover is slow, these cells are relatively small, fusiform (*fusus*, a spindle + *forma*, form) and more attenuated than when they are actively producing matrix. During periods of active growth, or during the repair of a wound in the tissue, these cells are larger, bulkier, and their cytoplasm is slightly more basophilic because of the increased number of cytoplasmic organelles involved in the synthesis of the matrix components. Although the standard convention is to refer to both the active and less active form of this cell as a fibroblast, a distinction is made by some histologists between the larger, active form termed the fibroblast and the smaller, less active form, termed the fibrocyte.

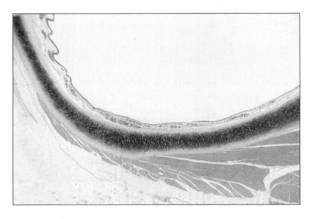

LOOSE CONNECTIVE TISSUE: CELLS
Slide #33: Trachea; 2 µm thick methacrylate section; eosin and toluidine blue stain; nonhuman primate.

Higher magnification images:
- (medium) tissues of the wall
- (high) fibroblast and plasma cell
- (high) fibroblast and plasma cell,
- (high) mast cell
- (high) mast cell
- (high) neutrophils and eosinophils
- (higher) neutrophils and eosinophils
- (high) macrophages
- (higher) macrophages and neutrophils
- (medium) lymphocyte

PLASMA CELL. Plasma cells are ovoid to spherical cells, up to 15 µm in diameter. The nucleus is usually eccentric (*ek-*, out + *kentron*, center) with dark heterochromatin distributed in peripheral clumps. This arrangement of the dark clumps of heterochromatin is said to give the nucleus the appearance of a clock face, whereas the complementary pattern of pale euchromatin looks like a cartwheel. Plasma cells are responsible for producing antibodies in the body. The cytoplasm is basophilic because of the high content of ribosomes that are necessary for the production of the antibodies. The prominent central pale region, called the cytocentrum (*cyto-*, cell + *kentron*, center), marks the location of the Golgi apparatus in which the antibodies are packaged for release. There are no secretion granules in the cytoplasm because the antibodies are released continuously as they are synthesized.

EOSINOPHIL (PME). Eosinophils are distinctive because of the bright pink–stained granules contained within their cytoplasm, which stains pale pink in this tissue section. In both peripheral blood and connective tissue, the eosinophil is the only cell whose cytoplasm contains such eosinophilic granules. The 2 or 3 segments characteristic of its nucleus may not all be visible in the tissue section. The eosinophil responds to inflammatory reactions, providing the means to inactivate the agents of inflammation. It also responds to parasitic infections in the body.

NEUTROPHIL (PMN, poly). Neutrophils have multisegmented nuclei and, in this tissue section, pale pink–stained cytoplasm. The neutrophil's specific granules are not visible in an H&E stained section, just as they are not visible in a peripheral blood smear stained with Wright's stain. Most PMNs in this tissue section are contained within blood vessels, from which they can leave in great numbers when necessary, as in an infection or inflammatory reaction.

LYMPHOCYTE. Lymphocytes are normally present in connective tissue where their role involves scouting and patrolling for potentially harmful antigenic substances. When appropriately stimulated they produce clones of effector and memory cells. Plasma cells are the effector cells produced through antigen–dependent proliferation of the B-lymphocytes. Like the lymphocytes identified in the peripheral blood, these cells have a high nucleus-to-cytoplasm ratio. That is, there is relatively little cytoplasm associated with the nucleus. As in the peripheral blood, it is not possible to differentiate among the various types and subtypes of lymphocytes without the use of immunocytochemical techniques designed to recognize the surface markers that are unique to each cell type.

In these tissue sections, clusters of lymphocytes reside just beneath the epithelium, monitoring that surface. Such clusters are referred to with the acronym MALT, which stands for mucosa–associated lymphoid tissue.

MAST CELL. Mast cells are comparatively large oval cells that are approximately 25 μm in diameter with a small oval nucleus. The key characteristic of the mast cell in a tissue section stained with toluidine blue is the presence of dense, reddish-purple, metachromatic (*meta-*, after + *chroma*, color) cytoplasmic granules. These granules contain histamine and heparin and other agents that when released are responsible for many of the symptoms associated with an allergy response.

MACROPHAGE. Macrophages can be most clearly identified in a standard H&E stained section when their morphology reflects their phagocytic function; otherwise they are less easily recognized. As with many other cells, macrophages can be definitively labeled with immunocytochemical or histochemical staining techniques. In this tissue section the macrophages are relatively large cells of irregular shape, 15 to 30 μm in length in the vicinity of the small blood vessels. The macrophage nucleus is oval with clumped heterochromatin, and the darkly pink cytoplasm contains numerous clear phagocytic vacuoles of various sizes. Because of the unique morphological features of this cytoplasm, it is possible to identify partial sections of macrophages.

Macrophages are part of the body's diverse collection of phagocytic cells derived from circulating monocytes. The collection is termed the mononuclear phagocyte system. Many of these macrophages have organ–specific names, like the alveolar macrophage in the lung, the microglial cell in the central nervous system, the Kupffer cell in the liver, and the osteoclast in bone. The tissue macrophage is also known as a histiocyte (*histo-*, web, tissue + -*cyte*, cell).

Mast cells are visible in their entirety in the spread preparation (Slide #7) of loose connective tissue since, like a blood smear, this is not a sectioned piece of tissue. This spread preparation was produced by placing a small piece of unfixed loose connective tissue on a microscope slide and gently stretching it into a thin flat sheet. The tissue was then fixed, washed, appropriately stained, and covered. Because of the nature of the spread preparations, it is possible to observe blood vessels arrayed as networks of anastomosing tubes and to view the relationship between the cells and the blood vessels.

This particular preparation was stained with only a basic dye, and so the cytoplasm of most cells is not stained and only their nuclei are visible. However, the basophilic granules in the cytoplasm of the mast cells stain well. The mast cells comprise a strikingly uniform population of distinct ovoid cells that are usually associated with the outer walls of small blood vessels. This location is typical for mast cells, whose granules contain several pharmacologically active agents that target the tissues of blood vessels, rendering them leaky as part of the inflammatory reaction.

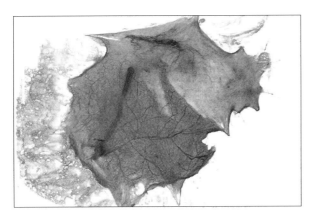

MAST CELL AND MACROPHAGE
Slide #7: Areolar Connective Tissue; spread preparation; methylene blue stain; rat

Higher magnification images:
- (medium) mast cells and blood vessels
- (high) mast cells and labeled macrophages
- (high) supravitally labeled macrophages

This tissue preparation has been supravitally (*supra-*, above + *vital*, life) stained to specifically label the population of macrophages. For this technique, the living animal received a series of intraperitoneal (*intra-*, within + *peritoneal*, which refers to the abdominal cavity) injections of a blue dye (trypan blue) that the macrophages phagocytose (ingest) as part of their role as resident tissue clean–up cells.

The macrophages in this preparation are thus labeled by phagocytosed dye particles. The dye particles are contained within phagosomes and residual bodies, components of the intracellular digestive system. Although the cytoplasm of the macrophages is unstained, the cytoplasmic domain of each macrophage can be determined by the distribution of the ingested dye particles. The shape of the macrophages, so defined, is usually irregular but varies among the cells. This irregularity in shape is consistent with a cell that crawls through the tissue seeking debris to phagocytose. The macrophage nucleus, identified by the concentration of blue particles in the unstained cytoplasm surrounding it, is typically ovoid.

ELECTRON MICROSCOPE IMAGES OF THE CELLS OF CONNECTIVE TISSUE
Several of the connective tissue cells are illustrated in the set of electron micrographs on the CD-ROM. The fine structural image of most of these cells is similar to the light microscope image, but provides additional details of the cell and its surrounding matrix.

FIBROBLAST. This fibroblast has a typically attenuated shape. Its relatively meager cytoplasm contains all the organelles associated with protein synthesis and secretion: rough endoplasmic reticulum, Golgi apparatus, secretion vesicles. The fibroblast is

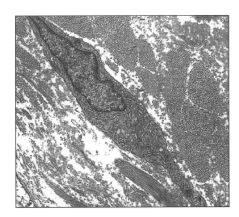

FIBROBLAST
Electron Micrograph #8: Fibroblast; rat.

Higher magnification images:
- type I collagen fibrils
- fibroblast organelles

involved in the synthesis and turnover of the matrix materials, and organizes the orientation of the fibrillar components in the matrix

Fibrils of type I collagen are dispersed in the matrix along with nonfibrillar matrix materials. In this plate, most of the collagen fibrils are transversely sectioned and appear as small circular profiles. The fibroblast synthesizes and secretes linear collagen molecules that are modified and assembled extracellularly. The polymer type I collagen fibrils have a characteristic 67 nm cross-banding pattern that results from the staggered array of the monomer collagen molecules. The smaller dark profiles adjacent to the fibroblast are fibrils being assembled from the collagen molecules. Type I collagen fibrils are strong, cable-like polymers that assemble together to form the collagen fibers that are visible in the light microscope.

PLASMA CELL. The plasma cell cytoplasm is packed with rough endoplasmic reticulum. Polyribosomes on the cytoplasmic surface of this membranous organelle are responsible for the cytoplasm's basophilia. Antibodies, synthesized in the rough endoplasmic reticulum, are packaged for secretion in the Golgi apparatus. This plane of section barely includes the Golgi apparatus, which is located in the cytocentrum, the cell's center. Since the Golgi apparatus has no ribosomes associated with it, the cytocentrum is pale in an H&E–stained light microscope preparation. There are no secretion granules in this cell because antibodies are not stored, rather they are released as they are generated.

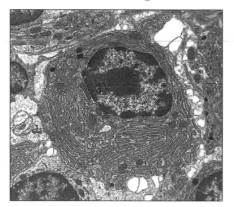

PLASMA CELL
Electron Micrograph #10: Plasma Cell; rat.

Higher magnification images:
- nucleus and rough endoplasmic reticulum
- cytocentrum of plasma cell
- rough endoplasmic reticulum

EOSINOPHIL AND MACROPHAGE. The ultrastructural image of the eosinophil reveals specific granules with unusual dense cores. The central dense core of the eosinophilic granules, termed the internum, contains major basic protein and a neurotoxin that are used to combat parasites. The internum is responsible for the characteristic refractile nature of the granules that is detected in an H&E–stained light microscope preparation. The outer portion of these specific granules, the externum, contains aryl sulfatase and histaminase in addition to other enzymes that counter the inflammatory reaction.

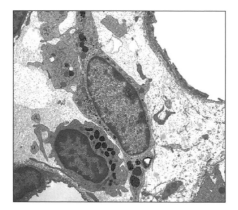

EOSINOPHIL AND MACROPHAGE.
Electron Micrograph #9: Eosinophil and Macrophage; rat.

Higher magnification images:
- macrophage cytoplasm
- granules and residual bodies
- fenestrated capillary

A macrophage is also illustrated in this electron micrograph. Its characteristic organelles include a Golgi apparatus and primary lysosomes as well as digestion vacuoles and residual bodies. The large residual bodies that are electron dense (i.e., appear black) in the electron micrograph correspond to the vacuoles that appear empty in the light microscope preparations.

MAST CELL. The ultrastructure of a mast cell reveals numerous electron dense granules packed in the cytoplasm, an image consistent with the light microscope image. These granules contain pharmacologically active agents that are responsible for initiating many aspects of the inflammatory response. The chemicals in the granules are collectively termed primary mediators, and include histamine, heparin, chondroitin sulfate, and neutral proteases. The granules also contain an eosinophil chemotaxic factor that attracts eosinophils to the site of inflammation. The packing of these negatively charged chemicals into the granules is responsible for the metachromasia that characterizes these granules. The cell's plasma membrane possesses numerous receptors for immunoglobulin E (IgE) and, following primary exposures to allergens, many IgE antibodies become bound to the cell's plasma membrane. Subsequent exposure to the appropriate allergens results in a very rapid response: the mast cell degranulates and synthesizes a secondary set of mediators of inflammation. Some of these secondary mediators are synthesized from membrane arachidonic acid precursors, and include leukotrienes and prostaglandins.

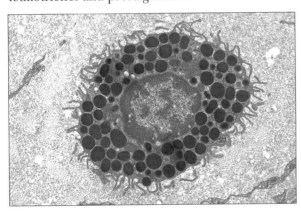

MAST CELL
Electron Micrograph #26: Mast Cell; rat.

ADIPOSE TISSUE

WHITE FAT CELLS. Adipose tissue is a special loose connective tissue that is dominated by unilocular (white) adipocytes. The name of these cells is based on the cell's content of one large droplet of lipid. Examine the subcutaneous (sub-, below + cutis, skin) layer (the hypodermis; hypo-, under + dermis, skin) of skin in this tissue section. In adipose tissue, the fat cells are individually held in place by delicate reticular fibers and they cluster in lobules bounded by fibrous septa. Unilocular fat cells can be very large cells,

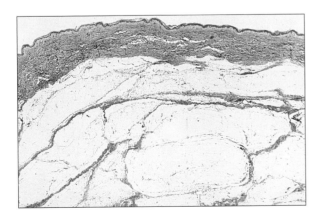

UNILOCULAR ADIPOCYTES IN WHITE FAT
Slide #82: Abdominal Skin; 15 μm paraffin section; H&E stain; human.

Higher magnification images:
• (high) white fat cells

nearly 150 mm in diameter. The large droplet of lipid displaces the small dark nucleus such that it becomes a flattened semilunar structure pushed against the edge of the cell. Because of the size of these cells, relative to the thickness of the section, the nucleus may not always be present in the section. The interior of these fat cells is unstained because the techniques of standard tissue preparation dissolve out the lipids, leaving a thin rim of eosinophilic cytoplasm that typically loses its round shape during tissue processing.

In connective tissue proper, as illustrated in the following spread preparation (Slide #9), unilocular adipocytes are dispersed among the other cells. Such adipocytes usually appear in small clumps near blood vessels, which is an understandable location since the source, and dispersion, of material stored in these adipocytes depends on transportation by the vascular system. This spread preparation has been specifically prepared to demonstrate white fat cells: the lipid has not been dissolved out by the usual tissue processing solvents and it has been stained with a fat-soluble dye. Compare the diameters of these cells to the size of the nuclei in the surrounding tissue and the red blood cells within the lumen of the capillaries.

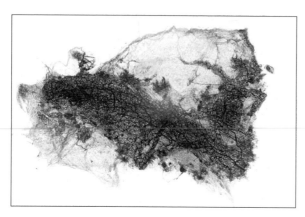

UNILOCULAR FAT CELLS:
Slide #9: Areolar Connective Tissue; spread preparation; Sudan IV stain for lipid; nonhuman primate.

Higher magnification images:
* (medium) unilocular adipocytes and capillaries

BROWN FAT CELLS. Brown fat tissue is a specialized type of adipose tissue that plays an important part in regulating body temperature. It has a limited distribution in the child, and occurs only in small amounts in the adult human. Substantially more brown fat is present in animals that hibernate than in humans.

Multilocular adipocytes are present in this tissue section of mixed white and brown adipose tissue from a young nonhuman primate. The individual multilocular adipocytes are frothy–appearing cells because the lipid, which is normally stored in multiple small droplets, has been leached out during tissue processing. The spherical nuclei are centrally or eccentrically located within the cell. Compared to unilocular white fat cells, the cytoplasm of the multilocular brown fat cell is relatively abundant and strongly stained because of the numerous mitochondria present. The mitochondria are involved in the oxidation of the stored lipid, but because they are unable to carry out oxidative

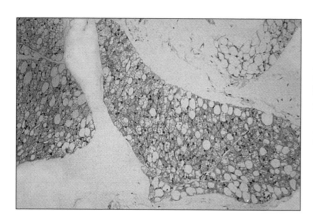

MULTILOCULAR FAT CELLS
Slide #49: Adipose Tissue; 2 mm, H&E stain; nonhuman primate.

Higher magnification images:
* (high) multilocular and unilocular adipocytes

phosphorylation, the energy produced is released in the form of heat, not captured in adenosine triphosphate (ATP). Brown adipose tissue is extremely well vascularized; blood is warmed when it passes through the active tissue.

FIBERS OF CONNECTIVE TISSUE MATRIX

COLLAGEN. The collagen fibers visible in standard light microscope preparations of connective tissue proper are largely bundles of the ubiquitous type I collagen fibrils. The collagen stains with eosin and is visible as fibrous pink–stained material in the extracellular matrix. Type I collagen is the principal form of collagen in the dermis and the capsules of organs. The collagen fibers in the matrix are assembled and organized under the direction of the fibroblast to best withstand the tensile forces applied to the tissue. The fine structure of collagen fibers is visible in Electron Micrograph #8, which illustrates the fibroblast.

RETICULAR FIBERS. The distribution of reticular fibers can be observed in this tissue section of a lymph node treated with a silver stain. Reticular fibers are type III collagen and they naturally attract silver salts. In the absence of a counterstain, the black-staining reticular fibers are seen to form a fine branching latticework that serves as a flexible scaffolding to support the resident cells. Within the interstices of this fibrous meshwork the unstained lymphocytes appear as yellowish cells. In an H&E stain, the reticular fibers stain pink, but because of their delicate size and geometry, they are not easily visualized without a special stain like this silver stain.

Reticular tissue refers to a class of delicate connective tissue present in highly cellular organs in which the principal fiber type is the reticular fiber, not the larger, coarser, more ubiquitous type I collagen fiber. In this delicate reticular tissue, fibroblasts may be termed reticular cells.

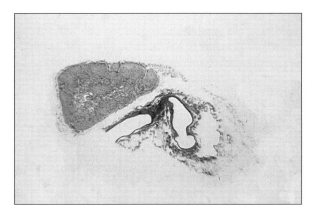

RETICULAR FIBERS
Slide #70: Lymph Node; 15 µm paraffin section; silver stain; nonhuman primate.

Higher magnification images:
- (medium) lymph node, reticular stain
- (high) reticular fibers

STROMA AND PARENCHYMA. The general term for the supporting network of an organ or gland is stroma (*stroma*, bed). The term for the specific cells that characterize the gland or organ is parenchyma (*parenche-*, to pour in beside). In the lymph node above, the stroma is reticular tissue and the principal parenchymal cells are lymphocytes. Reticular tissue forms the stroma of the liver and the spleen as well as lymphoid, hemopoietic, and adipose tissues.

ELASTIC FIBERS. This following spread preparation has been stained with Verhoeff's stain specifically to demonstrate the elastic fibers. Elastic fibers are naturally eosinophilic like collagen, and require a special stain to differentiate them from the reticular and collagen fibers in a tissue section. With a special stain for elastin, the elastic fibers in this preparation are dark, thin strands. Broken or snapped elastic fibers are seen to have kinked or curled ends.

With their respective special stains, both the reticular and the elastic fibers stain black. However, it is easy to differentiate between them if you consider how the geometry of the fibers in the tissue reflects their different functions. Elastic fibers typically ramify throughout a tissue that is subject to distorting tensile forces; the elastic recoil of these fibers enables the tissue to recover when the force is released. The amount of elastic tissue varies with the physical requirements of the tissue. Elastin may be in the form of fibers as in this spread preparation, or in sheets, as in the walls of blood vessels. Reticular fibers, in contrast to the elastic fibers, form delicate supporting networks in highly cellular organs and tissues. Although reticular tissue allows for an organ's change in volume (as in a swollen lymph node) it does so without storing recoil energy.

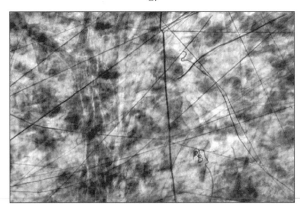

ELASTIC FIBERS
Slide #8: Areolar Connective Tissue; spread preparation; Verhoeff's stain for elastic fibers; nonhuman primate.

There is no higher magnification image.

This spread preparation has been stained only with Verhoeff's stain. Collagen fibers are the large unstained coarse bundles of varying widths. Although individual collagen fibrils do not branch, collagen bundles can branch.

This tissue section of skin is stained with Verhoeff's stain. Observe the black-stained elastic fibers in the dermis and the hypodermis. The elastic fibers in the superficial region of dermis are more delicate than the coarser elastic fibers of the deeper layers of the dermis.

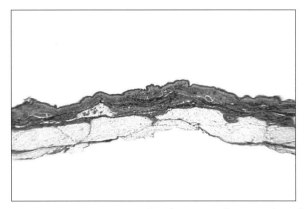

ELASTIC FIBERS IN A TISSUE SECTION
Slide #83: Thin Skin; 10 µm; Verhoeff's elastin stain; nonhuman primate.

Higher magnification image:
- (medium) epidermis, dermis and hypodermis

In electron micrographs, elastin stains poorly and is typically amorphous, with no distinct fibrils in the sense of collagen fibrils. An example of elastin is illustrated in the wall of the blood vessel illustrated in Electron Micrograph #14 in the CD-ROM.

CLASSIFICATION OF CONNECTIVE TISSUE

Connective tissues are classified as either general connective tissues or special connective tissues. The general connective tissues include the ubiquitous connective tissues that occur in and around other tissues, carrying nerves and vessels and maintaining three–dimensional structural relationships. The special connective tissues are ones that have special structural, metabolic, or physiological functions. They are found with a more limited distribution, usually only where those functions are required.

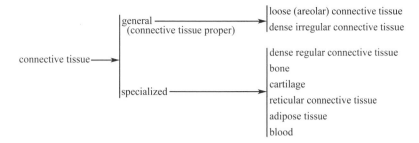

<table>
<tr><td rowspan="2"></td><td>general</td><td>loose (areolar) connective tissue</td></tr>
<tr><td>(connective tissue proper)</td><td>dense irregular connective tissue</td></tr>
</table>

connective tissue

general ———————————→ loose (areolar) connective tissue
(connective tissue proper)   dense irregular connective tissue

specialized ———————————→ dense regular connective tissue
                              bone
                              cartilage
                              reticular connective tissue
                              adipose tissue
                              blood

LOOSE (AREOLAR) CONNECTIVE TISSUE. The tissue underlying the epithelial lining of the trachea is a loose connective tissue. This tissue is characterized by having a variety of cells interspersed singly or in small groups among the fine fibers of the extracellular matrix. The extracellular matrix of the loose connective tissue stains less strongly with eosin than does the matrix of the dense connective tissue that surrounds the cartilage in this tissue section because it has fewer and smaller collagen fibers. Many small blood vessels and lymphatic vessels characterize the areolar connective tissue.

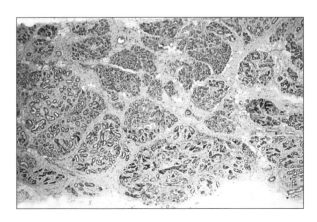

LOOSE OR AREOLAR CONNECTIVE TISSUE
Slide #33: Trachea; 2 μm methacrylate section; eosin and toluidine blue stain; nonhuman primate.

Higher magnification images:
- (medium) tissues of the wall
- (high) lamina propria

DENSE IRREGULAR CONNECTIVE TISSUE. Dense irregular connective tissue courses among the individual lobules of the mammary gland in this next tissue section. The dense and loose designations of connective tissue refer to ends of a continuum that is based largely on the relative numbers of cells and fibers present in the tissue. Dense irregular connective tissue is characterized by the presence of coarse, irregular bundles of collagen and few cells, primarily fibroblasts, whereas loose has more cells than fibers, a greater variety of cells, and the bundles of collagen are finer and more dispersed than those of dense irregular connective tissue. The connective tissue that immediately surrounds the secretory alveoli of the mammary gland, within the lobules, is a loose connective tissue.

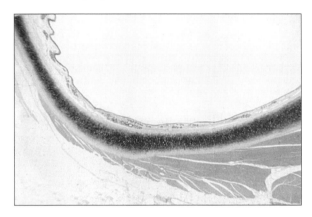

DENSE IRREGULAR CONNECTIVE TISSUE
Slide #89: Mammary Gland; 10 μm paraffin section, H&E stain; human.

Higher magnification image:
- (medium) loose and dense irregular connective tissue

Terms used to describe location within a structure like the mammary gland, which is organized into lobules (*lob-*, lobe; *-ule*, designating a diminutive), are interlobular (*inter-*, between) referring to a location between the lobules, and intralobular (*intra-*, within) referring to a location within the lobule. The dense connective tissue in this section of mammary gland is interlobular and the loose connective tissue is intralobular.

DENSE REGULAR CONNECTIVE TISSUE. This category of connective tissue is located in the body where it functions to resist strong tensile forces. Tendons, ligaments, aponeuroses, and fasciae are all examples of dense regular connective tissue. Observe the following tissue sections of tendon oriented in longitudinal and transverse planes of section. This poorly vascularized tissue is comprised principally of collagen bundles oriented in line with the principal direction of the pulling forces. Fibroblasts, often called tendonocytes in this tissue, are dispersed among the fiber bundles. The long axis of the flattened dark fibroblast nucleus is oriented parallel to the fiber bundles.

The tissue section of tendon in longitudinal section provides a comparison between the dense regular connective tissue of the tendon and the dense irregular connective tissue that surrounds the tendon. The irregularly interweaving coarse collagen bundles and the number of blood vessels in the latter tissue are two notable differences between the regular and the irregular dense connective tissue.

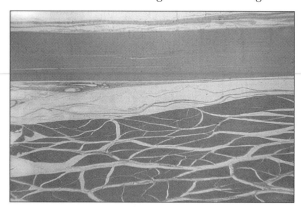

DENSE REGULAR CONNECTIVE TISSUE
Slide #13: Tendon; longitudinal section; 3 μm methacrylate section; H&E stain; nonhuman primate.

Higher magnification image:
• (medium) dense regular connective tissue

The transversely sectioned tendon illustrates clearly the regular distribution of the fibroblast nuclei as well as the very low density of blood vessels. The transversely sectioned skeletal muscle adjacent to the tendon is better vascularized than the tendon, reflecting the difference in the metabolic requirements of these two tissues.

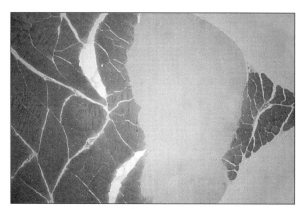

DENSE REGULAR CONNECTIVE TISSUE
Slide #14: Tendon and Muscle; transverse section; 3 μm, H&E stain; nonhuman primate.

Higher magnification image:
• (medium) dense regular connective tissue

6. CARTILAGE AND BONE AND BONE HISTOGENESIS

Cartilage and bone are specialized connective tissues that function as supporting materials with mechanically sophisticated physical properties. Cartilage is a semisolid, flexible, compressible, and resilient tissue; bone is a somewhat rigid, mineralized tissue that is able to withstand compressive and tensile forces equally well. Because of their special biomechanical properties, the distribution of cartilage and bone is restricted to locations in the body where these properties are required. Understanding the composition and organization of the matrix is key to appreciating the mechanical properties of these tissues. It is also important to recognize that both bone and cartilage are very dynamic tissues, responding with growth or matrix modification to changes in the mechanical forces imposed upon them.

This chapter examines both the matrix of cartilage and bone and the resident cells that synthesize and maintain the matrix. A key to understanding the structure and function of the resident cells requires considering a fourth dimension, the dimension of time, in the interpretation of these two-dimensional tissue sections.

The second part of this exercise examines the histogenesis of bone, both the initial formation of bone and the processes by which bone remodels itself in response to maturation, growth, and changing mechanical requirements. It is natural to think of bone as a static material, like the steel infrastructure of a building. However, bone tissue is not only able to respond to growth and changing physical demands, but also it houses the body's mobilizable store of calcium, a mineral that is critical to many physiologic functions.

The matrix provides one basis for the classification of the various categories of cartilage and bone. The following diagrammatic overview focuses on the matrix to categorize the tissues examined in this exercise. The first distinction between these two supporting tissues is based on whether the matrix is vascularized and mineralized.

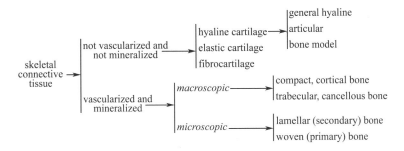

The following cells are examined in this exercise. The common word root for structures associated with cartilage is derived from the Greek word *chondrion*, meaning gristle or cartilage. The word cartilage is based on the Latin word *cartilago*, also meaning gristle or cartilage. The common word root for structures associated with bone is derived from the Greek word *osteon*, meaning bone.

> chondrocyte (*chondro-*, cartilage + *-cyte*, cell)
> osteocyte (*osteo-*, bone + *-cyte*, cell)
> osteoblast (*osteo-*, bone + *-blastos*, germ, seed)
> osteoclast (*osteo-*, bone + *-klastos*, broken)
> osteoprogenitor cell (*osteo-*, bone + *-progenitor*, a precursor)
> bone lining cell (a descriptive term for this cell's location)

Both cartilage and bone are usually ensheathed in a dense connective tissue envelope that provides the means for attachment of other tissues of the body to these skeletal tissues. The names of these are simple translations of the word roots.

perichondrium (*peri-*, around + *chondrion*, cartilage)
periosteum (*peri-*, around + *osteon*, bone)

In both bone and cartilage, the cells reside in a small cavity in the matrix called a lacuna (*lacuna*, pl. *lacunae*), a Latin word meaning a small hollow or lake. In bone the lacunae are interconnected by a vast system of tiny canaliculi (*canaliculus*, pl. *canaliculi*), a word derived by combining the Latin diminutive ending to the Latin word for canal.

CD-ROM Notice: The images examined in this chapter are listed numerically on the CD-ROM according to microscope slide number as they might be in a standard histology laboratory. Several of the numbered slides have multiple versions and all of the versions are included. In the case of the three tissue sections of the embryo head (#22), the three different lead–in images (I, II, and III) are linked to the same higher magnification images. On the other hand, for the compact bone (#27), the sets of linked images are different for the two lead in images (I and II). For the bone modeling and remodeling slides (#26), there are two different versions of the tissue section #26 and each one is used to illustrate different processes. To avoid confusion resulting from selecting the wrong nested series of images, read the label on the CD-ROM list carefully and compare them with the images in this Guide.

CARTILAGE

The extracellular matrix in cartilage consists largely of type II collagen fibrils dispersed in a ground substance of large, highly hydrated proteoglycan aggregates. Unlike bone, cartilage contains no nerves or blood or lymphatic vessels. The nutrients required to support the metabolism of the chondrocytes are carried by diffusion through the matrix. The appearance and nature of the matrix fibrillar material traditionally serve as the basis for the classification of cartilage types as hyaline, elastic or fibrocartilage. Hyaline cartilage is the most common type of cartilage.

The following structures and features of cartilage are named according to their appearance or functional significance.

interterritorial matrix (*inter-*, between; *matrix*, womb)
territorial matrix
isogenous group (*iso-*, equal + *genesis*, production)

HYALINE CARTILAGE: IMMATURE

The three different versions of this tissue section illustrate the location of cartilage in the growing embryo head: cartilage forms the flexible structures supporting the tissues of the nasal cavity. In these sections, as typical for embryonic cartilage, the growing cartilage matrix has a very high water content and thus is very lightly and homogeneously stained. The matrix lacks visible fibrous structure because the type II collagen fibers are fine and organized in a feltlike meshwork. Type II collagen fibrils do not assemble into bundles as do type I collagen fibrils.

The perichondrium is composed of dense connective tissue and surrounds the cartilage tissue. This enveloping layer consists mostly of type I collagen fibers that blend outward into the surrounding connective tissue. On the side of the perichondrium adjacent to the cartilage tissue, the perichondrium becomes more cellular and, at the perichondrium–cartilage junction, its fibers and cells blend into cartilage tissue. The

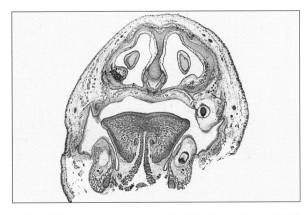

HYALINE CARTILAGE: IMMATURE
Slide #22: Fetal Head I; transverse section; H&E
stained 12 μm paraffin section; dog.

Higher magnification images:
- (medium) perichondrium
- (high) chondrocytes

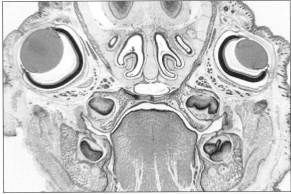

HYALINE CARTILAGE: IMMATURE
Slide #22: Fetal Head III; transverse section; H&E
stained 12 μm paraffin section; rat.

Higher magnification images:
- (medium) perichondrium
- (high) chondrocytes

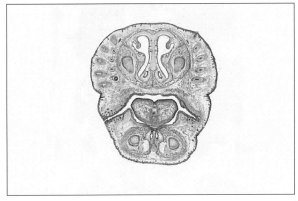

HYALINE CARTILAGE: IMMATURE
Slide #22: Fetal Head III; transverse section; H&E
stained 12 μm paraffin section; rat.

Higher magnification images:
- (medium) perichondrium
- (high) chondrocytes

perichondrium is imprecisely subdivided into two layers: an outer fibrous layer and an inner cellular layer. The cells residing within the outermost fibrous perichondrium are fibroblasts, but the cells at the perichondrium—cartilage junction are bipotential mesenchyme–derived cells capable of differentiating into chondroblasts as growth requires. In this tissue the fibroblasts and the bipotential stem cells are distinguished one from the other largely by their location in the perichondrium.

The resident cells of cartilage tissue are chondrocytes. The relatively inactive chondrocytes can be distinguished from the immature cells that are actively synthesizing cartilage matrix. The latter, which are referred to as chondroblasts by some histologists, are the smaller less mature cells residing deep to the perichondrium. Chondrocytes and chondroblasts both reside in lacunae in the fiber-reinforced, porous, gel-like matrix. In these preparations the chondrocytes appear dark and shrunken as a result of less-than-ideal fixation. Because of the nature of the cartilage matrix, standard fixatives penetrate slowly, allowing the deeply embedded chondrocytes to deteriorate before they can be properly preserved by the fixative.

MATURE HYALINE CARTILAGE

The cartilage of the mature trachea is easily located in this image. In this preparation the cartilage of the tracheal ring has a different appearance than that in the fetal heads. This is partly because the mature cartilage matrix is considerably less hydrated than the embryonic cartilage, meaning there is less dispersion of the polyanionic (negatively charged, therefore basophilic) proteoglycan aggregates in the matrix. Closer inspection also reveals the superior fixation of this tissue and its resident cells.

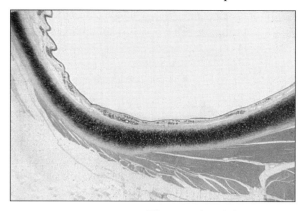

MATURE HYALINE CARTILAGE
Slide #33: Trachea; eosin and toluidine blue stain; 3 μm methacrylate plastic section; nonhuman primate.

Higher magnification images:
- (medium) cartilage
- (high) perichondrium
- (higher) chondrocytes

The matrix of this mature cartilage is not stained evenly. The intensely basophilic matrix surrounding the chondrocytes is referred to as the territorial matrix, and the interterritorial matrix is the paler material in between the groups of chondrocytes. The difference in staining occurs because of the uneven distribution of the principal components of the matrix: increased basophilia is because of increased concentrations of the glycosaminoglycan aggregates in the matrix and few collagenous fibrils in the immediate vicinity of the chondrocytes. Sometimes a narrow, very basophilic zone lines the lacuna, and this is termed the capsule of the chondrocyte, but there is no special encapsulating material between the chondrocyte and the matrix.

The chondrocytes in this tissue section are more variable in shape and size than those in the embryonic cartilage. In more central (deep) regions of this cartilage, chondrocytes have an oval to rounded shape and occur in clusters termed isogenous groups. Isogenous groups represent daughter cells produced by the mitotic division of chondrocytes. In the periphery of this tissue, subjacent to the perichondrium, chondroblasts are flattened and isolated. The fixation of this tissue has preserved the resident chondrocytes and chondroblasts well, providing a clear indication of their typically viable state in this tissue. These cells usually contain lipid droplets within their cytoplasm. Some of the clear spaces in the chondrocyte cytoplasm correspond to areas where glycogen has been dissolved during tissue processing. Glycogen is present in these cells to support their largely anaerobic glycolytic metabolism.

This tissue section illustrates the two modes of growth that characterize growing cartilage. Because of the flexibility of its matrix, cartilage can grow from within as well as by adding to its surface. In its inner regions this cartilage is undergoing interstitial growth (*interstitium*, from *inter-*, within + *sisto*, to stand): the chondrocytes divide and the daughter cells produce matrix, gradually enlarging the tissue from within. The second mode of growth, is termed appositional (*ap–, at or to* + *positus*, placing) and it occurs just beneath the enveloping perichondrium. The bipotential cells of the cellular perichondrium differentiate into chondroblasts and synthesize matrix, adding to the surface. It may seem counterintuitive that the these two modes of growth are so clearly illustrated in this slower growing mature cartilage in comparison to that in fetal cartilage. This apparent discrepancy occurs because of the speed of the growth process in the fetal cartilage. Mitotic division and separation of the daughter cells occurs quickly in the much more rapidly growing fetal cartilage, whereas the slower rates of the mature cartilage enable the capturing of the stages in time.

ARTICULAR CARTILAGE

The free surfaces of bones that face joint cavities are covered by a special layer of hyaline cartilage. Cartilage is an ideal material for this location because of its inherent resiliency. This tissue section is a patella (kneecap) and the tendon within which it has formed.

Articular cartilage is securely bound to the surface of the bone and has no perichondrium on its free surface. It is a special form of hyaline cartilage that is further modified to withstand the mechanical forces to which it is uniquely subjected. To withstand surface wear and friction, additional type II collagen fibrils are aligned within the matrix underlying the free surface of the cartilage; this extra collagen renders this superficial region of matrix slightly more eosinophilic and flattens the chondrocytes in their lacunae. To withstand compressive forces, collagen fibrils in the outer region are arrayed in arches with straight bundles of fibrils extending radially into the cartilage below. Although these radial bundles of collagen are not visible, the slightly vertical columns of chondrocytes, arrayed perpendicular to the surface, reflect their presence. Articular cartilage is anchored to the irregular surface of the underlying bone by a narrow zone of mineralized cartilage, and the surfaces of these two mineralized tissues interlock like three-dimensional puzzle pieces. This mineralized matrix is not compatible with the life of the chondrocyte because these cells depend on the hydrated matrix for metabolic support. The enlarged lacunae within the zone of mineralized matrix reflect the fact that the matrix has condensed as mineralization displaces the bound water, and the chondrocytes are dying. A basophilic line, or series of lines, termed the tidemark marks the interface between nonmineralized cartilage and the narrow region of mineralized cartilage matrix adjacent to the bone.

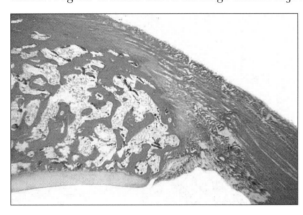

ARTICULAR CARTILAGE
Slide #31: Patella; H&E stained 3 µm methacrylate plastic section, nonhuman primate.

Higher magnification image:
  • (medium) articular cartilage

ELASTIC CARTILAGE

Elastic cartilage is a modified form of cartilage that occurs in those regions of the body where the firm support of cartilage requires added elasticity. Elastic cartilage is found in the epiglottis, the Eustachian tubes, and the external meatus of the ear.

The tissue section of the epiglottis (slide #29) is oriented with its free surfaces in the pharyngeal cavity and its base in the wall of the pharynx. The matrix of elastic cartilage is fundamentally similar to that of hyaline cartilage, consisting of cells, collagenous fibrils (type II), and ground substance, but with the addition of a dense meshwork of elastic fibers. The chondrocytes of elastic cartilage synthesize all the components of the matrix.

The Verhoeff's stain reveals elastic fibers that are especially numerous in the matrix. Without an elastic stain, that is, with a standard H&E stain, this cartilage appears somewhat more cellular and its matrix slightly more eosinophilic than hyaline cartilage. Observe the patches of matrix in this tissue section that have few elastic fibers. These regions represent protective sleeves of inelastic matrix that surround the blood vessels and nerves that traverse the plate of elastic cartilage.

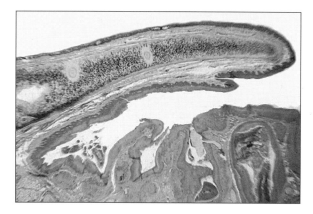

ELASTIC CARTILAGE
Slide #29: Epiglottis; Verhoeff stained 10 μm paraffin section, nonhuman primate.

Higher magnification image:
- (medium) elastic cartilage

FIBROCARTILAGE

Fibrocartilage exists in areas where the flexible structural support of cartilage is augmented by superior tensile strength of type I collagen, or where the notable tensile strength of a tendon is augmented by a supporting matrix. In this tissue section, fibrocartilage occurs at the insertion of a large tendon into bone. Examine the fibrocartilage located in the zone between the tendon, which is recognized by its very flattened fibroblasts, and the bone into which the tendon inserts. There is a gradual transition between the dense regular connective tissue of the tendon into fibrocartilage. The relatively sparse, ovoid chondrocytes are arranged singly, in groups, or in rows between the bundles of type I collagen. There is no perichondrium.

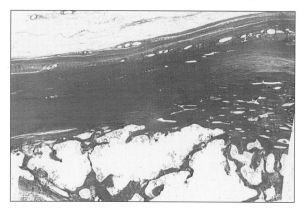

FIBROCARTILAGE
Slide #32: Patella; H&E stain; demineralized 3 μm methacrylate plastic section; nonhuman primate.

Higher magnification images:
- (medium) fibrocartilage and tendon
- (medium) fibrocartilage and bone

BONE

In bone, specific names describe certain macroscopic and microscopic structures and features. There are several eponyms that persist in this vocabulary despite efforts to replace the names with more descriptive ones.

> compact bone or cortical bone (*cortex*, pl. *cortices*, bark)
> cancellous bone, also spongy bone or trabecular bone (*cancellus*, a grating or lattice)
> trabecula, pl. trabeculae (*-ula*, diminutive of *trabs*, a beam)
> Haversian canal (after C. Havers 17th century English anatomist)
> Volkmann's canal (after A. Volkmann 19th century German physiologist)
> osteon, also called Haversian system (*osteon*, bone)
> interstitial lamellae (*inter-*, between + *-stitum*, standing; *lamella*, diminutive of *lamina*, a plate)
> inner and outer circumferential lamellae (*circum-*, around + *fer-*, bearing)
> cementing lines (refers to apparent cementing function of these lines)
> Howship's lacuna, also subosteoclastic compartment (after J. Howship,

18th–19th century British surgeon)
endosteum (*endo-*, within + *osteon*, bone)

TECHNICAL CONSIDERATIONS. Bone's mineralized matrix necessitates special treatment to enable the preparation of microscope tissue sections. Specifically, the mineral must be removed and this is accomplished by immersing the pieces of bone in dilute acid solutions or in chelating agents. The demineralized matrix of bone is about 95% collagen and the decalcified bone can be embedded and processed as any other histological tissue. An alternative method for examining bone tissue involves abrading or grinding flat pieces of mineralized bone until they become translucent. Although the resident cells are not preserved in these ground bone sections, the mineralized matrix and system of delicate channels that interconnect the lacunae are clearly apparent.

MACROSCOPIC CHARACTERISTICS OF BONE
Adult bone is designed to provide maximum strength with a minimum of weight and material. At a macroscopic level, two architectural types of bone can be grossly identified with the unaided eye. The first is cancellous bone, also termed spongy or trabecular bone. Cancellous bone is the lattice-like, internal arrangement of bony bars, plates and arches. This bony arrangement functions as the structural support to bone, dispersing the forces applied to its surface. The second type of bone is termed compact bone, also called cortical bone, and this arrangement of bone appears solid to the naked eye. In the adult, the matrix of this compact bone has a highly organized microscopic architecture that functions to maximize the strength of bone. The bones of the adult skeleton are composed of both compact and trabecular bone, and the relative proportions vary depending on the bone's location, health, and physical requirements. The cavity enclosed by the trabeculae and solid walls of bone is the marrow space, or cavity, and it contains the red or yellow bone marrow.

BONE MATRIX
These two following tissue sections are both of a transversely sectioned long bone with the marrow cavity in its center. There is typically no cancellous bone in the diaphysis, or shaft, of a long bone.

A fibrous sheath, the periosteum, covers all outside surfaces of a bone except on its articular surfaces and areas of tendon and ligament insertion. The periosteum is composed of two well-defined layers: an outer dense fibrous layer, and an inner cellular layer. In bone that is not actively growing, the inner cellular layer is relatively thin and the sheath is termed a mature periosteum. The endosteum is the single cell layer that lines the marrow cavity: the cells of the endosteum are either osteoblasts or bone lining cells. All inner surfaces of bone are covered by this layer of cells, and in a mature adult over 90% of these inner surfaces are covered by the squamous bone lining cells.

The matrix of most adult bone tissue is organized into microscopic plywood-like layers of mineral–impregnated collagen sheets. The mineral is a substituted calcium

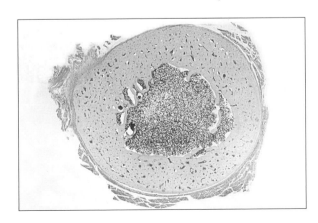

BONE MATRIX
Slide #27: Compact Bone I, Femur; H&E stained 12 µm demineralized paraffin section; human child.

Higher magnification image:
• (medium) periosteum and outer circumferential lamellae

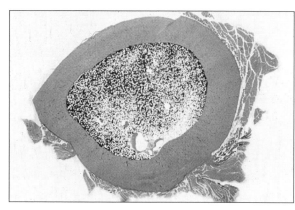

BONE MATRIX
Slide #27: Compact Bone II, Femur; H&E stained
12 μm demineralized paraffin section; human child.

Higher magnification images:
- (medium) compact bone
- (high) osteons
- (high) lamellar patterns

hydroxyapatite, and the collagen is type I collagen. Much of the mineral impregnates the individual collagen fibrils, improving the strength of the bone matrix at a molecular level.

The lamellae of bone assume various patterns in the wall of the diaphysis. This lamellar organization of the matrix maximizes the strength of the bone. Most of the compact wall in adult bone contains hundreds of highly structured, cylindrical osteons, also termed Haversian systems. The osteon is the basic structural unit of adult compact bone. Each roughly cylindrical osteon is about 1 mm in diameter and consists of concentric lamellae of bone matrix surrounding a lumen. Each lamella is a thin sheet of collagen whose fibrils are oriented in a spiral pattern that is pitched according to the stress and strain the osteon must withstand; the direction of the spirals alternate in adjacent lamellae. The lumen of the osteon is called the Haversian canal; it is approximately 50 μm in diameter and it carries the blood vessels and nerves of bone. Osteons tend to run longitudinally, parallel to the long axis of the bone, although they can branch and anastomose. In these tissue sections of transversely sectioned long bones most osteons are transversely sectioned.

Not all neurovascular channels in bone have radially concentric lamellae surrounding them; channels that open to the periosteum or marrow cavity or that interconnect adjacent Haversian canals are termed Volkmann's canals. Between adjacent osteons are the remnants of older Haversian systems; these are referred to as the interstitial lamellae.

In the peripheral region of the bone, beneath the periosteum, the bone matrix is organized into outer circumferential lamellae. Again, the layers are discernable because the fibrils of collagen comprising each lamellar sheet are oriented at different angles in adjacent sheets. During growth in diameter, the circumferential lamellae are deposited by the osteoblasts beneath the periosteum. Lamellae of the inner (marrow) aspect of the bone, subjacent to the endosteum, are called inner circumferential lamellae.

Fine basophilic cementing lines may be apparent at the perimeters of the osteons, cementing them in place. Cementing lines also occur among sets of lamellae in the inner and outer circumferential lamellae where, like the rings of a tree, they demarcate periods of circumferential growth. Observe how the amount of growth during such demarcated growth periods is not the same on all circumferential surfaces of the bone. Such differences in the relative thickness of added bone can occur in response to changing mechanical forces to which the bone is subjected.

Osteocytes reside in lacunae, the somewhat flattened holes in the mineralized matrix that are located between consecutive lamellae. The dark, condensed appearance of these bone cells in these tissue sections is an artifact of fixation; in living bone the role of osteocytes is extremely important for calcium metabolism and for the bone's response to mechanical stress.

MINERALIZED BONE. In this tissue section, the lacunae and canaliculi, once occupied by the osteocytes and their processes, are empty and appear black. This preparation of mineralized bone illustrates very clearly the arrangement of the many lacunae in the bone and the extensive pattern of the canaliculi emanating from the lacunae. In living bone, processes of the osteocytes interconnect with each other at gap junctions within these canaliculi.

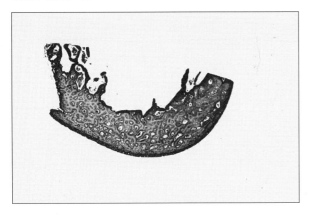

MINERALIZED BONE
Slide #28: Bone; ground mineralized section; human.

Higher magnification images:
- (medium) osteons
- (high) canaliculi

THE CELLS OF BONE

This next tissue section is a transverse section of an actively growing bone. A large central marrow space containing very active red bone marrow is enclosed within the bone. At this early stage in bone development, this bone is called the primary spongiosum; it is not categorized as either trabecular or compact bone. The periosteum is very thick, and like the previously viewed periosteum, it has an outer dense fibrous layer and inner cellular layer of osteoprogenitor cells. The apparent activity of this inner cellular layer indicates this as an active periosteum, in contrast to the periosteum of the more mature bones. The irregular pale basophilic islands of matrix visible within the pink-stained bone matrix are calcified cartilage matrix, remnants of the original cartilage model of this bone. This particular tissue section is a transverse section through a bone like that on Slide #24, which is to be examined later in this exercise.

Five different cells types can be identified in sections of bone. Four of these cells are different functional states of one cell type and each cell can be identified by its functionally significant, distinct morphology and location.

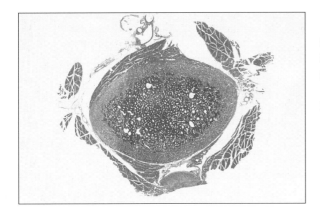

CELLS OF BONE
Slide #20: Bone; H&E stained 4 µm demineralized methacrylate section; rat humerus.

Higher magnification images:
- (medium) periosteum and osteoprogenitor cells
- (high) osteoblasts and bone lining cells
- (high) osteoclasts

OSTEOBLASTS. Osteoblasts are the cells primarily responsible for the synthesis of the organic bone matrix. Because this bone is still actively growing, there are a great number of osteoblasts. The osteoblasts are large, bulky, relatively basophilic cells, arranged in sheets along surfaces of the bone, most prominently here on the various irregular surfaces bordering the marrow cavity. These cells are not epithelial cells, but they are interconnected with gap junctions, enabling intercellular communication. Since bone matrix is rigid, bone can only grow by being deposited onto existing surfaces. Most of the bone matrix is intensely eosinophilic, but just beneath the layer of osteoblasts is a zone of newer bone that stains much lighter because it has not yet become mineralized. This pale premineralized matrix material is known as osteoid (*osteo-*, bone + *-oid*, form). It usually takes several weeks for osteoid to become fully mineralized.

BONE LINING CELLS. Bone lining cells form a single layer of squamous cells on bone surfaces. These cells are not actively synthesizing matrix, but are dormant and able to be activated as needed. It is not inconsistent to find an osteoid seam beneath the bone lining cells because the deactivation of osteoblasts into bone lining cells occurs more quickly than does the mineralization of osteoid. These squamous cells form an important ion barrier separating the bone matrix from tissue fluid. Bone lining cells cover all surfaces of bone that are not actively growing, including the interior walls of Haversian canals.

OSTEOCYTES. Osteocytes are individually entrapped in lacunae within the substance of the bone and their processes are located in the canaliculi that interconnect the lacunae. Osteocytes are derived from osteoblasts that become surrounded with matrix when the polarity of their osteoid secretion becomes reversed. Once entrapped, they maintain gap-junction mediated communication with other osteocytes and osteoblasts by means of their attenuated processes that extend within the canaliculi. In living bone they are capable of low levels of synthesis and osteolysis (*osteo-*, bone + *lysis*, dissolution).

OSTEOPROGENITOR CELLS. The osteoprogenitor cells in the cellular periosteum are multipotential cells that can give rise to osteoblasts as needed, either as part of normal growth or during the repair of bone fractures. Since osteoblasts themselves rarely divide, these cells are the principal source of osteoblasts. Osteoprogenitor cells also occur on the marrow side of bone in sites of active or potential bone formation. In mature bone, osteoprogenitor cells are stem cells and not a prominently numerous population of cells.

OSTEOCLASTS. Osteoclasts are distributed on the outer surface of bone in this tissue section. These cells are principally responsible for the breakdown and removal of bone. They are large, irregular multinucleated cells that are polarized in morphology and function. A ruffled border of highly elaborated membrane faces the bone and is the site for the localized demineralization and extracellular enzymatic digestion of bone. The small depression in bone in which some osteoclasts reside is termed Howship's lacuna, or the subosteoclastic compartment. Osteoclasts are not derived from the same cell line as the other cells of bone, rather they arise from the asynchronous fusion of monocytes that migrate to the bone and form these syncytial units as needed.

THE MICROSCOPIC ORGANIZATION OF BONE MATRIX

With regard to the microscopic organization of the bone matrix, it is either woven bone or lamellar bone. Woven bone is also termed primary or immature or bundle bone, whereas lamellar bone is also termed secondary or mature bone. In woven bone, the collagen forms bundles that intertwine around the osteocytes; in lamellar bone, the collagen is layered in sheets.

The first bone to appear during the formation of new bone, or in the repair of fractures, is woven bone. This immature bone is later replaced by stronger, structurally superior lamellar bone. Primary bone grows more rapidly than lamellar bone and it is less mineralized and more cellular than mature bone. Be aware that the macroscopic designation of compact vs. trabecular bone is completely independent of this microscopic designation of the organization of the bone matrix. Bone that appears to the unaided eye as either compact or trabecular bone, can be microscopically organized as either woven or lamellar bone or a mixture of the two. In the adult, most bone matrix is organized into lamellae.

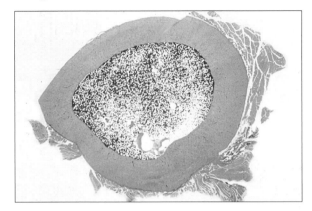

COMPACT: WOVEN AND LAMELLAR BONE
Slide #27: Bone; H&E stained 4 μm demineralized paraffin section; human.

Higher magnification images:
- (medium) wall
- (medium) lamellar and woven bone

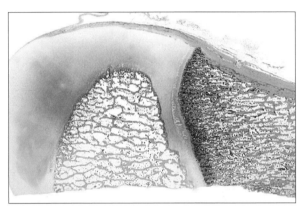

TRABECULAR: WOVEN AND LAMELLAR BONE
Slide #26: Bone; H&E stained 4 μm demineralized paraffin section; human.

Higher magnification image:
- (high) lamellar and woven bone

BONE HISTOGENESIS

The two forms of osteogenesis are classified according to the tissue in which the bone initially develops: intramembranous bone formation (*intra-*, within + *membrana*, a covering membrane) occurs in a well–vascularized primitive connective tissue and endochondral bone formation (*endo-*, within + *chondros*, cartilage) occurs in a preexisting cartilage model.

INTRAMEMBRANOUS OSTEOGENESIS

The developing cranial vault is an example of intramembranous bone development. Each membranous bone begins its development at an ossification center, a richly vascularized region where multipotential mesenchymal cells proliferate. Osteoblasts differentiate from mesenchymal cells in these centers. The osteoblasts initiate matrix formation by laying down the eosinophilic organic matrix, osteoid. Definitive matrix results from the impregnation of the osteoid by calcium salts. The nascent surfaces of bone tissue are surrounded by osteoblasts that continue to form bone, some of them surrounding themselves completely with matrix to become the entrapped osteocytes. The delicate trabeculae increase in length and become thicker and more compact as bone is added to their surfaces. The primitive connective tissue surrounding the trabeculae becomes organized into a periosteum as mesenchymal cells differentiate into fibroblasts. Some mesenchymal cells persist in this bone, becoming the population of osteoprogenitor cells that reside in the cellular periosteum and bone marrow cavity.

At the midline of the developing cranial bones in these tissue sections, in the region of the midsagittal suture, the initial stage in intramembranous bone formation is represented: partially differentiated mesenchymal cells are seen adjacent to the delicate surfaces of newly formed bone. There is no preexisting cartilage model, just a well vascularized primitive connective tissue. In regions of cranial bone located lateral to this midpoint, development has progressed further: the bone is thicker and osteoblasts are entrapped within the matrix. The periosteum is forming. In this tissue section, intramembranous bone formation is also generating both mandible and maxillary bones.

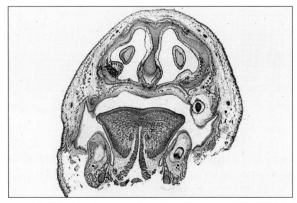

INTRAMEMBRANOUS OSTEOGENESIS
Slide #22: Embryo Head I; H&E stained 4 μm paraffin section; dog.

Higher magnification images:
- (medium) cranial suture
- (high) osteoblasts

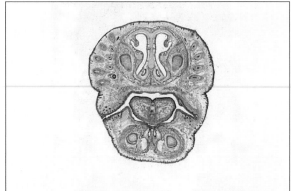

INTRAMEMBRANOUS OSTEOGENESIS
Slide #22: Embryo Head III; H&E stained 4 μm paraffin section; rat.

Higher magnification images:
- (medium) cranial suture
- (high) osteoblasts

ENDOCHONDRAL OSTEOGENESIS

Most bones of the skeleton arise from preexisting hyaline cartilage models. Cartilage is an ideal material for the bone model because it can grow rapidly while still maintaining its supporting functions. Cartilage provides the provisional matrix and continues to grow until the bone completes its growth. The chondrocytes of bone models are unlike those of other hyaline cartilage because they are able to initiate changes that result in the mineralization of the matrix. Mineralization renders the matrix incompatible with the life of the chondrocyte and the chondrocytes die, leaving behind the delicate scaffolding of calcified cartilage matrix. The mineralized cartilage matrix provides a surface upon which bone can be laid down, but it is easily eroded and eventually completely replaced by mature bone.

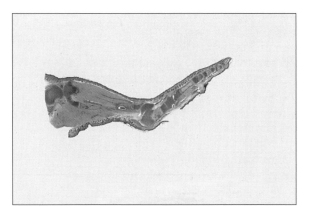

ENDOCHONDRAL OSTEOGENESIS
Slide #23: Bone Formation; H&E stained 4 μm demineralized methacrylate section; rat limb.

Higher magnification images:
- (medium) endochondral bones
- (medium high) primary center of ossification
- (high) bone collar
- (high) chondrocytes

Beginning with a cartilage model, the first step in its replacement by bone is the formation of a periosteal bone collar, which actually forms intramembranously beneath the perichondrium (henceforth, the periosteum) in the region of the diaphysis of the cartilage model. Ossification is initiated in a primary ossification center, which in long bones is located within the shaft of the diaphysis. The secondary ossification centers of a developing long bone appear subsequently in each epiphysis.

The early stages of endochondral bone formation are illustrated in this tissue section of growing rat limb bones. Primary centers of ossification are evident in all the bones in this limb, with the proximal bone models being more advanced than the distal ones. Near the ends of each model, the cartilage and chondrocytes appear normal, but in the direction toward the center of the cartilage model, the progression of transformational stages is evident. Initially the chondrocytes become hypertrophied and the intervening matrix becomes calcified and compacted. The chondrocytes near the center of the model have died, leaving irregular cavities. By this time, a bud of blood vessels has penetrated the periosteum and invaded the previously avascular calcified cartilage. Osteoblasts differentiate from the osteoprogenitor cells that accompany the blood vessels into the model and proceed to differentiate into osteoblasts. Osteoblasts lay osteoid down upon the remnant spicules of calcified cartilage. Bone builds up upon these surfaces and the resulting trabeculae become the primary spongiosum of the new bone. Cartilage is added to the ends of this still–growing bone model and the replacement by bone progresses from the center toward these ends.

GROWTH IN LENGTH

The epiphysis is the rounded expanded end of the long bone (*epi-*, upon + *-physis*, growth). In the secondary center of ossification, growth and replacement by bone proceeds radially within the epiphysis. The plate of cartilage remaining between the primary and secondary centers is the epiphyseal plate, or growth plate, illustrated in the following tissue section, Slide # 24. The alternative names of this region are based on the location and function, respectively. Elongation of long bones proceeds from the epiphyseal plates, with cartilage proliferating (via interstitial growth) in the distal end of the epiphyseal plate and endochondral bone being deposited principally on the diaphyseal side of the plate. When final growth in length is achieved, the plate undergoes ossification, resulting in a bony union of the epiphysis and diaphysis (*dia-*, between + *-physis*, growth).

Endochondral ossification in a long bone typically occurs at both ends of the primary center of ossification. Because the growth occurs along the long axis of the bone, the succession of phases appears in an ordered series of transverse zones in the growth plate. Starting from the ends of the cartilage and progressing toward the primary center, these regions of the epiphyseal plate are as follows:

zones of the epiphyseal plate	morphological characteristics
zone of resting cartilage	hyaline cartilage with standard appearance
zone of proliferation	proliferating chondrocytes with daughter cells arranged into columns oriented parallel to the long axis of the cartilage model
zone of maturation and hypertrophy	columns of hypertrophied chondrocytes with compacted columns of matrix between cell columns
zone of calcifying cartilage and degenerating chondrocytes	blood vessels and osteoprogenitor cells occupying spaces left by the the degenerating chondrocytes
zone of resorption and ossification	osteoblasts from the primary center deposit bone on the exposed columns of calcified cartilage

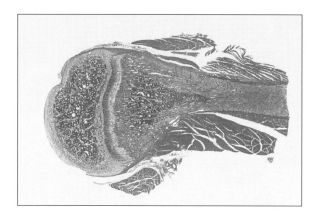

EPIPHYSEAL PLATE
Slide #24: Epiphyseal Plate; H&E stained 4 μm demineralized methacrylate section; rat humerus.

Higher magnification images:
• (medium) epiphyseal plate
• (high) zones of proliferation and hypertrophy
• (high) zones of degeneration and ossification

BONE MODELING

Bone modeling is the process by which the shape, position, or size of the rigid bone is altered by the simultaneous removal of bone on one surface by osteoclasts and the laying down of bone on the other surface by osteoblasts. Examples of bone modeling are provided in the tissue sections of the epiphyseal plate and the fetal head.

In the tissue section of the growth plate, the newly–formed bone of the metaphysis is being modeled or shaped. The epiphyseal plate is located at the broad end of the metaphysis, which is the funnel-shaped portion of bone located between the diaphysis and the epiphysis. The new bone must be reshaped to the diameter of the diaphysis. Osteoclasts remove bone from the outer wall of the metaphysis while osteoblasts build up the bone on the inner side of the wall.

In the tissue section of the fetal head, the shape and the position of the growing jaw bone is altered to accommodate the growing tooth and the growing embryo head. Bone is being removed by osteoclasts from within the developing tooth socket, while osteoblasts simultaneously build up bone on the other side of the developing mandible.

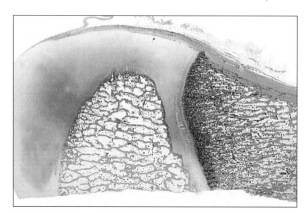

BONE MODELING
Slide #26: Bone; H&E stained 4 μm demineralized paraffin section; human.

Higher magnification images:
• (medium) metaphysis
• (high) osteoclasts

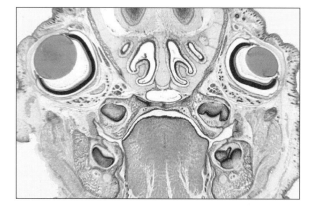

BONE MODELING
Slide #22: Fetal Head II, transverse section; H&E stained 12 μm paraffin section; rat.

Higher magnification Images:
• (low) two teeth
• (medium) developing mandible
• (high) modeling

BONE REMODELING

Bone remodeling is the process by which woven, old, or structurally inferior bone is replaced by new lamellar bone. It involves the sequential removal of bone by osteoclasts followed by the laying down of bone by osteoblasts.

In this tissue section, immature bone is being replaced by the structurally stronger lamellar bone. First, osteoclasts drill enlarged channels termed resorption tunnels, or cavities, through the bone. The osteoclasts are accompanied by blood vessels and osteoprogenitor cells. When the tunnel is approximately 1 mm in diameter the osteoclasts recede and the osteoprogenitor cells differentiate into osteoblasts and lay down the sheets of alternating spirals of collagen beginning on the interior surface of the tunnel. Some of the osteoblasts are trapped as osteocytes, but they retain contact with other osteocytes by their gap–junction connected processes within the canaliculi. The osteoid is laid down in sheets until the lumen reaches a diameter of approximately 50 μm. At this stage, the osteoblasts convert to bone lining cells, leaving the blood vessel and nerve in the newly formed Haversian canal. The subsequent mineralization is a relatively slow process that takes several weeks.

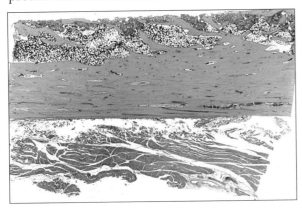

BONE REMODELING
Slide #26: Bone, longitudinal section; H&E stained 12 μm demineralized paraffin; human.

Higher magnification images:
- (medium) resorption tunnel
- (medium) new osteon

7. BONE MARROW AND HEMOPOIESIS

Hemopoietic tissue resides within the central cavities of bones, comprising the bone marrow. At birth the bone marrow of nearly all bones is actively generating blood cells; with time, active hemopoiesis becomes reversibly restricted to the marrow of a few bones of the axial skeleton. This chapter examines a tissue section of actively hemopoietic tissue within the central cavity of a young bone.

All the cells of peripheral blood arise from a single pluripotential hemopoietic stem cell (PHSC). This stem cell accounts for approximately 0.1% of the cells in bone marrow. Mitotic division of the PHSC generates more PHSCs as well as two populations of multipotential hemopoietic stem cells, one committed to generating lymphocytes and the other committed to generating myeloid cells — erythrocytes, granulocytes, monocytes, and platelets. These multipotential hemopoietic stem cells can replicate themselves as well as generate unipotential progenitor cells that are each committed to producing a single blood cell type.

With standard histological stains all of these stem cells, from the PHSC to the progenitor cells, look like small lymphocytes and they circulate between the marrow and the peripheral blood. Although morphologically indistinguishable from each other, these variously committed hemopoietic cells bear unique surface markers and it is possible to differentiate among them — and separate them for harvesting — on that basis. The unique surface markers enable the precise regulation of blood cell production: a variety of natural growth factors act on specific stem cells, progenitor cells, and precursor cells.

Precursor cells arise from the progenitor cells. Unlike their predecessors, the precursor cells have recognizable morphological characteristics. Most of these precursor cells undergo a series of morphologically distinct stages of terminal differentiation, producing the mature cells that circulate in peripheral blood. It is these stages of terminal differentiation that are examined in this exercise.

Bone marrow is relatively easily examined for the purpose of clinical diagnosis. Typically, an aspirated sample of marrow is smeared on a microscope slide and analyzed. The various terminally differentiating cells are categorized and differentially counted, and their morphological features observed. Like peripheral blood, irregularities in relative numbers and aberrant morphology have valuable diagnostic significance.

Terminal differentiation involves the progressive transformation of a young, immature committed precursor cell into the mature cell. The stages in the progressive differentiation are named according to morphological characteristics. Understanding the name helps place the cell in the correct stage of the developmental continuum. The continuum followed by the differentiating cells of the erythrocyte series and the continuum followed by the differentiating cells of the granulocyte series are described in the following pages.

With regard to common word roots, the Greek word *erythros* means red. The cells of the erythrocyte series are also termed normoblasts, a name derived from the Latin *normalis* meaning normal, or according to pattern. The terms erythroblast and normoblast are both used for the stages in the terminal differentiation of the cells leading to mature erythrocytes.

> erythrocyte series (*erythros*, red + *-cyte*, cell)
> > proerythroblast or pronormoblast (*pro-*, before + *erythros*, red + *blastos*, germ)
> > basophilic erythroblast or basophilic normoblast (*bas-*, base + *phileo*, to like, love)

polychromatophilic erythroblast or polychromatophilic normoblast (*poly-*, many + *chroma*, color)

orthochromatic erythroblast or orthochromatic normoblast (*ortho-*, correct + *chroma*, color)

reticulocyte (*reticulum*, a small net + *-cyte*, cell)

granulocyte series (*granulum*, granule + *-cyte*, cell)

myeloblast (*myelo-*, bone marrow + *blastos*, germ)

promyelocyte (*pro-*, before + *myelo-*, bone marrow + *-cyte*, cell)

neutrophilic, eosinophilic, and basophilic myelocyte (*myelo-*, marrow + *-cyte*, cell)

neutrophilic, eosinophilic, or basophilic metamyelocyte (*meta-*, between + *myelo-*, marrow + *-cyte*, cell)

neutrophilic band stage

megakaryocyte (*megas*, big + *karyon*, nut, nucleus + *-cyte*, cell)

BONE MARROW TISSUE SECTION

RED BONE MARROW

The tissue section of decalcified bone illustrates the stroma and parenchyma of red bone marrow. The marrow stroma consists of reticular fibers, reticular cells, macrophages, and blood vessels. The stromal cells provide structural support and, in addition, supply many factors for growth and differentiation of the hemopoietic cells.

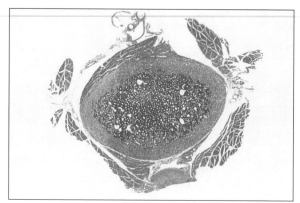

RED BONE MARROW
Slide #20: Bone; H&E stain; demineralized 4 µm methacrylate section; rat.

Higher magnification images:
- (medium) bone marrow
- (high) megakaryocyte

The large blood vessels in this tissue section are sinusoids. They are open and cleared of blood cells because this tissue was fixed by vascular perfusion. Normally, these sinusoids are kept from collapsing by pressure that builds up because the central veins that drain these sinusoids are of smaller diameters. Blood cell formation occurs outside the lumens of the vessels and the terminally differentiated cells enter the peripheral circulation by traversing migration pores in the endothelial cells that line the sinusoids.

Pluripotential and multipotential hemopoietic stem cells look like small lymphocytes and are present in the marrow in very small numbers. Most of the morphologically identifiable cells populating the marrow are blood cells in their terminal stages of differentiation. In normal marrow, granulocyte precursors outnumber erythrocyte precursors in a ratio of about 3:1. This ratio reflects not the relative numbers of these cells in the peripheral blood, but differences in the relative life spans of granulocytes and erythrocytes: fewer of the much longer–lived erythrocytes are produced to maintain their 99% composition level in peripheral blood. Within each series of terminal differentiation, the relative numbers of cells in stages toward the mature end of the developmental sequence are increased. In infections and disease, these relative numbers can shift toward the immature end of the sequence.

The developing blood cell most easily identified in this tissue section is the megakaryocyte, the cell that produces platelets. The fully differentiated megakaryocyte is a very large cell, 50–100 µm in diameter, with a single complex multilobed nucleus that may contain up to 64 times the normal haploid number of chromosomes. Megakaryocytes are typically located adjacent to the abluminal side of the blood sinusoids from which position they release platelets (as proplatelets) into the blood.

Monocytes are generated in the marrow. The stages of terminal differentiation are not particularly morphologically distinct and they resemble those seen in the circulation; promonocytes appear to contain more azurophilic granules than typical monocytes. Terminally differentiating monocytes represent approximately 2% of the nucleated cells in the marrow.

Lymphocytes have much the same appearance in the bone marrow as in peripheral blood. The B-lymphocytes undergo proliferation and terminal differentiation in the bone marrow and are released into the circulation as immunologically competent cells. Lymphocytes comprise about 10%–24% of the nucleated cells in bone marrow.

YELLOW BONE MARROW

Compare the bone marrow in this tissue section with that in the previous tissue section. This is an older bone that has begun a conversion to yellow marrow. The reticular cells accumulate lipid and become unilocular fat cells. The conversion of red to white marrow is reversible.

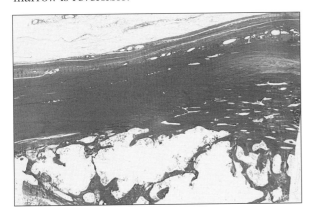

YELLOW BONE MARROW
Slide #32: Patella; H&E stained 4 μm demineralized paraffin section; nonhuman primate.

Higher magnification image:
- (medium) adipocytes

BONE MARROW SMEAR

CD-ROM Notice: The linked images illustrating the bone marrow cells in stages of terminal differentiation are listed below the standard lead-in image.

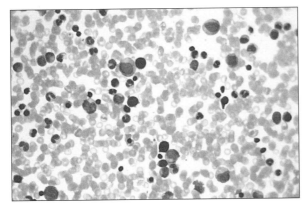

BONE MARROW SMEAR
Slide #18: Bone Marrow; smear; Wright's stain, human.

Higher magnification images:
- (high) myeloblasts
- (high) erythroblast series
- (high) erythroblast series
- (high) neutrophilic myelocyte
- (high) promyelocyte and erythroblasts
- (high) neutrophilic series
- (high) basophilic myelocyte
- (high) eosinophilic myelocyte and promyelocyte
- (high) granulocyte series

The terminal stages of differentiation of the blood cells of bone marrow are identified based on progressive nuclear and cytoplasmic characteristics and these morphological features become the basis for their names. These cells are typically viewed in a bone marrow smear.

This diagrammatic overview of the cells in bone marrow is organized with respect to key morphological characteristics.

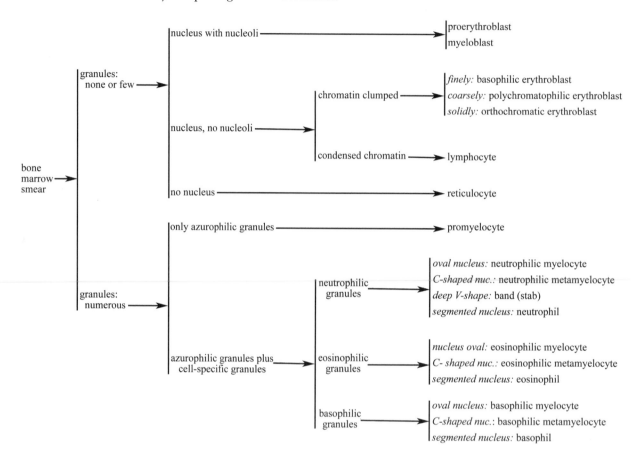

ERYTHROID SERIES

The key to recognizing the stages in terminal differentiation of the erythroid cells lies in recognizing the progression of changes that occur in the nucleus and in the cytoplasm of the precursor cell. These progressive changes are illustrated graphically below. Basically, the nucleus of the precursor is large with dispersed chromatin and multiple nucleoli that reflect its production of ribosomes; at the end of differentiation, the nucleus is absent. The cytoplasm of the precursor cell begins with very blue coloration, reflecting the concentration of polyribosomes, and in the final stage the cytoplasm is eosinophilic because of the concentration of hemoglobin. Stages in the

cell type:	proerythroblast	basophilic erythroblast	polychromatophilic erythroblast	orthochromatic erythroblast	reticulocyte	erythrocyte
nuclear chromatin:	very dispersed	fine clumps	coarse clumps	nearly solid	extruded	
cytoplasmic coloration:	very blue	blue	patchy blue and grey	grey		

terminal differentiation of the erythroid series are named according to the progressive shift in coloration of the cytoplasm as ribosomes are replaced by hemoglobin.

The first recognizable stage is the proerythroblast, 12–20 μm in diameter, a precursor cell distinguishable from other blast cells by its intensely basophilic cytoplasm. This coloration is because of the staining of ribonucleoprotein (RNP) by methylene blue, combined with staining of hemoglobin by eosin, since a small amount of hemoglobin is already present. The round nucleus has a fine chromatin network and 3–5 pale gray nucleoli. The cytoplasm is uniform and without granules.

Daughter cells enter the basophilic erythroblast stage, which is represented by several generations of cells. These initially measure approximately 15 μm in diameter but diminish in size with each succeeding division. The chromatin is finely clumped, giving the nucleus a characteristic cracked appearance. A nucleolus may be present.

The polychromatophilic erythroblast is a later stage; cells are smaller than the preceding ones and the nuclear chromatin appears very coarsely clumped. These cells are still able to undergo mitotic division, but they are the last stage able to do so. The color of the cytoplasm is variable and often blotchy, depending on relative proportions of RNP and hemoglobin present.

An orthochromatic erythroblast has cytoplasmic coloration like that of the reticulocyte. The nucleus is very condensed (pyknotic, from *pyknos*, thick) and ready for extrusion. Enucleation (*enucleo*, to remove the kernel; from *e*, out + *nucleus*, kernel) often occurs while the young erythrocyte passes into the marrow sinusoids. The reticulocyte is the final stage of terminal differentiation and looks like a typical red blood cell but is termed a reticulocyte because it retains residual traces of ribosomes and cytoplasmic membranes in its cytoplasm. These cytoplasmic remnants are stainable by exposing fresh cells to cresyl blue prior to Romanovsky staining. The number of reticulocytes in a normal peripheral blood smear is low.

GRANULOCYTIC SERIES

The key to recognizing the stages in terminal differentiation of the granulocyte series lies in understanding the progression of nuclear changes and the progressive changes in the populations of cytoplasmic granules. These changes are illustrated graphically below. Basically, the nucleus of the precursor cell is large with dispersed chromatin and containing multiple nucleoli; in the terminal stage, the nucleus has become condensed and segmented. The cytoplasm of the precursor cell has no cytoplasmic granules; subsequently azurophilic granules are produced, followed by a switch to the production of the cell-specific granules. Once the cell–specific granules are evident, the named stages include designation of the specific granulocyte line.

cell type:	myeloblast	promyelocyte	specific myelocyte (*specific*=neutrophilic, eosinophilic, or basophilic)	specific metamyelocyte	band (neutrophil only)	mature granulocyte
nucleus:	dispersed chromatin with nucleoli		oval to slightly indented	C- or V- shaped	horseshoe shape	progressively more segmented
cytoplasmic granules:	none	only azurophilic granules	azurophilic granules plus increasing numbers of neutrophilic, eosinophilic, or basophilic granules			

Terminal differentiation of granulocytes begins with the myeloblast, a precursor cell approximately 12–20 μm in diameter, with a large nucleus containing 3 to 5 very prominent nucleoli and no cytoplasmic granules. It has light blue cytoplasmic coloration and a high nucleus-to-cytoplasm ratio. It may have cytoplasmic blebs at its cell periphery.

The promyelocyte stage is characterized by large numbers of azurophilic granules in the cytoplasm. The promyelocytes are among the largest cells present in the marrow, excluding the megakaryocytes. The chromatin is finely dispersed and one or more nucleoli are usually present to generate ribosomes.

The three granulocytic lines begin to be morphologically distinguishable from each other in the myelocyte stage. It should be noted that the myeloblast and the promyelocytes are committed unipotential cells, even though it is not possible to identify to which particular granulocyte line in this Wright's stained smear. At the beginning of the specific myelocyte stage, azurophilic granule production ceases and is followed by generation of the cell–specific granules. These specific granules appear initially over the Golgi area and later disperse throughout the cytoplasm. Thus a neutrophilic myelocyte is first recognizable by a clear, pale area in the Golgi region, and early eosinophilic myelocytes have pink-stained granules in the same region. As myelocytes continue to divide and differentiate, the cytoplasm loses its bluish cast owing to progressive dilution of ribosomes by the specific granules. The basophilic series is thought to differentiate in a similar manner, but intermediate stages are infrequent.

The metamyelocyte stage is characterized by marked nuclear indentation (forming a shallow C- or V- shape) and leads progressively to further segmentation of the nucleus that is highly developed only by cells of the neutrophilic series. Azurophilic granules are greatly reduced in number because the myelocytes continued to undergo mitotic division after production of the azurophilic granules has ceased. Metamyelocytes no longer undergo mitotic division. The band stage of the neutrophilic line has a horseshoe–shaped nucleus with early signs of constriction. This nuclear shape marks the limit of nuclear constriction for most eosinophils and basophils, whereas neutrophils progress to a further segmented polymorphonuclear stage.

8. Nervous Tissue and Neuromuscular Junction

The body's nervous system functions to receive, integrate, and send signals about the internal and external environment in order to direct and coordinate the activities of other tissues and organs in the body. The principal tissue of this system is nervous tissue, and the principal cells are neurons. As a consequence of their very special function, neurons are characterized by an unusual, highly polarized and extremely attenuated shape. Very long cellular processes extend from the cell body that houses the cell's metabolic center. For the histologist, this shape means that an entire neuron is rarely seen in standard tissue sections; we view only parts of entire neurons.

This chapter examines the various parts of neurons and their supporting cells in the spinal cord and peripheral nervous system. To illustrate the neurons and the relationships between them and their supporting cells, this exercise examines these cells along a continuum from the macroscopic to the microscopic to the ultrastructural view. Key to appreciating the unique shape of the neurons is appreciating that their shape reflects a morphological adaptation to their function as receivers/integrators/relayers of signals that help to coordinate the sensory input with motor output in the body. Understanding the morphology provides the structural framework for understanding the normal physiology of the nervous system and the pathology of diseases that affect neurons, the nervous system, and motor systems of the body.

The diagrammatic overview below illustrates the relationships among the nervous system structures examined in this exercise. The cell bodies of neurons reside in specific locations in the central and peripheral nervous system. The neuronal processes, some specialized for receiving signals and others specialized for relaying signals, can extend long distances away from the cell body. This exercise focuses on the components located in the peripheral nervous system.

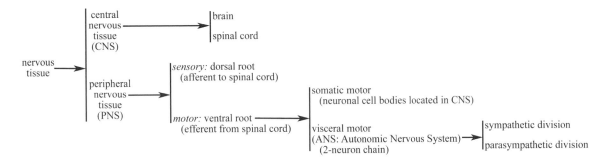

As a reflection of the morphological and functional specialization of neurons and their parts, the various parts of the neuron are named. Greek and Latin word roots are common, and understanding the translation will help the retention and recall of the terms. The following are parts of the neuron and the word derivations of the names.

> neuron (*neuron*, a nerve)
> soma, pl. somata (*soma*, body)
> perikaryon (*peri-*, around + *keryon*, kernel)
> axon hillock (*hillock*, a small elevation)
> dendrite (*dendr-*, tree)
> axon (*axon*, axis)

axon terminal

synapse (*synapsis*, a connection)

Many common structures encountered in nervous tissue have eponyms that persist today. The individuals so recognized were all active in the late 19th century when the technology for the high-resolution compound microscope became available and enabled their remarkable observations.

Nissl substance and Nissl bodies (after Nissl, a German neurologist, 1860—1919)

Node of Ranvier (after Ranvier, a French pathologist, 1835–1922)

Schmidt–Lanterman cleft (after Schmidt, a 19th century American anatomist and pathologist and Lanterman a 19th century American anatomist)

Schwann cell (after Schwann, a German histologist and physiologist, 1810—1882)

myenteric plexus of Auerbach (after Auerbach, a German anatomist, 1828—1897)

submucosal plexus of Meissner (after Meissner, a German histologist, 1829—1905)

The following cells are illustrated in this section. Relate the function of each item to its structure and its location in the central or peripheral nervous system.

anterior horn cell; lower motor neuron (name refers to the location and functional category, respectively)

neuroglial cells (*neuro-*, neuron + *-glia*, glue)

sensory ganglion cell (*ganglion*, pl. *ganglia*, a swelling or knot)

visceral motor ganglion cell (*viscus*, pl. *viscera*, the internal organs; *ganglion*, a swelling or knot)

REFERENCE DIAGRAM OF SLIDE LOCATIONS

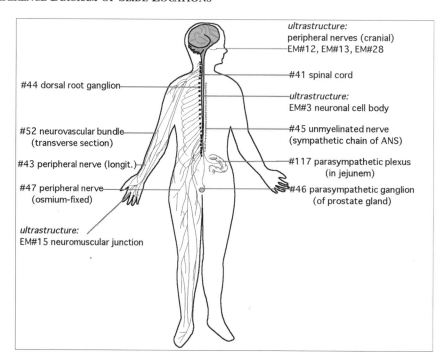

NEURONS AND GANGLIA

The following structures are illustrated in this section. Recognize the functional significance of each of them.

> white and grey matter of CNS (central nervous system)
> neuropil (*neuro-*, neuron + *pilos*, felt)
> ventral, or anterior, root (refers to anatomical location in animal and man, respectively)
> dorsal, or posterior root (refers to anatomical location in animal and man, respectively)
> dorsal root (spinal) ganglion (*ganglion*, pl. *ganglia*, a swelling or knot)
> autonomic ganglion (*autos*, self + *nomos*, law)
> parasympathetic ganglion (*para-*, alongside or near + sympathetic)

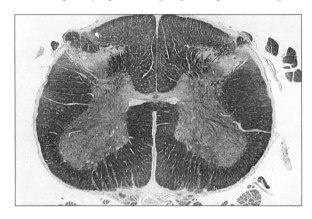

ANTERIOR HORN CELLS (CNS)
Slide #41: Spinal Cord; cresyl violet and luxol fast blue stain; 25 µm thick section; human.

Higher magnification images:
- (medium) spinal grey matter
- (high) neuronal cell bodies and neuroglia
- (high) neuronal cell bodies and white matter

NEURON

The spinal cord is the tapered columnar extension of the brain and resides within the vertebral canal. It is associated with pairs of spinal nerves that carry signals between the body and the central nervous system. Its internal structure is uniform and macroscopically visible. The terms white and grey matter refer to the appearance in fresh tissue of the densely packed myelinated axons and the H-shaped central core of neurons and their supporting cells, respectively. The bulging regions of grey matter visible in this transverse section are termed horns or columns. Observe how the spinal cord is bilaterally symmetric, but asymmetric along the dorsal (posterior) to ventral (anterior) axis. Both anterior/posterior and dorsal/ventral designations are used in descriptions of the spinal cord. Motor functions are centered in the anterior, or ventral, grey matter (termed anterior horns), whereas sensory and relay functions are centered in the posterior, or dorsal, grey matter (termed posterior horns).

Myelin is a cellular material that provides electrical insulation for many axons. It stains blue with luxol fast blue in this tissue section. Myelinated axons comprise the white matter in the periphery of the spinal cord. Almost all of these axons in the white matter are transversely sectioned because they are traveling to and from the brain.

NEURONAL CELL BODY. At low magnification look for the cell bodies (the somata) of the largest nerve cells, the anterior horn neurons. These cells are somatic motor neurons and their axons travel in the anterior roots and innervate skeletal muscle. These neurons are multipolar cells (*multi-*, many + *-polar*, poles; referring to a neuron with more than two cellular processes arising from it) with round euchromatic (pale) nuclei that contain a prominent nucleolus. In the perikaryal cytoplasm look for the violet colored Nissl bodies (or Nissl substance), which are clumps of ribosomes and rough endoplasmic reticulum that extend into the broadly tapered bases of dendrites. The axon hillock is an elevation from which the axon arises and it is free of Nissl substance. Dendrites cannot be visualized in this preparation because (*1*) they contain cytoplasm that does not stain with this histological stain and (*2*) they are small and very entangled with other dendrites and processes in the surrounding area.

The grey matter area surrounding the anterior horn cells is the neuropil, which is a dense intermingling of dendrites and axons and neuroglial cell processes. The small nuclei in the neuropil belong to the neuroglial cells of the central nervous system; these cells are the supporting cells of the central nervous system. The cytoplasm of the neuroglial cells is not stained in this tissue section.

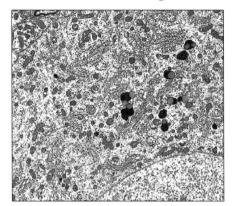

NEURONAL CELL BODY
Electron Micrograph #3: Cytoplasmic Organelles; perikaryal cytoplasm of a lower motor neuron from spinal cord of rhesus monkey.

Higher magnification views:
 • nuclear envelope and lipofuscin
 • Golgi complex or apparatus
 • rough ER and polysomes (Nissl substance)

Examine the ultrastructure of the perikaryal cytoplasm of a motor neuron in Electron Micrograph #3. Note that the neuropil comes into direct contact with the neuronal cell body and includes cellular processes of other neurons (axons and dendrites) as well as cellular extensions of the supporting cells (neuroglia) of the central nervous system. The motor neuron is characterized by a large round euchromatic (*eu-*, good + *chroma*, color) nucleus. The cytoplasm surrounding the nucleus (termed the perikaryal cytoplasm, in distinction from the axoplasm of axons and the dendroplasm of dendrites) contains a full complement of organelles and inclusions as a reflection of the cell body being the metabolic center of this very large cell. The clumps of rough endoplasmic reticulum are prominent, and correspond to the Nissl bodies seen in light microscope preparations.

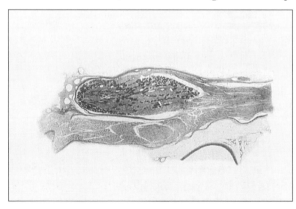

DORSAL ROOT (SPINAL) GANGLION
Slide #44: Dorsal Root Ganglion; Lee's stain; methacrylate-embedded; 3 μm thick; nonhuman primate.

Higher magnification images:
 • (high) dorsal root ganglion cells
 • (high) ventral root, myelinated axons

Observe the dorsal root ganglion in this tissue section. The term ganglion is used to describe a collection of neuronal cell bodies located outside the CNS, and this ganglion (in distinction to those of the autonomic nervous system) is associated with the dorsal root of the spinal nerve. Each dorsal root ganglion is grossly visible as a single swelling along each of the 31 pairs of dorsal roots associated with the spinal cord. It is a collection of large neuronal cell bodies belonging to the primary sensory neurons.

The primary sensory neurons of this ganglion are unipolar (*uni-*, one + *polar*, pole) meaning that this neuronal cell body gives rise to only one process. The spinal ganglion cell bodies are large, oval, and exhibit finely granular Nissl substance in the perikaryal cytoplasm. The neuronal nucleus is large and euchromatic (pale) and a nucleolus is prominent. Each neuronal cell body is completely surrounded by a single layer of enveloping cells, known as satellite cells. The satellite cells are Schwann cells, the same cell type that forms peripheral myelin. The single neuronal process leaves the capsule of satellite cells, acquires a myelin sheath, and bifurcates into a peripheral and a central process. The centrally directed axon carries sensory signals into the CNS and the distally directed axon becomes associated with a sensory receptor.

MYELINATED AXONS. This tissue section includes the purely motor ventral root subjacent to the ganglion. Centrally (to the left side of this section image) the dorsal and ventral roots are separated and carry signals to and from the spinal cord, respectively. Distally (to the right side of the section) the dorsal and ventral roots unite to form the spinal nerve. Examine the anterior (ventral) root. It is made up of heavily myelinated axons that originate from the lower motor neurons whose cell bodies are located in the anterior horn of the spinal cord. The axon appears as a grayish core within the myelin sheath, which appears thick, pink and frothy. Myelin has a high content of lipid and its bubbly appearance is attributed to lipid extraction that occurs during fixation of the tissue. The cells that produce the myelin sheaths are Schwann cells, the nuclei of which are scattered along the periphery of the sheaths. Myelin is a membranous sleeve wrapped around individual lengths of axons. It isolates the transmembrane flow of ions that propagates the electrical signals along axons into small spaces between sequential myelin segments. The interruptions in the tubular myelin sheath where adjacent Schwann cells meet are termed nodes of Ranvier. The lengths of myelin between these nodes define the internodal segments of a nerve fiber. Single paired "bubbles" in the myelin sheath are termed Schmidt-Lanterman clefts. Myelinated axons will be examined later in this exercise.

PARASYMPATHETIC GANGLION CELLS. Examine the parasympathetic ganglion located to the side of the prostate gland in this next tissue section, and contrast it with the spinal (dorsal root) ganglion of the previous one. The neurons within the ganglia of the autonomic nervous system provide motor innervation to smooth muscle and glands and receive synaptic input from the visceral motor neurons whose cell bodies are located in the spinal cord. Thus, unlike the somatic motor system, the visceral motor system has a two-neuron chain innervating the target cells. The autonomic ganglion neurons are multipolar and their cell bodies are angular in shape (unlike the round-to-oval profiles of dorsal root ganglion cell bodies). As a population, the soma size is considerably smaller than that of the primary sensory neuron in a spinal ganglion. Satellite cells are present but not as numerous around each cell body as in spinal ganglia, because it requires fewer cells to cover these smaller neuronal cell bodies. Observe that the nerve fibers in the bundles between the ganglia are unmyelinated.

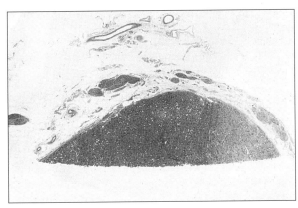

AUTONOMIC GANGLION
Slide #46: Parasympathetic Ganglion; Lee's stain; 3 μm thick methacrylate section; nonhuman primate.

Higher magnification images:
- (high) ganglion cell bodies and unmyelinated axons

Small, interconnected terminal ganglia of the parasympathetic nervous system are located in the walls of the digestive tract. They are visible in the wall of the jejunum in the following tissue section. There are two ganglia identified, both part of an extensive plexus (network) of axons; they differ in location and the muscles they innervate.

Observe the visceral motor neurons in the myenteric plexus of Auerbach, which is located between the two layers of smooth muscle in the muscularis externa, and in the submucosal plexus of Meissner, located within the submucosal connective tissue. Both ganglia receive their input from the preganglionic fibers of the parasympathetic division of the autonomic nervous system and innervate the smooth muscle of the digestive tract wall: neurons of Auerbach's plexus innervate the muscle layers of the muscularis externa, and thus function in peristalsis; neurons of Meissner's plexus innervate the thin layers of the muscularis mucosae, and influence the independent movement of the mucosa. Satellite cells do not encapsulate the neuronal cell bodies, but are present in the meshwork of supporting cells.

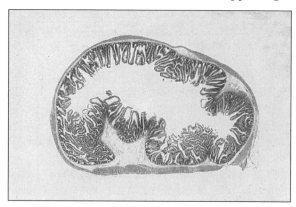

AUTONOMIC PLEXUS
Slide #117: Small Intestine, Jejunum; eosin and toluidine blue stain; 3 μm methacrylate section; nonhuman primate.

Higher magnification images:
- (medium) submucosal and myenteric ganglia
- (high) Meissner's submucosal plexus
- (high) Auerbach's myenteric plexus

PERIPHERAL NERVES

The following structures are associated with the axon and its supporting tissues.

peripheral nerve (*periphereia*, circumference; *nervus*, nerve)
nerve fascicle (*fasciculus*, a small bundle)
axon, myelinated and unmyelinated
mesaxon, internal and external (based on its similarity to mesentery)
internode of myelin (*inter-*, between + *nodus*, a knot)
neurofilaments and microtubules
endoneurium (*endo-*, in, within + *neuro-*, neuron)
perineurium (*peri-*, around + *neuro-*, neuron)
epineurium (*epi-*, on + *neuro-*, neuron)

MYELINATED AND UNMYELINATED FIBERS

Examine this tissue section of a neurovascular bundle (named because these peripheral nerves are bundled with the blood vessels) to see peripheral nerve structure. Within the peripheral nerve individual axons are transversely sectioned; most are myelinated and appear as small bluish-grey central spots within the myelin sheaths. The myelin sheaths

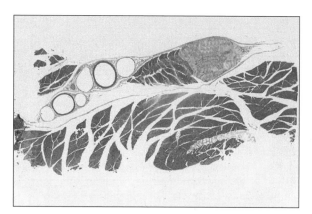

PERIPHERAL NERVES: TRANSVERSE SECTION
Slide #52: Neurovascular Bundle; H&E stain; 3 μm thick methacrylate section; nonhuman primate.

Higher magnification images:
- (medium) peripheral nerve fascicle

are stained lightly pink and sometimes have a peripheral Schwann cell nucleus. The individual nerve fibers (the term fiber refers to the axon plus its myelin sheath) are separated one from the other by fine reticular fibers that comprise the endoneurium. The delicate endoneurium fibers are not visible in this light microscope preparation, but are visible in electron micrographs. A number of these nerve fibers are gathered together much like the strands in a telephone cable to form fascicles, each of which is surrounded by a dense sheath, the perineurium. The perineurium is composed of several layers of squamous cells strengthened with collagen fibers to provide resistance to tensile forces. The perineurium is substantial enough to support delicate sutures used to repair severed peripheral nerves. A peripheral nerve may consist of only a single fascicle, but more commonly, a number of fascicles are bundled together within a dense connective tissue sheath, which is termed the epineurium.

The myelin sheath is better appreciated by examining the following tissue section in which the blue-stained myelin sheaths are more intact than what is typical of most light microscope preparations. In this tissue section the lipid molecules of the myelin have been fixed with an osmium fixative. Standard histological techniques do not preserve the lipid in myelin and typically the light microscopic image of myelinated axons bears little resemblance to the living, insulating sheath of axons. Notice the capillaries in this fascicle. The blood vessels look as pale as the nerve fibers because they have been cleared of blood; their walls are thinner than the myelin ensheathing the axons. Faintly stained mitochondria can be observed within the axoplasm.

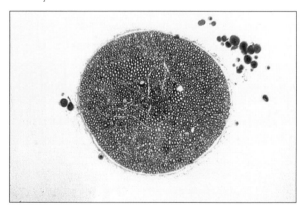

PERIPHERAL NERVE: TRANSVERSE SECTION
Slide #47: Sciatic Nerve; postfixed in osmium tetroxide and stained with toluidine blue; 2 μm araldite plastic section; mouse.

Higher magnification image:
  • (medium) myelinated axons and perineurium

AXON ULTRASTRUCTURE. An unmyelinated nerve fiber is a group of small axons bundled together by a chain of Schwann cells. The Schwann cells overlap within the fiber, so that the axon bundle at any given point may be associated with more than one Schwann cell. Observe how the small axons are embedded in membrane-lined grooves that deeply indent the surface of the Schwann cell. The principal constituents of the axoplasm are microtubules and neurofilaments. Several myelinated axons surround the unmyelinated axons in this image. Typically the unmyelinated axons are of considerably smaller

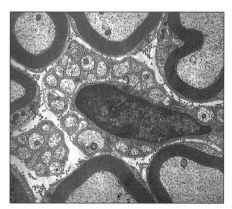

UNMYELINATED PERIPHERAL NERVE AXONS
Electron micrograph #12: Schwann Cell and Unmyelinated Axons (EM negative provided by Dr. Alan Peters.)

Higher magnification view:
  • Schwann cell processes and axons

diameter than the myelinated axons. Schwann cells have an external lamina, which like the basal lamina of epithelia consist of a lamina lucida and lamina densa. The external lamina covers all surfaces of the Schwann cell, but does not extend into the grooves. The fine collagen fibrils surrounding the nerve fibers constitute the endoneurium.

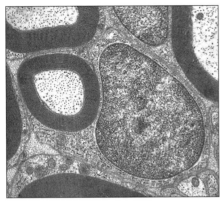

MYELINATED PERIPHERAL NERVE FIBER
Electron micrograph #13: Schwann Cell and Myelinated Axon.
(EM negative provided by Dr. Alan Peters.)

Higher magnification view:
• myelin, internal and external mesaxon

The myelin sheath results from the multiple wrapping of Schwann cell plasma membrane around the axon. The innermost and outermost ends of the spiral wrapping, where the two lips of the Schwann cell cytoplasm come together, are termed the internal and external mesaxon, respectively. There is one Schwann cell for each internodal length of the axon, and the Schwann cells do not overlap as they myelinate sequential axon segments. The axoplasm of the axon does not contain the variety of organelles found in the neuronal cell body; the principal constituents are mitochondria a few membranous vesicles, and microtubules and neurofilaments.

When the flat sheet of the Schwann cell wraps around the axon to form compact myelin, the cytoplasm is squeezed out and the cytoplasmic faces of the two membranes become apposed to each other. The extracellular faces of the Schwann cell plasmalemma also bind together. At higher magnifications, as in Electron Micrograph #28, a regular periodicity (of approximately 18 nm) is visible: the major dense lines alternate with intraperiod lines (or minor dense lines). The major dense lines correspond to the compacted inner cytoplasmic surfaces, whereas the intraperiod lines correspond to the joined external surfaces.

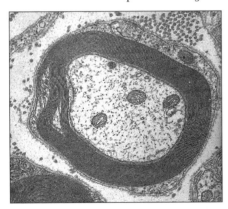

MYELIN SHEATH
Electron Micrograph #28: Myelin sheath.
(EM negative provided by Dr. Alan Peters)

Higher magnification views:
• myelin lamellae

The internodal length of myelin is interrupted by oblique clefts where the compaction of the Schwann cell membrane is lost. If you could unroll the membranes of myelin, the Schmidt-Lanterman cleft would represent a continuous narrow strip of Schwann cell cytoplasm passing between the innermost and outermost faces of the myelin sheath.

PERIPHERAL NERVE: LIGHT MICROSCOPY. In a peripheral nerve such as illustrated in Slide #43, the nerve fibers assume an undulating course. This appearance is typical for peripheral nerves given that nerve fibers cannot stretch, and extending them beyond their linear limits can have serious consequences, such as peripheral nerve axotomy. The axoplasm of the axons appears as central strands within the pale staining myelin sheath. Elongated Schwann cell nuclei are numerous, and relatively indistinguishable from the nuclei of the fibroblasts that are part of the endoneurium. The myelin has the bubbly appearance that results from the incomplete fixation of the lipid component of the sheath. The perineurium is not especially distinct because of its oblique plane of section in this preparation, although the epineurium is very prominent in this tissue section.

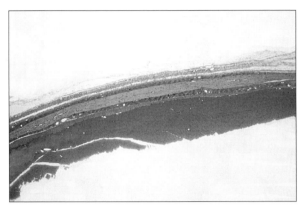

PERIPHERAL NERVE: LONGITUDINAL SECTION
Slide #43: Peripheral Nerve, longitudinal section; H&E stain; 3 μm thick methacrylate section; nonhuman primate.

Higher magnification images:
- (medium) nerve fascicle
- (high) myelinated fibers

In Slide #46, observe the small nerve fibers, the number of Schwann cells, and the perineurial sheath that surrounds each fascicle of nerve fibers in this tissue section. There is no thick fatty collar of myelin surrounding these axons, and the Schwann cells appear to be more closely packed than Schwann cells of myelinated peripheral nerves. In this preparation, some of the nerve bundles contain cell bodies of sympathetic ganglion cells that are typically clustered within ganglia that are interconnected by these fascicles of axons. In the autonomic nervous system, the axon of the first neuron in the two-neuron chain is thinly myelinated whereas the axon of the second neuron of the chain is unmyelinated.

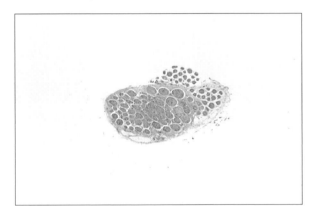

UNMYELINATED NERVE
Slide #45: Sympathetic Chain, from a region between ganglia; H&E stain, 15 μm thick paraffin section, human.

Higher magnification images:
- (medium) nerve fascicles
- (high) unmyelinated axons

Other examples of unmyelinated fibers are seen in Slide #46 (parasympathetic ganglia), examined previously in this chapter, where they are associated with the parasympathetic ganglia. The fibers of the autonomic nervous system represent the largest concentrations of purely unmyelinated and thinly myelinated nerve fibers in the body.

NEUROMUSCULAR JUNCTION

As a motor nerve approaches a muscle, the terminal branches of the axons emerge from their myelin sheaths and expand to form enlargements that are filled with synaptic vesicles. These synaptic vesicles contain the neurotransmitter acetylcholine, which can be released from the axon to stimulate the depolarization of the muscle. This specialized intercellular junction between the neuron and the muscle is termed a synaptic junction. The special enlarged endings of these motor neurons are called axon terminals. They contain mitochondria and some smooth endoplasmic reticulum, but no rough endoplasmic reticulum.

The following structures are specifically associated with the neuromuscular junction.

> motor end plate
> synaptic vesicle
> active zone of axon terminal
> synaptic cleft
> junctional folds

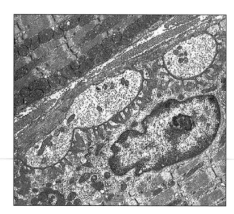

NEUROMUSCULAR JUNCTION
Electron Micrograph #15: Neuromuscular junction from rat tissue.

Higher magnification views:
- axon terminal and junctional folds
- Schwann cells and endomysium

The nerve terminal occupies a gutter or depression that indents the surface of the skeletal muscle fiber. To visualize this relationship between the nerve and the muscle fiber, think of placing your open hand, with fingers spread apart, onto a soft ball of bread dough, slightly indenting the surface. Your arm represents the motor neuron axon, and your coat sleeve (if you have one) is its myelin sheath. Your fingers and hand represent the axon terminals. Continuing with this analogy, the indented region on the bread dough left when you remove your hand corresponds to the specialized region of the muscle fiber membrane, called the motor end plate. The nerve ending and the muscle cell form a chemical synapse at this area of contact. In the region of the motor end plate, the extracellular gap between the axon and the indented surface is called the primary synaptic cleft. The sarcolemma of the muscle fiber forms invaginated folds within this cleft termed junctional folds, or secondary synaptic clefts. The crests of the folds are separated from the plasma membrane of the axon terminal by a cleft that is 60–100 nm wide. The external lamina of the muscle fiber occupies the cleft, and it follows the contours of the sarcolemma, even into the junctional folds.

An action potential traveling along the axon reaches the axon terminal and causes the synaptic vesicles to approach specialized densities in the membrane facing the cleft. These densities are termed active zones and the synaptic vesicles attach to the preterminal membrane at these spots and open, releasing the acetylcholine into the cleft. Acetylcholine receptors in the sarcolemma of the muscle fiber bind the acetylcholine, resulting in the depolarization and contraction of the muscle fiber.

A motor neuron located in the spinal cord innervates several muscle fibers. The neuron plus the collection of muscle fibers it innervates is termed the motor unit. The number of muscle fibers controlled by a single motor neuron varies, and ranges from about 10 muscle fibers to 100s of fibers. The size of the motor unit, that is, how many muscle fibers are associated with a single motor neuron, depends on the functional precision of the muscle innervated.

9. MUSCLE TISSUE

Muscle tissues are responsible for moving the body within space and altering the shapes of hollow structures within the body. Muscle cells are excitable elongate cells specialized to contract in length when appropriately stimulated. When they shorten, they move the tissues to which they are attached. An organizational overview of muscle tissue and its subtypes is represented diagrammatically as follows:

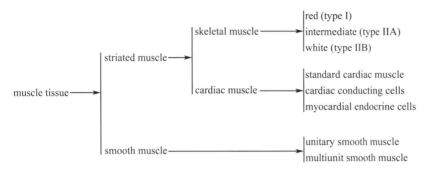

This hierarchical overview categorizing muscle first from the morphological perspective provides one way of thinking about muscle tissues. However, the student should recognize that in several ways, cardiac muscle is more like smooth muscle than skeletal muscle. For example, both cardiac and smooth muscle are individual cellular units (i.e., one cell/one nucleus); both are classified as involuntary muscle; and both have gap junctions that may electrically couple the myocytes. In contrast, the cellular units of skeletal muscle are large multinucleated fibers formed through the fusion of embryonic precursor cells; they are classed as a voluntary muscle; and gap junctions do not transmit depolarizing signals among them.

The following terms relate to the histology of muscle cells and fibers, and to become conversant on this topic it is important to be familiar with the location, function, and morphology of each of these terms. Word roots are provided to aid in your understanding and recall. Note that the principal word roots in this section are *sarco-*, the Greek root meaning flesh, and *myo-*, the Greek root meaning muscle.

skeletal muscle fiber or myofiber (*myo-*, muscle + *fiber*, fiber)
muscle fascicle (*fasciculus*, a small bundle)
epimysium (*epi-*, on, upon + *-mysium*, muscle)
perimysium (*peri-*, round about, above + *-mysium*, muscle)
endomysium (*endo-*, in, within, upon + *-mysium*, muscle)
sarcomere (*sarco-*, flesh + *-mere*, a part)
myofibril (*myo-*, muscle + *-fibril*, small fiber)
myofilament (*myo-*, muscle + *-filamentum*, a thread)
A and I bands (I and A refer to the appearance in polarized light: anisotropic and isotropic)
H band (from earlier term, Hensen's line, after 19th–20th century German anatomist)
Z and M lines (from German *Zwischenscheibe*, between disc; M stands for middle)
sarcoplasm (*sarco-*, flesh+ *-plasm*, a thing formed)
sarcolemma (*sarco-*, flesh + *-lemma*, husk)
sarcoplasmic reticulum (*reticulum*, small network)
terminal cisterns
t-tubule (t stands for transverse; *-ule*, diminutive of tube)

triad (*tri-*, three)
cardiac muscle cell or myocyte (*cardia-*, heart)
intercalated disc (*inter-*, between + *-calated*, proclaimed)
diad (*di-*, two)
sarcoplasmic cone
Purkinje fibers (after J. E. von Purkinje, 19th century Bohemian anatomist)
cardiac conducting cells
myocardial endocrine cells
smooth muscle cell or myocyte
caveola, pl. caveolae (*caveola*, a small pocket or recess)
dense bodies and dense plaques

CD-ROM Notice: The images on the CD-ROM examined in this chapter are listed numerically, by microscope slide number as they might be in a standard histology laboratory. Observe that Slide #36 is listed more than once because, as in a real laboratory exercise, it is used to demonstrate more than one structure. The lead–in images on the CD-ROM are labeled, and have links, that are appropriate for the tissue or structure being illustrated, and each is so designated in the list. To avoid confusion resulting from selecting the wrong nested series of images, read the label on the CD-ROM list carefully.

SKELETAL MUSCLE

Skeletal muscle fibers are large unbranched, multinucleated fibers that exhibit serially periodic cross striations. The individual cellular units are properly called fibers, not cells or myocytes, because they are multinucleated syncytial units (*syn-*, together + *cyt-*, cell) derived embryologically from immature cells known as myoblasts. The cytoplasm of a muscle fiber is termed sarcoplasm and its plasmalemma, the sarcolemma. The nuclei are pushed to the periphery of the fiber where they reside just beneath the sarcolemma. Skeletal muscle is innervated by somatic motor neurons, whose cell bodies reside in the central nervous system.

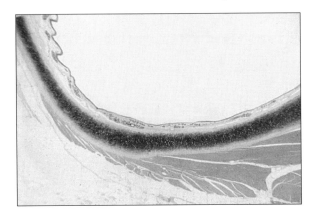

Skeletal Muscle
Slide #33: Trachea, 2 μm thick methacrylate section; H&E stain; nonhuman primate.

Higher magnification view:
• (medium) skeletal muscle fibers

Examine this light microscope tissue section to identify the cross-striations that characterize striated muscle. At a medium level of magnification, the dark A-bands and the light I-bands are readily apparent. Upon close inspection narrow dark Z-lines are seen to bisect the I-bands. The region from one Z-line to the next Z-line, approximately 2–3 μm in length, defines a sarcomere, which is the basic unit of contraction in a skeletal muscle fiber. Thus a sarcomere is composed of two half I-bands and a complete A-band. The light staining H-band that bisects the dark A-band is more easily seen in an electron micrograph.

Skeletal muscle ultrastructure. Compare the light microscope image of skeletal muscle with its ultrastructure. Observe that the banding pattern that is so characteristic in the light microscope image is attributed to the precise alignment of sarcomeres, which are linearly arrayed in long composite structures called myofibrils. The sarcomeres are formed from precisely arranged stable filaments, primarily myosin and actin. The ATP-fueled interaction of actin and myosin in the sarcomeres facilitate the rapid, complete, and powerful contraction that characterizes this form of muscle.

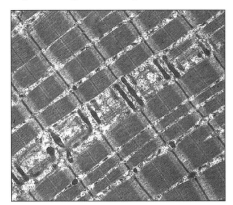

SARCOPLASM OF SKELETAL MUSCLE
Electron Micrograph #16. Skeletal Muscle Sarcoplasm; rat.

Higher magnification images:
- sarcoplasmic reticulum and mitochondria
- sarcomeres and triads

In the electron micrograph observe that the pale H-band is bisected by an M-line. A comprehensive histology text should be consulted for a detailed description of the precise arrangement and interaction of the actin and myosin filaments and the several associated proteins: the A-band is principally myosin polymers; the I-band is made up the thinner actin filaments and actin-associated molecules including troponin and tropomyosin and nebulin; the muscle corresponds to the center of the A-band that is free of interdigitating actin filaments; the M-line marks the middle stabilized region of the myosin filaments; and the Z-line anchors the actin filaments. A very large linear protein, termed titin, links the myosin to the Z-line and stabilizes the array of myosin filaments, as well as provides elastic recoil to the stretched sarcomere. With the expenditure of energy in the presence of calcium, the actin and myosin filaments interact and slide past each other to produce muscle contraction. Only the I-band and the M-band change width during contraction.

The myofibrils extend from one end of the muscle fiber to the other and comprise about 80% of the sarcoplasm (cytoplasm) of the skeletal muscle fiber. The balance of the sarcoplasm contains mitochondria, which provide the energy for contraction, the sarcoplasmic reticulum, which is a highly organized system responsible for sequestering the calcium that is released for the productive interaction of actin and myosin, and the t-tubules, which carry the depolarizing signal for contraction into the interior of the fibers. The triad is an organelle complex that represents the site where muscle fiber excitation is coupled to contraction; it is so named because it consists of two terminal cisterns (enlarged portions of the sarcoplasmic reticulum) associated with a t-tubule. In skeletal muscle, triads surround the myofibrils, two per sarcomere, specifically located at the interface of the A and I bands.

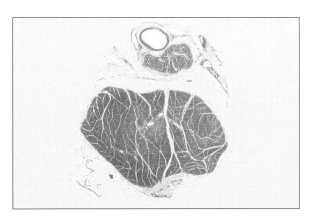

SKELETAL MUSCLE: TRANSVERSE SECTION
Slide #36: Lumbrical Muscle; 2 μm thick methacrylate section; H&E stain; nonhuman primate.

Higher magnification view:
- (medium) skeletal muscle fibers

LIGHT MICROSCOPE IMAGE. This is a transverse section of the lumbrical muscle, one of the intrinsic muscles of the hand. At the higher magnification, the transversely sectioned muscle fiber clearly reveals the peripheral position of the small dark nuclei. Observe the dense capillary network that typifies skeletal muscle. The numerous capillaries surrounding the muscle fibers are open and cleared of blood because this tissue was fixed by perfusion through its vascular system.

CONNECTIVE TISSUE INVESTMENTS

The connective tissue investments of muscle fibers are illustrated in this tissue section. A named skeletal muscle, like this one, is composed of individual fibers that are grouped into bundles of fibers termed fascicles. Each muscle fiber and each fascicle is ensheathed within a specific connective tissue investment that together enable the efficient conversion of muscle contraction to body movement. Endomysium refers to the reticular fiber investment of individual muscle fibers. The perimysium is a more substantial layer of connective tissue, with coarser bundles of collagen, and it surrounds the fascicles and carries the larger vessels and nerves of the muscle. The epimysium surrounds the whole muscle, anchoring it to fascia and tendons. In larger muscles, the epimysium corresponds to the deep fascia of gross anatomy. This small muscle does not have a very substantial epimysium.

Muscle spindles are complex sensory receptors that enable the smooth operation and constant adaptation of the muscles of the body to movement. They are elongate encapsulated structures composed of sensory fibers and small muscle fibers. They are located within the muscle and oriented parallel to its long axis.

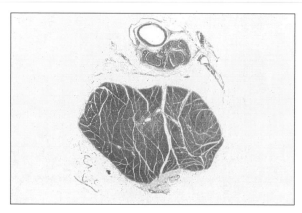

CONNECTIVE TISSUE INVESTMENTS
Slide #36: Lumbrical Muscle; 2 μm thick methacrylate section; H&E stain; nonhuman primate.

Higher magnification views:
- (medium) muscle fascicles and epimysium
- (medium) perimysium
- (medium) neurovascular structures and muscle spindles

SKELETAL MUSCLE FIBER SUBTYPES

Skeletal muscle fibers are subclassified into three types based on physiological, metabolic, and morphological criteria. Observe the three subtypes of skeletal muscle in the tissue section of the tongue that has been stained with PAS to demonstrate glycogen in the sarcoplasm of the muscle fibers. Red fibers, type I oxidative, have the lowest content of glycogen and therefore stain the least intensely with PAS. They tend to be the smallest fibers in a skeletal muscle. They are capable of repeated contraction without fatigue. White fibers, type IIB glycolytic, have the highest concentration of glycogen and are the most intensely stained in this preparation. White fibers tend to be the largest-diameter fibers in a skeletal muscle. They are capable of powerful contractions, but in contrast to the red fibers, they fatigue easily. Careful inspection of these transversely sectioned white fibers reveals the reticulated pattern of the glycogen distribution in the sarcoplasm surrounding the myofibrils. Intermediate fibers, type IIA, are intermediate with respect to the other fibers in terms of their size, metabolism and physiological characteristics.

Observe that each muscle fascicle consists of a mixture of red, white and intermediate fibers. This is typical of most muscles, although the relative numbers of each fiber

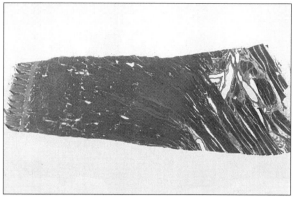

SKELETAL MUSCLE: FIBER SUBTYPES
Slide #37: Tongue; 4 μm thick methacrylate section; PAS stain; nonhuman primate.

Higher magnification view:
- (medium) skeletal muscle fibers, orientation
- (high) skeletal muscle fiber subtypes

type depend on the function of the muscle. The tongue, like most axial muscles, consists largely of red (appearing pale in PAS stain) and intermediate fibers. In standard H&E preparations these muscle subtypes are not readily distinguished from one another.

CARDIAC MUSCLE

The cardiac muscle cells of the heart are medium-sized, striated, and often branched. There is usually just one, but occasionally two, nuclei located centrally in the myocyte. The striations of cardiac muscle cells tend to be delicate and less obvious than those of skeletal muscle because the cardiac myofibrils are finer and they are not quite so packed together as the myofibrils of skeletal muscle. There is a very high density of mitochondria in cardiac muscle as a reflection of the cardiac myocyte's very high oxygen requirement. The mitochondria assemble in broad rows between the myofibrils. Myofibrils can be observed in these longitudinal sections as they course from one end of the myocyte to the other leaving a cone-shaped region of sarcoplasm on the fore and aft sides of the centrally located nucleus. These pockets of the sarcoplasm are termed sarcoplasmic cones.

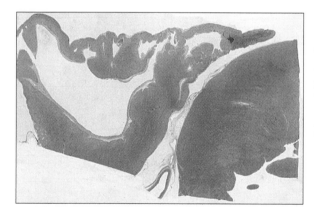

CARDIAC MUSCLE
Slide #63: Heart: Atrium and Ventricle; 2 μm thick methacrylate section; hematoxylin and toluidine blue–phloxinate; nonhuman primate.

Higher magnification view:
- (medium) cardiac muscle cells
- (high) intercalated discs

INTERCALATED DISC

Prominent intercellular junctions, called intercalated discs, are uniquely characteristic of cardiac muscle. These junctions connect contiguous cardiac muscle cells at a zigzag or stepped interface that appears in the light microscope image as a narrow, dark, irregular band oriented perpendicular to the long axis of the myocyte.

In an electron micrograph, the cardiac muscle cells appear similar to the skeletal muscle fibers except that they are smaller and they have a much higher numerical density of mitochondria. The substitution of a two-part diad (with only one terminal cistern of the sarcoplasmic reticulum associated with one t-tubule) for the triad of skeletal muscle constitutes another difference between these two striated muscle types.

The intercalated disc is a set of three intercellular junctions that are all visible in the

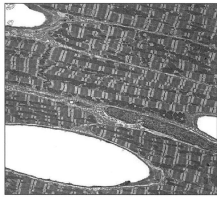

CARDIAC MUSCLE
Electron Micrograph #25: Cardiac Muscle; rat.

Higher magnification view:
• intercalated disc

electron micrograph: the fascia adherens, the desmosome, and the gap junction. The fascia adherens and the desmosome are both located where the intercellular interface between these two cells is oriented perpendicular to the direction of the force of contraction and they bind the contracting myocytes strongly together. The fascia adherens is located in the region where the myofibrils of one myocyte bind to the myofibrils of the next myocyte. The sheetlike fascia adherens links the actin components of two myofibrils, just as the encircling zonula adherens of an absorptive epithelium links the actin of the terminal webs of adjacent cells. Desmosomes are located between the myofibrils; they provide stronger intercellular attachment between the myocytes linking the intermediate filaments of the two contiguous myocytes. The gap junction is located in the region of the interface between the two myocytes where the two sarcolemmae are oriented parallel to the long axis of the cells. In this location the gap junction is not subjected to the same tensile forces as the other two intercellular junctions. This gap junction, also called a nexus, is the site where the depolarizing signal passes from one cell to the next, generating the waves of contraction that pass through the heart. The gap junction is formed from a series of complex transmembrane units termed connexons that are cylindrical and align between cells to form a 1.5 nm diameter channel. A gap of only 2–4 nm separates the two cells. These junctions mediate the chemical and electrical coupling of cells in a variety of tissues in addition to cardiac muscle.

CARDIAC CONDUCTING CELLS

Cardiac conducting cells constitute part of the impulse conducting system of the heart and their function is to coordinate the beating of the heart so that blood flows through its chambers in the proper sequence and volume. The conducting cells are modified cardiac muscle cells and as such, do contain myofibrils and are interconnected with gap junctions. However, these conducting myocytes contain more glycogen and fewer myofibrils than the standard ones, a modification that renders them lighter staining than the smaller surrounding cardiac muscle cells. The numerical density of gap junctions between these conducting cells is greater than that between standard

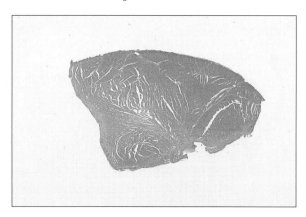

CARDIAC CONDUCTING CELLS
Slide #38: Cardiac Muscle I; 2 μm thick methacrylate section; H&E stain; human.

Higher magnification view:
• (low) cardiac conducting cells

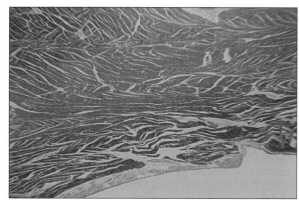

CARDIAC CONDUCTING CELLS
Slide #38: Cardiac Muscle II; 12 μm thick paraffin section; Phosphotungstic Acid Hematoxylin (PTAH) stain; human.

Higher magnification view:
• (medium) Purkinje fibers

myocardial cells, facilitating a more rapid conduction of the depolarizing signal from cell to cell. In most parts of the heart's conducting system, these modified cells are larger than standard cardiac myocytes; in the nodes of the cardiac conducting system (the SA node and the AV node), they tend to be smaller.

Two tissue sections illustrate the cardiac conducting cells. In the H&E stained section, the bundle of cardiac conducting cells are recognized by their location, staining characteristics and size. The second tissue section is stained with PTAH, a stain that stains myofibrils and thereby clearly illustrates the reduced myofibril content of the conducting fibers. The cardiac conducting fibers located in the subendocardial layer of the ventricles, as in this PTAH stained tissue section, are specifically called Purkinje fibers.

MYOCARDIAL ENDOCRINE CELLS

A functionally specialized category of cardiac muscle cells occurs predominantly in the walls of the atrium of the heart. They are the myocardial endocrine cells so named because in addition to being appropriately contractile, they contain special granules in the sarcoplasmic cone that are released in response to detected increases in blood volume. The granules contain the hormone atrial naturietic protein, which targets several tissues in the body, in particular cells in the kidney, which respond by increasing water loss. These modified cardiac muscle cells are part of a diffuse system of endocrine cells dispersed throughout the body.

SMOOTH MUSCLE

Smooth muscle cells, the myocytes in the walls of the blood vessels and visceral organs, are nonstriated, spindle-shaped cells with tapered ends. Each smooth muscle cell has a single centrally located nucleus that is long and narrow in the relaxed smooth myocyte but can assume a corkscrew shape when the smooth muscle cells contract maximally. Smooth muscle is innervated by visceral motor fibers, but contraction and relaxation can be initiated by a variety of additional factors, depending on the location of the muscle.

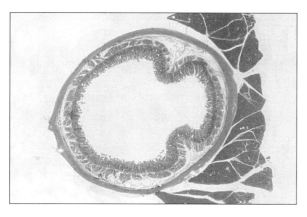

SMOOTH MUSCLE
Slide #116: Duodenum (small intestine); 2 μm thick methacrylate section; H&E stain; nonhuman primate.

Higher magnification view:
• (medium) muscularis externa

Observe the general appearance of smooth muscle in the muscularis externa of the duodenum where smooth muscle cells, because of the orthogonal arrangement in this layer, are both longitudinally and transversely sectioned. In smooth muscle tissue like the muscularis externa, the fusiform (*fusi-*, spindle + *-form*, shape) myocytes are packed closely together and staggered, with the tapered ends of some cells fitting against the thicker middle portions of adjacent cells. In longitudinal section the regularly dispersed nuclear profiles reflect this packing, whereas in transverse section, both staggered nuclei and intermingled large and small profiles of the tapered ends illustrate how the myocytes are packed.

Observe the low density of capillaries in this smooth muscle tissue section that has been fixed by vascular perfusion. Unlike cardiac and skeletal muscle, the metabolic requirements of smooth muscle are relatively low and the reduced density of capillaries reflects this difference.

The ultrastructure of smooth muscle reveals several functionally important features of smooth muscle that are not visible in the light microscope. The sarcoplasm is dominated by myofibrils that are not organized into sarcomeres. Muscle contraction occurs through the linked interaction of two cytoskeletal systems: the contractile proteins, principally actin and myosin, and the noncontractile, cable-like intermediate filaments. Both of these cytoskeletal systems link to the dense bodies and dense plaques in the smooth muscle sarcoplasm and sarcolemma, respectively. These electron-dense bodies contain the actin-binding α-actinin (like the Z-line of skeletal muscle) and anchor the contractile and intermediate filaments to each other and to the sarcolemma. The stable vesiclelike caveolae invaginating the sarcolemma represent another morphological characteristic of smooth muscle. The function of the caveolae is not known for certain.

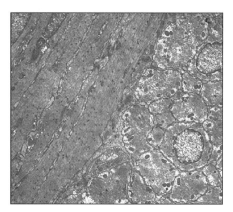

Smooth Muscle
Electron Micrograph #17: Smooth Muscle; muscularis externa; rat gut.

Higher magnification view:
- smooth muscle fibers and gap junctions
- caveolae, dense bodies and plaques, and nerve fibers

Unitary and multiunit smooth muscle

The two subcategories of smooth muscle are based on the functional arrangements of the myocytes. Smooth muscle like that in the wall of the gut in which the myocytes are closely packed together and electrically coupled with gap junctions is classified as the unitary type of smooth muscle. They act as a unit. A slow wave of contraction passes along the inner circularly spiraled sheet of myocytes and the outer longitudinally spiraled sheet of myocytes to move intestinal contents in a distal direction. The multiunit type of arrangement is illustrated in Electron Micrograph #14 where the more dispersed arrangement of individual myocytes of the wall of the blood vessel differs from the packed unitary type arrangement in the gut. The vascular smooth muscle cells are separated by elastic and reticular fibers and there are no gap junctions electrically coupling them. Multiunit myocytes are principally under the control of the nervous system, and can contract independently of other myocytes in the wall.

Individual smooth muscle cells in the walls of large arteries are enmeshed in elastic and reticular fibers that provide elasticity and support to the wall, respectively. In

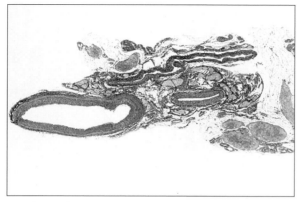

SMOOTH MUSCLE
Slide #53: Blood Vessels; 15 μm thick paraffin
section; Mallory's trichrome stain; human.

Higher magnification view:
• (medium) smooth muscle fibers

routine H&E staining, both the myocytes and the extracellular fibers stain pink, but with Mallory's trichrome stain as illustrated in this tissue section, it is easy to differentiate among them. The red-stained smooth muscle fibers are easily detected against the blue reticular fibers, the pale pink elastin, and the deeper blue collagen fibers of the vessel's outer wall. The smooth myocytes, not fibroblasts or reticular cells, synthesize and secrete the matrix material of the muscle layer of this vessel wall.

SMOOTH MUSCLE: OTHER ARRANGEMENTS

It is instructive to examine the variety of arrangements of smooth muscle cells in the body. By varying the arrangement and sizes of the fiber bundles, smooth muscle accomplishes a variety of movements. For example, in the wall of the gut the smooth muscle arranged in orthogonally oriented compact sheets is able to propel intestinal contents in a distal direction, by shortening and squeezing the tube in a cyclic manner. The encircling smooth muscle ensheathment in blood vessels plays no role in propelling the blood because the heart pumps the blood within this closed system of vessels, and so the smooth muscle of the blood vessel wall facilitates the two important tasks of (*1*) directing the flow of blood into various regions of the body and (*2*) controlling the pressure within the closed system by adjusting the tonic, inelastic state of contraction. In the wall of a hollow organ like the urinary bladder, smooth muscle reduces the size of the entire lumen in order to expel the luminal contents.

In this tissue section of the urinary bladder the interlacing bundles of smooth muscle in the wall are sectioned in transverse, oblique and longitudinal planes of section. Simultaneous contraction in all these directions moves all regions of the wall toward the lumen, reducing its size and emptying the bladder.

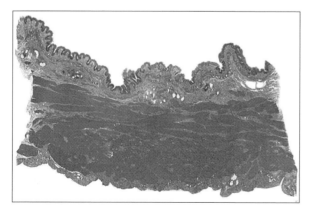

SMOOTH MUSCLE ARRANGEMENT
Slide #165: Urinary Bladder, contracted; 2 mm thick
methacrylate section; hematoxylin and toluidine
blue–phloxinate; nonhuman primate.

Higher magnification views:
• (medium) inner wall
• (medium) outer wall

The arrector pili muscles associated with the hair follicles of the skin are isolated long and narrow smooth muscle fascicles. They originate high in the dermis and insert deeper, in the wall of the hair follicle. Contraction of this muscle causes the hair to become erect, sometimes causing a buckle in the skin known as a goose bump.

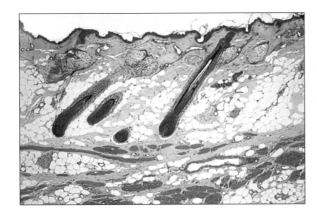

SMOOTH MUSCLE ARRANGEMENTS
Slide #88: Scalp; 2 μm thick methacrylate section;
Lee's stain; nonhuman primate.

Higher magnification view:
  • (medium) hair follicle

SKELETAL AND SMOOTH MUSCLE

The esophagus marks the beginning of the alimentary canal. In most of the alimentary canal the muscularis externa consists entirely of smooth muscle and it is under the control of the autonomic nervous system. However, the first part of the esophagus is under voluntary control, and its muscularis externa is composed of skeletal muscle. The muscle of the musclularis externa changes from voluntary skeletal muscle to involuntary smooth muscle in a proximal to distal direction. In the middle third of the esophagus length, both smooth muscle cells and skeletal muscle fibers are intermixed in the muscularis externa. By the final third of the esophagus, the muscularis externa is entirely smooth muscle.

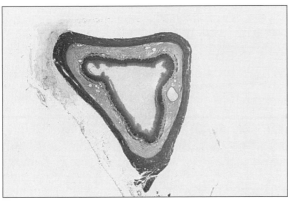

SKELETAL AND SMOOTH MUSCLE
Slide #109: Esophagus, 2 μm thick methacrylate
section, Lee's stain; nonhuman primate.

Higher magnification views:
  • (medium) inner circular layer
  • (high) outer longitudinal layer

    This tissue section provides an opportunity to compare directly the smooth and skeletal muscle in longitudinal, oblique, and transverse planes of section. As illustrated in this tissue section, the skeletal muscle fibers are considerably larger in diameter than smooth muscle cells. Compare the diameters, striations, and location of the nucleus within the respective cellular units.

10. INTEGUMENT

Integument refers to the skin and structures that are derived from the skin, such as the nails, hairs, and several types of glands. Skin covers the entire external surface of the body, forming nearly 10% of the total body mass. Unlike many other organs of the body, the functional importance of skin as an organ is easily overlooked and underestimated. It provides a self–renewing interface between the body and the environment; it functions as a major sense organ; it protects the body against chemical, mechanical, and thermal damage, as well as damage from sun and water. It is absorptive and secretory, and provides a barrier against invasion by potentially harmful organisms and materials, and, if breached, it provides defense and repair mechanisms.

A person's skin serves as a means of nonverbal communication, some quite involuntarily. Skin is of cosmetic importance, and changes associated with normal maturation and aging are reflected in the skin and its appendages. A person's general state of health is reflected in the appearance and condition of the skin, and examination of the skin is valuable for diagnosing far more than dermatological disorders.

The skin is a composite of all the basic tissue types. As an organ it clearly demonstrates, both macroscopically and microscopically, the relationship between structure and function. Although basically similar over the entire body, the skin shows local variation in thickness, degree of keratinization, pigmentation, sizes and numerical density of hairs, frequency and types of glands, extent of vascularization, and innervation. Many of these features are examined in this chapter.

The tissues that comprise the skin have organ–specific names that designate location, morphology or function. The word integument is derived from the Latin prefix *in*, meaning on, plus the root from *tego*, meaning to cover. The Greek word *derma*, meaning skin, is the common root for the principal layers of this organ. A diagrammatic overview of these layers, with the relevant word roots, follows.

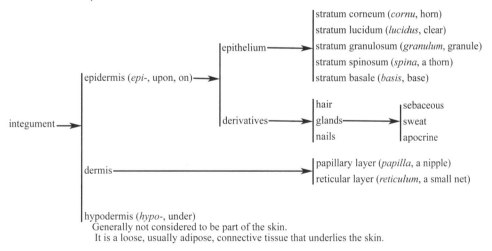

The epidermis is a keratinized stratified squamous epithelium. The principal cell type is the keratinocyte, which proliferates and differentiates before being desquamated from the free surface. A small number of additional cells with specific function and morphology contribute to the population of cells in the epidermis.

> keratinocyte (*keras*, horn + -*cyte*, cell)
> melanocyte (*melas*, black + -*cyte*, cell
> Langerhans cell (after P. Langerhans, a 19th century German anatomist)
> Merkel cell (after F. Merkel, a 19th–20th century German anatomist)

The following geometric patterns are identified at the interface of the epidermis and the dermis.

interpapillary pegs or rete pegs (*inter-*, between + *papilla*, a nipple; *rete*, a net)
dermal papilla or dermal ridge (*derma-*, skin; *papilla*, a nipple)

The following sensory receptors and glands are examined in this exercise.

Meissner's corpuscles (after G. Meissner, a German histologist)
Pacinian corpuscles (after F. Pacini, a 19th century Italian anatomist)
eccrine sweat gland (*ec-*, out of + *krino*, to secrete)
sebaceous gland (*sebum*, tallow)

> **CD-ROM Notice**: The images examined in this chapter are listed numerically on the CD-ROM by microscope slide number as they might be listed in a standard histology laboratory. Observe that some slides have more than one version, each designated with Roman numerals, and both are used for illustration. The labels and linked images are different for each lead–in image. To avoid confusion resulting from selecting the wrong nested series of images, read the label on the CD-ROM list of slides carefully.

REFERENCE DIAGRAM FOR SLIDE LOCATIONS

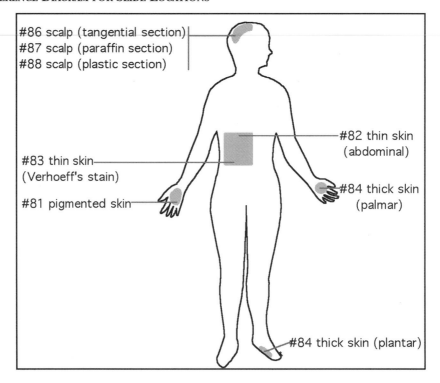

#86 scalp (tangential section)
#87 scalp (paraffin section)
#88 scalp (plastic section)

#82 thin skin (abdominal)

#83 thin skin (Verhoeff's stain)

#84 thick skin (palmar)

#81 pigmented skin

#84 thick skin (plantar)

SKIN

The body's skin is composed of two tissue layers: the epidermis, which is a stratified squamous keratinized epithelium and the dermis, an underlying bed of connective tissue. These two layers and the derivatives of the epidermis, the hair, nails and glands, constitute the integument.

The hypodermis is a deeper, loose connective tissue layer, which frequently contains large amounts of adipose tissue, and is not considered to be part of the skin. The hypodermis corresponds to the superficial fascia of gross anatomy, and the amount of fat in this layer is affected by body location, gender, age, and the physical and nutritional state of the individual.

The hypodermis provides the body not only with a reservoir of stored lipid to be used as an energy source, but also provides the body with insulation and protective padding. As a reflection of these latter functions, the adipocytes located in those areas of hypodermis that function as insulation or protection are among the last to be depleted when the body taps its adipocytes for energy. The hypodermis of the palm of the hand represents one location where the hypodermis provides protective padding and is not readily depleted as other stores of fat are used to support nutritional needs.

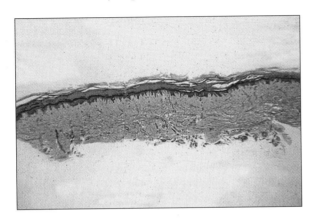

SKIN
Slide #84: Thick Skin I; H&E stained 12 µm paraffin section; human.

Higher magnification image:
 • (medium) layers of the epidermis

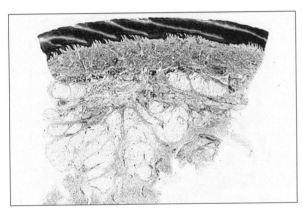

SKIN
Slide #84: Thick Skin II; hematoxylin stained 20 µm paraffin section; human.

Higher magnification image:
 • (medium) layers of the epidermis

EPIDERMIS

The stratified squamous epithelium in both of these tissue sections illustrates the five cellular layers. Like all epithelia, the epidermis contains no blood vessels. The principal cells of the epidermis are keratinocytes and the layers of the epidermis mark the progressive differentiation of the keratinocytes from their genesis in the deepest layer to the nonnucleated keratin-filled cells of the surface. Because the epidermis is constantly undergoing renewal, some cells may appear transitional from one type to another. The layers are as follows:

STRATUM BASALE. The deepest layer is a single layer of cuboidal to low columnar cells resting on the basement membrane. These cells are mitotically active, but since mitotic activity in the skin generally occurs at night, specimens collected during the day do not reflect the high level of proliferation that characterizes the cells in this layer. This layer is firmly attached to the underlying connective tissue by means of hemidesmosomes and an undulating interface.

STRATUM SPINOSUM. The second layer consists of multiple layers of cells that range in shape from polyhedral to somewhat flattened. Spiny "intercellular bridges" that span broad intercellular gaps are diagnostic of this layer. The bridges are cytoplasmic extensions of the keratinocytes filled with tonofilaments and joined by a desmosome. Tonofilaments (*tono-*, tone, tension + *filum*, a thread) are bundles of cytokeratin filaments. Thus the cells of the epidermis are very strongly bound to each other and can resist substantial mechanical distortions without being pulled apart. The stratum spinosum varies in thickness: it has an undulating deep interface with the stratum basale, but is smooth on the side adjacent to the stratum granulosum.

STRATUM GRANULOSUM. The third layer of the epidermis contains keratinocytes whose cytoplasm contains irregularly shaped keratohyalin granules (*keras*, horn + *hyalos*, glass). This layer is three to five cells thick and the cells are somewhat flattened. The keratinocyte nucleus is undergoing degenerative change. The keratohyalin granules are associated with the tonofilaments, which continue to accumulate in the cells as differentiation progresses. Additional granules (termed lamellar or membrane-coating granules) in these cells contain material that is secreted to create the intercellular glycolipid sheets that contribute to the skin's water barrier. This barrier is a two-way permeability barrier, controlling what passes out of, as well as into, the epidermis and underlying tissues.

STRATUM LUCIDUM. The fourth layer consists of flattened, poorly stained cells arranged three to five cells thick. The cells have no nuclei and individual cells are difficult to discern. The cells are believed to be incompletely keratinized transitional cells. This layer is typically found only in the thick skin of the palms and soles of the feet.

STRATUM CORNEUM. The fifth layer is the most superficial layer and consists of closely packed, overlapping flattened cells from which the nucleus is absent. These cellular entities represent the final product of keratinocyte differentiation. The cytoplasm of the keratinocytes has been completely replaced by a filamentous substance, keratin, embedded in an interfibrillar matrix. In thick skin, this layer may be about 50 cells thick, whereas in thin skin it may be only a few cells thick. The thickness of this layer can be increased in response to repeated abrasive activity upon the surface of the skin. The dead cells are sloughed from the surface after loosening the intercellular attachments.

The epidermis of a thick skin, like that which covers the soles of the feet and the palms of the hands, consists of all the layers described. The layers of a thin skin, like the abdominal skin and the skin of the scalp, both to be observed later in this chapter, differ from thick skin in that the stratum granulosum is at best only two cells thick, a stratum lucidum is missing, and the stratum corneum is considerably thinner.

The following tissue section illustrates a pigmented skin in which the keratinocytes in the basal layer are heavily pigmented with golden-brown melanin granules, or melanosomes (*melas*, black + *soma*, body). The keratinocytes do not generate these melanosomes; rather, melanocytes, which reside in the basal layer among the keratinocytes, synthesize and transfer melanin-containing granules to the cytoplasm of

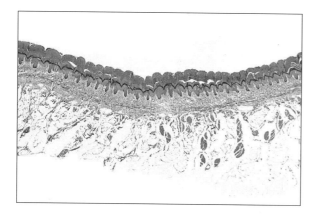

PIGMENTED SKIN; DERMAL LAYERS
Slide #81: Thick Skin, pigmented; H&E stained 10 μm paraffin section; human.

Higher magnification images:
- (medium) epidermis and dermis
- (high) melanocytes and keratinocytes
- (medium) dermis and Pacinian corpuscles
- (high) Meissner's corpuscle
- (high) Meissner's corpuscle and capillaries
- (medium) Pacinian corpuscle and sweat gland

the keratinocytes. In this H&E-stained section the melanocytes are shrunken and surrounded by a clear ring. Pigmentation of human skin can be intrinsic and genetically determined as well as reversible, based on environmental or hormonal influences. Racial variations in pigmentation are not due to differences in the numerical density of melanocytes, but rather because of the size and the activity of these cells.

Two additional cell types are present in the epidermis but not specifically illustrated in these tissue sections. One is the Merkel cell, which also appears as a cell in the basal cell layer with clear cytoplasm. Merkel cells are innervated by myelinated sensory fibers and are particularly numerous in regions of the skin that are sensitive to touch, like the fingertips. The second usual epidermal resident is the Langerhans cell. These cells are antigen-presenting cells that are dispersed in the basal and spinous layers of the epidermis. They are key elements in the skin-associated lymphoid tissue (SALT) that functions in immune surveillance and response, including the rejection of skin grafts. Langerhans cells can migrate out of the epidermis and participate in transporting antigenic materials to lymph nodes. Both of these cell types can be specifically stained with special stains and immunocytochemical techniques, but are difficult to identify with certainty in a standard light microscope preparation like this one.

DERMIS

The interface between the epidermis and dermis is uneven, and the magnitude of irregularity depends on where the skin is located. The downward projections of epidermis into dermis are called interpapillary or rete pegs, and in three dimensions they form a complex network of ridges. The complementary upward projections of the dermis are termed dermal papillae, or dermal ridges. The interdigitation of these two tissues contributes to the firmness of attachment between them. The depth of the interdigitation is greater in thick skin than thin skin, and greatest in skin subjected to strong frictional forces.

The dermis is a connective tissue that physiologically supports the skin with nerves, blood vessels, and lymphatic vessels. Blood flow in the dermis serves the nutritional needs of the cells of the dermis and epidermis, but also provides important thermoregulatory functions for the whole body. Capillaries loop up into the dermal papillae delivering blood close to the cells in the stratum basale and spinosum. The capacity of the complex network of dermal blood vessels and vascular plexuses can be changed substantially in response to requirements to conserve or disperse body heat.

The dermis can be subdivided into two layers, papillary and reticular. The more superficial papillary layer includes the ridges that protrude into the epidermis; it is composed of a closely woven mesh of thin collagen and elastic fibers. The deeper reticular layer comprises the major part of the dermis and consists of coarse, densely interwoven fibers. It is classified as a dense irregular connective tissue and the typical connective tissue cells are somewhat sparse. The primary direction of the collagen fibers is parallel to the skin's surface. There are occasional networks of elastic fibers. The number and arrangement of the collagen bundles give the skin its tensile strength, whereas the elastic fibers provide elastic recoil. The density, arrangement, and nature of these fibers vary with location, age, gender, and nutritional state of the body.

SENSORY RECEPTORS. Meissner's corpuscles are encapsulated sensory receptors located in the tips of the dermal papillae where they serve as tactile receptors for fine touch. They are oval structures composed of delicate cells that spiral around nerve endings that terminate in the corpuscle. These supporting cells are probably modified Schwann cells. The numerical density of these receptors varies in different locations of the body, being more frequent, for example, in the skin of the finger tips than in the skin of the back and shoulders.

Pacinian corpuscles are located deep in the reticular dermis or in the hypodermis. These large (1–4 mm in diameter) receptors are sensitive to pressure, coarse touch, and vibration. In a well-fixed tissue section, the distinct spherical corpuscles resemble the cut surface of an onion. In some tissue sections, as illustrated in this tissue section, the delicate concentric lamellae are apparent but the corpuscle has become shrunken and distorted, giving it an artifactual stellate profile.

SWEAT (ECCRINE) GLANDS. This tissue section is abdominal skin, a thin skin. Observe the thinness of the epidermis relative to that of thick skin, as well as the absence of a stratum lucidum and the decreased frequency and size of the dermal ridges.

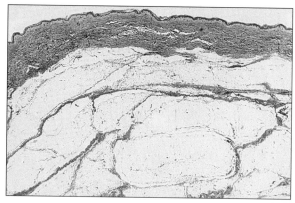

THIN SKIN

Slide #82: Thin Skin; H&E stained 10 μm paraffin section; human.

Higher Magnification Images:
- (medium) papillary and reticular dermis
- (medium high) sweat gland

The sweat glands are highly coiled secretory tubules that reside in the dermis. Isolated profiles of the spiraling sweat gland ducts are illustrated traversing the dermis between the gland and the surface upon which the watery secretion is delivered. The gland cells form a simple epithelium of pale pyramidal or cuboidal cells. In favorable planes of section, it is possible to see the peripherally located, spindle-shaped nucleus of the myoepithelial cell whose role it is to squeeze the tube and move sweat into the lumen. The secretory portion of the simple coiled tubule is continuous with the excretory duct, which is lined with a stratified (two layers) cuboidal epithelium.

ELASTIC FIBERS. Verhoeff's stain for elastin highlights the elastic fibers in the dermis. The elastic fibers in the papillary layer are delicate and ones in the reticular layer are more coarse. Elastic fibers are also present in the hypodermis.

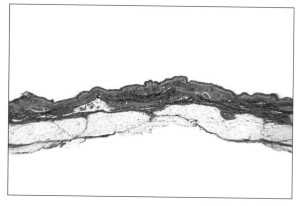

ELASTIC FIBERS

Slide #83: Thin Skin; Verhoeff's stain; 12 μm paraffin section; human.

Higher magnification image:
- (medium) dermis and epidermis

HAIR

Hairs are filamentous keratinized structures produced by a specialized invagination of the epidermis, the hair follicle. The density of hairs varies with region of the skin, as does the hair's shape, coarseness, length, and rate of growth. The following parts of the hair are examined in this exercise.

hair papilla (*papilla*, a nipple)
hair shaft
hair follicle (*folliculus*, a small sac)

internal and external root sheaths
glassy membrane
arrector pili muscle (*arrector*, that which raises; *pilus*, hair)

The hair shaft extends its free end above the skin; its deep end is enclosed within the tubular hair follicle. The follicle is typically oriented oblique to the surface of the skin. The length of the follicle ranges from shorter ones (about 1 mm) that extend only into the dermis to longer ones (about 3 mm) that extend into the hypodermis. The base of the hair follicle is expanded into the hair bulb, which is indented by a bulge of well vascularized connective tissue termed the dermal papilla. The cells in the lower half of the expanded hair bulb contain mitotically active keratinocytes; these multipotent cells comprise the germinal matrix that gives rise to the hair as well as to the cells of the inner root sheath. Melanocytes occur among the keratinocytes at the apex of the dermal papilla and provide the melanosomes that are responsible for hair color.

The tubular hair follicle originates as an ingrowth of the epidermis with which it is continuous. It is surrounded by a connective tissue investment termed the dermal sheath. The unusually thick basement membrane that is located between the dermal sheath and the follicle is the glassy membrane. The epithelial sheath of the follicle is subdivided into an internal and external root sheath. The cells of the external root sheath are continuous with the stratum basale of the epidermis.

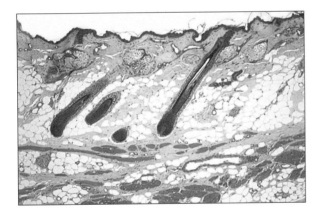

HAIR
Slide #88: Scalp; Lee's stain; 4 μm plastic section; nonhuman primate.

Higher magnification images:
- (medium) hair follicle
- (high) hair bulb
- (high) hair shaft
- (high) sebaceous glands

Both the hair shaft and the follicle are concentrically layered structures. The hair shaft has three layers: the medulla, cortex, and cuticle. Innermost of the layers is the medulla, a narrow core that is composed of moderately keratinized cells. Surrounding the medulla is the highly keratinized thick cortex that forms the bulk of the hair shaft. The cuticle is the hard, thin keratinized layer that covers the outside of the hair. Within the follicle, the hair is surrounded by an inner root sheath, which also has three concentric layers. These layers are an innermost cuticle of the inner root sheath, surrounded by Huxley's layer, and lastly the outermost Henle's layers. These three internal root sheath layers are not labeled in the tissue images. The cells of the internal root sheet are generated in the germinal matrix, migrate upwards as the hair grows, and eventually disintegrate at about the level of the sebaceous gland ducts, leaving space for the sebum.

The narrow bundle of smooth muscle fibers, called the arrector pili muscle, is responsible for elevating the hair. Its origin is high in the dermis and it inserts into the dermal root sheath in a level slightly above the middle of the follicle. Sebaceous glands are saccular structures situated within a region of dermis located in the angle between the arrector pili muscle and the hair follicle. These glands are branched alveolar glands and their short ducts empty into the neck of the hair follicle. The secretion, sebum, is produced by a holocrine type of secretion; cells generated in the periphery of the gland differentiate as they move toward its center and degrade into a complex oily secretion. Sebum provides a protective coating for hairs and contributes to the surface lipids of skin. In some areas of the body, where hair follicles are absent, sebaceous glands open directly on the skin.

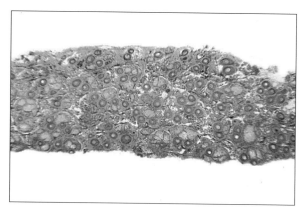

HAIR: TRANSVERSE SECTION
Slide #86: Scalp; H&E stain; 10 μm paraffin section; human.

Higher magnification images:
- (medium) dermis level
- (medium) hypodermis level

The concentric layers of the hair, the epidermal root sheaths and the dermal sheath are well illustrated in this tissue section that is oriented in a plane parallel to the surface of the scalp.

11. CIRCULATORY SYSTEM

The circulatory system functions to pick up, transport, and deliver gases, nutrients, hormones, cells, and other materials throughout the body. It consists of several continuous component parts each with a basically tubular shape that is modified to carry out a function subservient to the central purpose of the system — exchange across the walls of the capillaries and the postcapillary venules.

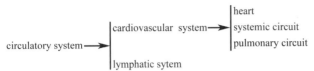

The closed circuit of vessels (the arteries, capillaries, veins) and in–line pump (the heart) constitute the cardiovascular portion of the circulatory system. The pulmonary system is a short-run, high-volume, closed system of vessels (and pump) that is part of the body's circulatory system and is examined as part of Chapter 18: Respiratory System. Although the blood traveling in the systemic and the pulmonary circuits does not mix, all blood flows sequentially through both circuits. The lymphatic vascular system is a separate unidirectional series of capillaries, vessels, and ducts that is open-ended and drains lymph from the tissues and delivers it to the cardiovascular system. A hierarchical overview of the structures examined in this Chapter is illustrated in the following chart.

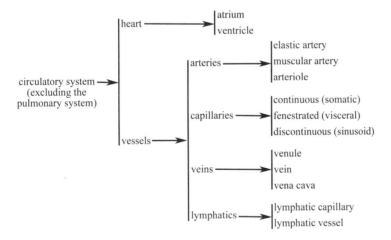

The walls of the vessels are structurally modified to carry out the functions required of them. In order to discuss the walls of the systemic circuit, it is necessary to recognize and understand the structural components and their system–specific names. The concentric layers of the walls of blood vessels are known as tunics.

tunica intima (*tunica*, a coat; *intima*, inmost)
tunica media (*tunica*, a coat; *media*, middle)
tunica adventitia (*tunica*, a coat; *adventitia*, coming to)
lamellar units (*lamella*, diminutive of *lamina*, thin plate or leaf)
internal elastic lamina (*lamina*, thin plate or flat leaf)
external elastic lamina
vasa vasorum (*vasa*, a vessel; *vasorum*, of a vessel)
nervi vascularis (*nervi*, nerves; *vascularis*, related to vessels)
vein valves

REFERENCE DIAGRAM FOR SLIDE LOCATIONS

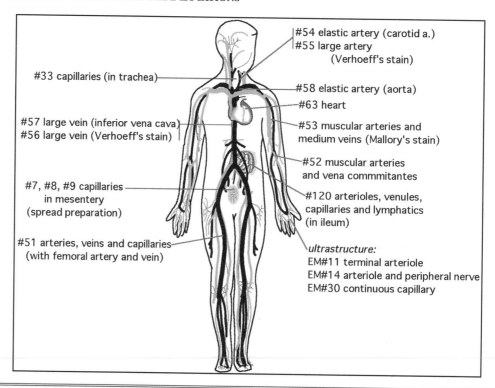

#54 elastic artery (carotid a.)
#55 large artery
            (Verhoeff's stain)

#33 capillaries (in trachea)

#58 elastic artery (aorta)
#63 heart

#57 large vein (inferior vena cava)
#56 large vein (Verhoeff's stain)

#53 muscular arteries and
medium veins (Mallory's stain)

#52 muscular arteries
and vena commmitantes

#7, #8, #9 capillaries
    in mesentery
(spread preparation)

#120 arterioles, venules,
capillaries and lymphatics
(in ileum)

#51 arteries, veins and capillaries
(with femoral artery and vein)

ultrastructure:
EM#11 terminal arteriole
EM#14 arteriole and peripheral nerve
EM#30 continuous capillary

CD-ROM Notice: The images examined in this chapter are listed numerically on the CD-ROM by microscope slide number as they might be listed in a standard histology laboratory. Note that some microscope slides are listed more than once because there is more than one tissue section with that number and both versions are used for illustration. To avoid confusion resulting from selecting the wrong nested series of images, compare the lead–in images with those illustrated in this guide and read the label on the CD-ROM list carefully.

COMMENTS ON TISSUE PREPARATION

The tissue sections illustrated in this exercise reflect the fact that the appearance of a given structure can vary significantly with differences in fixation, sectioning, and staining. To interpret the visual images of these structures, bear in mind how the solid organs and tissues were processed and how those histological techniques influence the images.

The choice of histological stains clearly influences what can be seen in a tissue section. For example, there are three principal elements in the wall of a vessel, each with important functional significance: elastin, reticular fibers, and smooth muscle. Each of these, however, is acidophilic and stains pink with eosin in a standard H&E preparation. To be able to distinguish clearly among these three elements, special histological stains may be used. Elastin, which provides the critical elasticity in the wall of a healthy vessel, is specifically demonstrated with a Verhoeff stain. Mallory's trichrome stain is used to distinguish between smooth muscle and collagen (including reticular) fibers, staining muscle red and collagen blue. A silver stain specifically highlights reticular fibers. Being able to distinguish among these three components is important if you desire to demonstrate unequivocally that genetics, disease, or injury may have compromised one or all of them.

This exercise also illustrates differences in appearance attributable to mode of fixation. It should not be surprising that the appearance of vessels in a tissue section that has been fixed by immersion in a fixative solution differs from that of vessels fixed by the perfusion of a fixative through the body's own vascular system. In the former, muscles in the walls of the arteries are contracted, the arterial lumens are small and the walls particularly thick. The thinner–walled veins in such immersion–fixed material are often collapsed, and are likely to contain blood cells. In contrast, when material is fixed by perfusion, the vessels are cleared of blood and the arteries are typically dilated as a result of the perfusion pressure. In the perfusion–fixed material examined in this exercise, there is less difference between the artery and vein wall thickness with respect to lumen diameter than there is in the immersion–fixed material. In general, tissues fixed by perfusion are better and more evenly preserved than tissue fixed by immersion because the fixative in the former has been delivered directly to the deep tissue before postmortem deterioration can occur.

Finally, this laboratory illustrates differences in the appearance of vessels attributable to tissue section thickness. The spread preparations approach the maximum thickness for light microscope examination. These spreads are whole mounts of loose connective tissue that have been prepared by stretching a piece of unfixed mesentery or fascia onto a microscope slide and subsequently fixing it and selectively staining it. The small vessels in a spread preparation can be viewed as the interconnected tubes they are.

BLOOD VESSELS

As noted, the basic pattern of the entire cardiovascular system is that of a three–layered tube, and that wall pattern is modified according to the function of the part. The tunica media is the layer that exhibits the greatest functionally–related morphological modification.

ELASTIC ARTERIES

Elastic arteries are the first functional and morphological category of vessels arising from the heart. In a sense, these arteries function as an auxiliary pump, preventing the blood pressure from dropping to zero in the diastolic phase of the cardiac cycle. The force of the heart's contraction not only propels blood forward, but also produces an expansion of the highly elastic walls of these vessels, which upon elastic recoil continues the propulsion of the blood forward in circulation. For this reason, elastic arteries are functionally termed conducting arteries.

Slide #54, illustrated below, is a tissue section of an elastic artery stained with the Lee's stain. Elastic material stains lightly against the more darkly staining smooth muscle cells. Three tunics comprise the wall of the elastic artery as with all arteries.

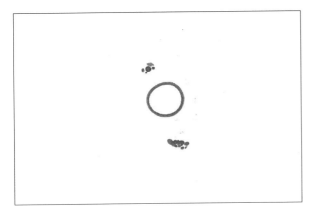

ELASTIC ARTERY
Slide #54: Carotid Artery; Lee's stain; 3 µm methacrylate section; nonhuman primate.

Higher magnification images:
- (medium) wall
- (high) lamellar units

The tunica intima is the innermost of the layers. As part of this layer, elongate endothelial cells line the lumen, arranged with their long axes parallel to the flow of blood. The subendothelial layer of loose connective tissue is relatively thin in this tissue section, and it includes elastic fibers and some smooth muscle cells. This subendothelial layer typically becomes thicker with advancing age. Although relatively unimpressive looking, the tunica intima is clinically important because it is the principal site of the vascular pathology associated with atherosclerosis.

The second of the tunics is the tunica media and it is the thickest layer in the wall of an elastic artery, with many encircling elastic membranes and fibers interspersed among scattered smooth muscle cells and reticular fibers. The elastic membranes have gaps and holes, like slices of Swiss cheese, that permit the unrestricted passage of tissue fluid among the tissues of the wall. The media of the elastic artery is comprised of a series of structural units termed lamellar units. These are composite layers consisting of one elastic lamella and its associated smooth muscle, collagen, and elastic fibers. A large elastic artery may have 50 or more such lamellar units comprising its wall. Aneurisms may occur when the tunica media fails, as when the elastic material is improperly formed or damaged.

The tunica adventitia is often thin, with the collagenous fibers moderately organized into longitudinal spirals. The tunica adventitia typically serves as a casing to restrict excessive expansion of the vessel wall. There is no distinct external elastic membrane.

Elastic material stains black with Verhoeff's stain, and the lamellar units of the wall of the elastic arteries are particularly apparent after staining with Verhoeff's stain. Recognize how section thickness can affect what you see in a tissue section. The gaps that were visible in the elastic lamellae of the previous 2 μm plastic section are not visible in the lamellae of this one because this tissue section is considerably thicker and the small holes are obscured within the section.

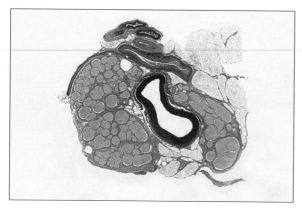

ELASTIC ARTERY
Slide #55: Large Artery; Verhoeff's stain; 12 mm paraffin section; human.

Higher magnification image:
• (medium) wall of elastic artery

This large vessel (Slide #55) is an elastic artery and its tunica media is made up of thick elastic laminae packed with relatively little intervening smooth muscle and reticular fibers. The amount of smooth muscle and reticular fibers in the lamellar units varies according to the location and function of the vessel and its mechanical requirements. Lamellar units in the walls of those vessels that require relatively more elasticity contain more elastic material, fewer reticular fibers and fewer smooth muscle cells.

The elastic artery in this tissue section is accompanied by numerous large nerve fascicles. Nerves and vessels typically travel together in the body. The small longitudinally sectioned vessel in the connective tissue associated with this elastic one is a muscular artery. Its tunica media is principally smooth muscle.

The following pair of tissue sections (Slide #58) were sectioned from the same block of tissue and stained to demonstrate different components of the wall: the section stained with Verhoeff's stain specifically illustrates the elastic lamellae and fibers. It is a thinner tissue section than the previous Verhoeff's stained tissue, so the elastic does not seem so densely packed. Filamentous elastic fibers are visible among the elastic lamellae. The section stained with H&E illustrates the smooth muscle cells that are loosely dispersed in the extracellular matrix of the wall. In contrast, smooth muscle cells in the tunica media of muscular arteries (to be viewed subsequently) are very closely packed together. It should be noted that the smooth muscle cells are responsible for synthesizing all of the elastin, collagen, and nonfibrillar extracellular matrix in the media of the vessel; there are no fibroblasts or reticular cells in the media.

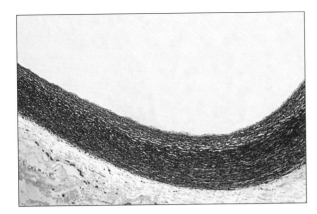

AORTA
Slide #58: Aorta; Verhoeff's stain; 3 μm plastic section; human.

Higher magnification image:
 • (medium) wall

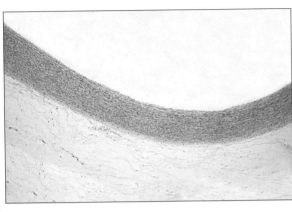

AORTA
Slide #58: Aorta; H&E stain; 3 μm methacrylate section; nonhuman primate.

Higher magnification image:
 • (medium) wall

MUSCULAR ARTERIES AND MEDIUM VEINS

Most of the named arteries of the body are muscular arteries. As a category, muscular arteries range in size from large ones with many layers of encircling smooth muscle in the media to small ones with as few as three layers of smooth muscle. An artery with fewer than three layers of smooth muscle in the media is typically classified as an arteriole.

Functionally, muscular arteries are categorized as distributing vessels. They are responsible for distributing the blood into regions of the body as it is needed (as to the muscles during physical exercise) and away from regions where the need for blood is reduced (as away from the stomach after a meal has been digested). The wall of the muscular artery is dominated by the tunica media, which is composed largely of encircling smooth muscle cells. Vasoactivity, in the form of vasodilation and vasoconstriction, is principally controlled by the autonomic nervous system. Thus, the nervi vascularis in the wall of the vessel are branches of the autonomic nervous system.

The two tissue section images linked to the image below (Slide #55) are not from this Verhoeff's stained tissue section but they illustrate the gradual transition that occurs

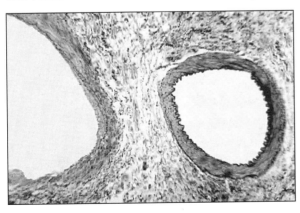

ELASTIC TO MUSCULAR ARTERY
Slide #55: Large Artery; Verhoeff's stain; 12 μm paraffin section; human.

Higher magnification images:
 • (medium) wall of elastic artery
 • (medium) wall of muscular artery

from the elastic to the muscular artery. With increasing distance from the heart, and changing mechanical needs, the amount of elastic material in the tunica media diminishes and the lamellar units contain increased amounts of nonelastic material. In large muscular arteries, elastic lamellae are no longer present within the tunica media. A robust internal elastic lamina (membrane) and poorly developed external elastic laminae border the all–muscle tunica media. As the muscular arteries become smaller in diameter, the external elastic lamina disappears, leaving only the prominent internal elastic lamina in place. The internal elastic lamina is present through to the smallest of arterioles.

Most arteries travel in the body accompanied by one or more veins, although all veins do not travel in the company of arteries. Generally when traveling together, arteries and veins of similar size category accompany each other traveling to and from the heart. Pulsation of the artery helps move the blood in the veins, and vein valves prevent backflow. Veins are functionally categorized as the capacitance vessels of the cardiovascular system. The total volume of the venous compartment is greater than that of the arterial system because of both the greater diameter of the veins, and the greater total length of veins. Typically about 70% of the body's blood is contained at one time within the veins.

The wall structure of muscular arteries and medium veins is illustrated in a series of tissue sections. These sections demonstrate some of the variation in appearance attributable to differences in tissue preservation, mode of fixation, and staining. The description of the walls of these vessels follows the description of the tissue sections.

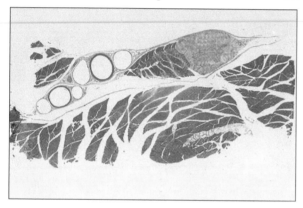

MUSCULAR ARTERY AND MEDIUM VEIN
Slide #52: Neurovascular Bundle; H&E stain; 2 μm methacrylate section; nonhuman primate.

Higher magnification images:
- (medium) wall of artery and vein
- (medium high) artery wall
- (high) vein valve

This tissue section above (Slide #52) illustrates two transversely sectioned muscular arteries (the radial and ulnar arteries) and accompanying venae commitantes (singular: vena commitans, meaning companion vein). The tissue was fixed by the perfusion of fixative through the vessels, causing the lumens to be distended and cleared of blood.

This following tissue (Slide #51) was fixed by immersing the piece of fresh tissue in fixative. There are at least five pairs of muscular arteries and companion veins in this tissue section. Although the pairs of vessels are of different caliber, the walls of the

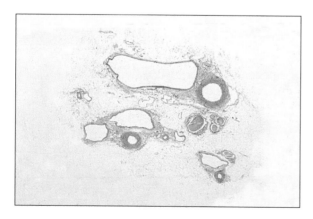

MUSCULAR ARTERY AND MEDIUM VEIN
Slide #51: Muscular Arteries; H&E stain; 12 μm paraffin section; human.

Higher magnification images:
- (medium) wall of muscular artery and vein
- (medium) medium muscular artery and vein

muscular arteries are, in each pair, thicker than those of veins, and the arterial lumens are smaller. The especially thick wall is attributed to the fact that the smooth muscle in the arterial wall contracts when exposed to the fixative, making the lumen smaller and rounder, and the wall thicker than the companion vein's. There are fewer muscle cells in the walls of the veins. As a result, the veins in this form of preparation have large, usually irregular lumens and relatively thin walls. This difference in the thickness of the vessel walls is apparent when you handle fresh arteries and veins.

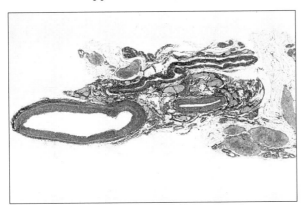

MUSCULAR ARTERY AND MEDIUM VEIN
Slide #53: Artery and Vein; Mallory's trichrome stain; 12 μm paraffin section; human.

Higher magnification images:
• (medium) large artery wall
• (high) small muscular artery

This third tissue section (Slide #53) illustrates vessels fixed by immersion and stained with Mallory's trichrome stain, which stains smooth muscle cells red, reticular fibers and collagen blue and elastic material pink. The reticular fibers are an important stromal component of the vessel wall because they envelop the smooth muscle and translate smooth muscle contraction into vasoconstriction. The stromal tissues in the tunica media and tunica intima are synthesized, secreted, and maintained by the resident smooth muscle cells.

The small Mallory-stained muscular artery illustrated in the second linked image has approximately 5 layers of smooth muscle in its tunica media. This vessel is oriented in such a way that the smooth muscle is cut in both transverse and longitudinal planes of section. Because blood vessels like this one have only a limited ability to stretch linearly, their path through tissue is tortuous and images like this one are not uncommon.

TUNICS. Examine the muscular arteries present in each of these three tissue sections. The three coats (tunics) typical of the walls of all muscular arteries are as follows:

TUNICA INTIMA. This tunic composed of flattened endothelial cells and subendothelial connective tissue is sometimes quite thin, but it increases in thickness with advancing age. A prominent internal elastic lamina separates the intima from the media. The internal elastic lamina is a thick perforated elastic sheet between the intima and the media; it has a pronounced serpentine form when the vessel is contracted, but is smooth when the vessel is dilated.

TUNICA MEDIA. This tunic composed of circumferentially arranged smooth muscle ranges in thickness from that in a large muscular artery, which has 20 to 40 layers, to that in the small muscular artery that has approximately 3 to 20 layers.

TUNICA ADVENTITIA. This tunic is composed of dense connective tissue. The tunica adventitia of a muscular artery may be quite thick, sometimes thicker than the media. It serves as an outer casing for the muscular artery and blends into the surrounding connective tissue, securing the vessel in place. Large muscular arteries have a poorly defined external elastic membrane that is continuous with the fibroelastic inner region of the adventitia, giving it a thick appearance. Small systemic blood vessels, termed the vasa vasorum, penetrate the adventitia of the larger muscular arteries but do not ramify among the muscle fibers of the tunica media.

VEIN WALL TUNICS. The walls of the veins tend to be simpler and more variable than those of arteries. Basically, the tunica intima of veins is often poorly developed; in most large veins the intima may include scattered encircling smooth muscle and indistinct elastic fibers in the subendothelial layer. A netlike internal elastic membrane may be present. The vein's tunica media is weakly developed, with 1 to 12 layers (in small to large veins) of smooth muscle loosely arranged in circular spirals. The thickest part of the vein wall is typically the fibroelastic tunica adventitia. There is no external elastic membrane.

Small and medium veins have valves that insure the unidirectional flow of blood within them. The frequency of the valves along the length of the vein depends on the location of the vein in the body. For example, valves occur more frequently within the veins of the legs than within the veins of the arm. The valves are composed of a pair of semilunar folds of the tunica intima.

ARTERIOLES AND VENULES

Arterioles are the smallest arteries and are typically classified as those vessels with fewer than three layers of smooth muscle in the media. They function as the resistance component of the cardiovascular system. The constriction and tone of the smooth muscle are the principal determiners of blood pressure in the body. The muscles are innervated by sympathetic nerves of the autonomic nervous system.

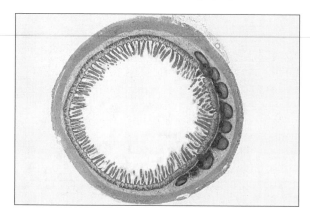

ARTERIOLES, VENULES, AND CAPILLARIES
Slide #120: Ileum; H&E stain; 2 µm methacrylate section; cat.

Higher magnification images:
- (medium) small muscular artery and vein
- (high) arteriole, venule and capillary
- (high) arteriole and venule
- (high) arteriole and lymphatic capillary

This tissue section (Slide#120) is from a perfused preparation so most of the arterioles are cleared of blood. The tunica intima of the arterioles is thin, and the internal elastic membrane is usually distinct. Arterioles have no external elastic membrane, and the fibroelastic tunica adventitia blends into the connective tissue within which they are embedded.

The veins of smallest diameter are venules. Venules are most easily identified when they accompany an arteriole. The wall of the smallest venules often consists of little more than an endothelial cell. These small venules can be distinguished from capillaries based on their lumen size and shape, which is usually greater than 25 µm in diameter and irregular. Generally, the venule's tunica intima consists of the endothelium and its basement membrane with no distinct subendothelial layer or internal elastic membrane. Larger venules may have one to three layers of loosely arranged smooth muscle constituting the tunica media and a tunica adventitia of mostly longitudinal collagen fibers.

Capillaries (to be examined in detail subsequently) are tiny vessels that appear in tissue sections as little more than a simple ring of a diameter approximately equal to that of a red blood cell, less than 10 µm. Frequently, a red blood cell is trapped within the lumen. The nucleus of the endothelial cell might not be included in the section.

Electron Micrograph #14 illustrates a segment of the wall of a small transversely sectioned arteriole and an associated peripheral nerve that is traveling alongside it. The

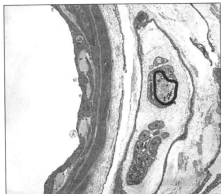

ARTERIOLE
Electron Micrograph #14: Arteriole and Peripheral Nerve; rat.

Higher magnification images:
- intima and media
- peripheral nerve

vessel wall is somewhat constricted and the endothelial cells are individually bunched, rather than buckled into the lumen. Four endothelial cells contribute to this small segment of the lumen and intercellular junctions bind the cells together. These endothelial cells are not small cells, as this section may suggest, but rather in this transversely sectioned vessel the endothelial cells are arranged with their long axes oriented parallel to the flow of blood, which is hydrodynamically superior to an encircling arrangement of endothelial cells. The cytoplasm of the endothelial cells reveals mitochondria and free ribosomes, the standard organelles necessary to support the variety of extremely important metabolic functions attributed to these cells. There are few caveolae in the endothelial cells because transendothelial transport is not a major function of the arteriole. Pockets of amorphous extracellular elastin are located between the endothelial cells and the smooth muscle; the elastin constitutes the internal elastic lamina. Direct intercellular contact between the endothelial cell and the smooth muscle cell of the media provides a means of communication, as when luminal contents influence a vasoactive response. Two layers of smooth muscle cells form the tunica media of this arteriole. The dense filamentous nature of the myocyte cytoplasm and the caveolae of the sarcolemma are characteristic of smooth muscle cells. An attenuated fibroblast process encircles the outer aspect of the vessel as part of its poorly developed adventitia. The adventitia is continuous with the surrounding loose connective tissue. A small peripheral nerve travels with this small vessel. The nerve consists of a myelinated axon and a cluster of unmyelinated axons enclosed by a single cellular layer of perineurium.

This following electron micrograph (#11) illustrates a terminal arteriole whose circumference is incompletely enveloped by a smooth muscle cell. Parts of three endothelial cells line the lumen, suggesting the endothelial cells at this level of the vascular tree are, as in the larger vessels, elongated along the long axis of this vessel. The basal lamina of the endothelial cell and that of the smooth muscle cell fuse and provide structural support for the vessel wall. The endothelial cell is clearly involved in transendothelial transport, as indicated by the presence of numerous caveolae in its cytoplasm. Caveolae are stable vesicles that shuttle across the thin endothelium,

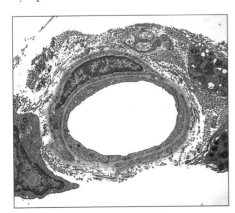

TERMINAL ARTERIOLE
Electron Micrograph #11: Terminal Arteriole; nonhuman primate.

Higher magnification images:
- smooth muscle and nerve
- intercellular junction
- caveolae

opening on the luminal and abluminal surfaces to collect and deliver dissolved material.

Unmyelinated axons like those in the small bundle in this micrograph innervate the smooth muscle of an arteriole wall. The terminal arterioles, like this one, serve primarily to control the flow of blood into the capillary bed and the scattered muscles in their walls are primarily influenced by local metabolic factors.

A pericyte is a cell similar to the smooth muscle cell of this micrograph but the pericyte differs from the smooth muscle cell with respect to both morphology and function. The long axis of the pericyte is oriented parallel to (not perpendicular to, as with the smooth muscle cells) the long axis of the vessel, and small secondary processes may encircle the vessel. Pericytes are multipotential cells that can proliferate and differentiate when stimulated by injury or growth factors. They can give rise to endothelial cells and smooth muscle cells that for

VENA CAVA

Typical large veins, as seen in the previous tissue sections, have a relatively thin tunica intima, a media that is composed of several layers of spirally–arrayed smooth muscle that are separated by collagen fibers, and an adventitia of collagen and elastic fibers that is usually the thickest tunic. The tunica media of veins is thinner and more loosely organized than the media of artery with which it is paired.

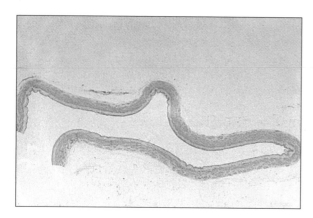

VENA CAVA
Slide #57: Vena Cava; H&E stain; 2 μm methacrylate section; human.

Higher magnification images:
- (medium) vein wall
- (high) vein wall

The vena cava is somewhat unusual in comparison to other large veins because it has longitudinal bundles of smooth muscle in its wall. Other, but not all, large veins in the body (such as the iliac, portal, renal and adrenal veins) also have longitudinal smooth muscle in the wall. In fact, in the renal vein and parts of the inferior vena cava virtually all of the musculature is arranged longitudinally. These named veins have an intima that tends to be thicker than that of standard arteries and veins. In the majority of these special large veins, a media is very thin or absent. However, the two human vena cava tissue sections illustrated here both have only a slightly thickened intima, and a tunica media that is thin and composed of loosely arrayed spiraling smooth muscle. A

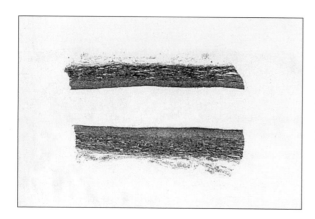

VENA CAVA
Slide #56: Vena Cava; Verhoeff's stain; 12 μm paraffin section; human.

Higher magnification image:
- (medium) vein wall

very thick tunica adventitia makes up the greatest part of the vena cava wall. Of this tunica adventitia, the innermost region is composed principally of collagen fibers (and some elastin), the middle region has bundles of longitudinal smooth muscle and the outer region is composed of collagen and elastic fibers.

TABLE 11.1 MORPHOLOGICAL CHARACTERISTICS OF SYSTEMIC VESSELS AND HEART

ORGAN	FUNCTION	LAYERS:		
		tunica intima	tunica media	tunica adventitia
HEART	*pump*	endocardium (endothelium, thin subendothelial connective tissue, fibroelastic subendocardium)	myocardium (cardiac muscle)	epicardium (visceral pericardium and subepicardial connective tissue)
ELASTIC ARTERY	*conduct*	endothelium, thin to thick subendothelial connective tissue, a few longitudinal smooth muscle fibers	40–60 spiraling fenestrated sheets of elastic laminae alternating with layers of smooth muscle/collagen/ elastic fibers	thin to well-developed, fibrous connective tissue
MUSCULAR ARTERY	*distribute*	internal elastic lamina endothelium, subendothelial connective tissue, some longitudinal smooth muscle	large vessels: external elastic lamina smooth muscle with some elastic fibers	fibroelastic connective tissue
ARTERIOLE	*regulate pressure*	internal elastic lamina endothelium, thin or no subendothelial connective tissue	fewer than 3 layers of smooth muscle	thin, merges with surrounding connective tissue
CAPILLARY	*exchange*	endothelium (occasional pericytes)	none	none
VENULE	*exchange, return*	endothelium, some pericytes	0–3 layers of smooth muscle	very thin, merges with surrounding connective tissue
VEIN	*return*	endothelium, valves, little subendothelial connective tissue,	spiraling smooth muscle, thinner and more loosely organized than artery's media	relatively thick, longitudinal collagen and elastic fibers
VENA CAVA	*return*	endothelium, subendothelial connective tissue	poorly developed or absent, 3–12 loose layers of spiraling smooth muscle	very thick, inner fibroelastic connective tissue, middle longitudinal bundles of smooth muscle, outer fibroelastic connective tissue
HEART	*pump*	endocardium	myocardium	epicardium

THE HEART

The heart is the pump of the circulatory system. It is a four–chambered organ, combining the pumps (ventricles) and receiving chambers (atria) for the closed circuit of pulmonary vessels as well as the closed circuit of systemic vessels into one structure. Blood in the right ventricle of the heart is pumped to the lungs for respiration; the oxygenated blood returns from the lungs to the left atrium of the heart and flows into the left ventricle where it is pumped into the systemic circulation. Deoxygenated blood from the body returns to the right atrium, and flows into the right ventricle where the route repeats. A system of valves in the heart insures the proper direction of flow, and the cardiac conducting cells coordinate the contractions of the cardiac cycle.

Structurally, the heart is a three-layered tube like the rest of the system. The following terms relate specifically to its layers. The combining word root relating to the heart is *cardi-* from the Greek word for heart. The word atrium comes directly from the Latin word (*atrium*) meaning entrance hall, and the Latin word *ventriculus* means a small belly.

epicardium (*epi-*, upon + *cardi-*, heart)
subepicardial layer (*sub-*, beneath)
endocardium (*endo-*, within + *cardi-*, heart)
subendocardial layer (*sub-*, beneath)
myocardium (*myo-*, muscle + *cardi-*, heart)
pericardium, visceral and parietal layers (*peri-*, around + *cardi-*, heart; *viscus*, pl. *viscera*, the internal organs; *paries*, wall)
coronary arteries (*corona*, a crown or garland)

The three layers of the heart are designed similar to the rest of the cardiovascular system: innermost is an endothelium-lined endocardium with a distinct subendocardial layer; a middle muscular layer is the thickest of the three layers; and an outermost layer accommodates the organ's large systemic vessels. As a reflection the difference in the relative forces of contraction produced by the atrium and the ventricle, the myocardium of the former is thinner than that of the latter. This difference is illustrated in the tissue section.

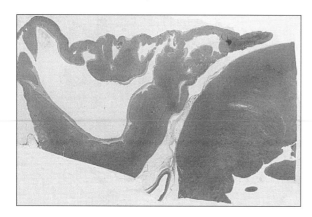

ATRIUM AND VENTRICLE
Slide #63: Heart; hematoxylin & toluidine blue-phloxinate stain; 2 μm methacrylate section; nonhuman primate.

Higher magnification images:
- (high) endocardium
- (medium) myocardium
- (medium) epicardium
- (high) epicardium

The heart resides within the pericardial cavity, which is entirely lined by a serous membrane termed the pericardium. This serous membrane is reflected over the surface of the heart, where it is termed the visceral pericardium. That portion of the serous membrane that lines the inner wall of the pericardial cavity is termed the parietal pericardium. These two serosal surfaces are normally separated by a thin film of fluid that allows the heart to beat with minimal friction.

The endocardium of the heart consists of a lining endothelium and a layer of loose subendothelial connective tissue. Smooth muscle fibers are scattered within this underlying connective tissue among the fibroblasts. A thick layer of subendocardial fibroelastic connective tissue binds the endocardium to the connective tissue that surrounds the cardiac muscle fibers in the wall of the heart. In the ventricle, the Purkinje fibers travel in the subendocardial layer.

The middle layer is the myocardium and it is composed of very well-vascularized cardiac muscle. The cardiac muscle cells are aggregated into well-organized sheets and bundles, although the arrangement of such is more visible macroscopically than microscopically. In the light microscope tissue section, the cardiac muscle cells are assembled in large, intricately intermingled bundles.

The epicardium is the external coat of the heart. It is the visceral pericardium and consists of a mesothelium and an underlying thin fibroelastic layer. The epicardium overlies a layer of variable thickness termed the subepicardial areolar connective tissue. The subendocardial layer becomes quite thick in areas where large coronary vessels travel within it. In obese individuals excess fat accumulates in this layer and puts added strain on the heart.

SYSTEMIC AND LYMPHATIC CAPILLARIES

Capillaries are functionally classified as exchange vessels given that they represent the site in the cardiovascular system where oxygen, carbon dioxide, metabolites, and other substrates pass between the tissues and the blood. The morphology of the capillary walls reflects the relative amount, control, and rate of exchange that occurs across them. Relevant terminology includes the following:

caveolae (*cavum*, a hole + *-ola*, diminutive, meaning small)
fascia occludens (*fascia-*, a band; *occludens*, closing up)
fenestration (*fenestra*, window)
capillary bed
pericyte (*peri-*, around + *-cyte*, cell)

CAPILLARIES

Examine these areolar tissue spread preparations to view the capillary bed. These are pieces of loose connective tissue that have been teased apart, so the blood vessels are seen as anastomosing systems of tubes. The large bubbles associated with the vessels are unilocular fat cells. Using the red blood cells as a unit of measure, observe that the diameter of capillary lumen is no greater than that of a red blood cell, whereas the diameter of a postcapillary venule lumen is equivalent to two or more erythrocyte diameters. During preparation of this tissue, the arterioles constrict, forcing the blood into the postcapillary venules. The density of a capillary bed varies with the tissue: tissues with high metabolic requirements (e.g., cardiac muscle) have an extensive, dense capillary bed, whereas those with low metabolic activity (e.g., tendon) have fewer capillaries.

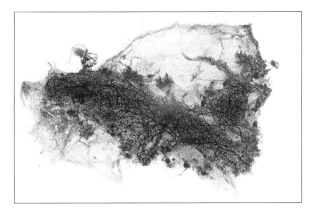

CAPILLARY BED
Slide #9: Areolar Tissue; spread preparation; Sudan IV; rat.

Higher magnification image:
• (medium) capillary bed

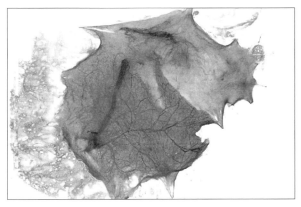

CAPILLARIES AND ARTERIOLE
Slide #7: Areolar Tissue; spread preparation; azure II; rat.

Higher magnification images:
• (medium) vascular bed
•(high) arteriole

In these tissue sections arterioles are recognized by a picket fence-like arrangement of the two sets of cell nuclei that comprise their walls. Since the cytoplasm of the cells is not stained, nuclei of the endothelial cells are not obscured by the encircling smooth muscle. The long axes of the endothelial cell nuclei are oriented parallel to the long axis of the vessel, whereas the nuclei of the smooth muscle cells are oriented perpendicular to the long axis of the vessel.

FENESTRATED CAPILLARY. This type of capillary exist where the volume of exchange across the wall of a capillary is greater than that permitted by continuous capillaries. This class of capillary is also called visceral capillary because this type is located in the mucosa of the alimentary canal, in exocrine and endocrine glands, in the medulla of the thymus and, as here, the kidney.

The name of this capillary is derived from the presence of small pores, about 60 nm in diameter, in the endothelium termed fenestrations. Fenestrations usually appear clustered together in patches in the wall of the capillary; the amount of the wall that bears such pores varies with the location of the capillary and amount of exchange occurring across the wall. The glomerular capillaries of the kidney represent a site where a substantial volume of exchange occurs, and the entire circumference of the glomerular capillary is fenestrated. In most vessels, the fenestration is bridged by a thin, complex diaphragm of nonmembranous material that controls the passage of material across the opening. The glomerular capillaries are unusual in that no diaphragms bridge their fenestrations.

Other examples of fenestrated capillaries are illustrated in Electron Micrographs #9 and #19.

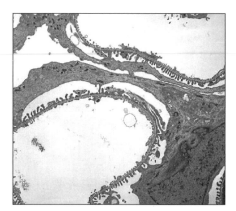

FENESTRATED CAPILLARY
Electron Micrograph #24: Glomerular Capillary; rat kidney.

Higher magnification images:
  • fenestrations
  • basal laminae

CONTINUOUS CAPILLARY. Capillaries of this class are located in tissues where exchange across the endothelial wall is more restricted than it is in the fenestrated capillaries. These capillaries are referred to as somatic (*soma*, body) capillaries because they are located in all the muscle tissues. They are also present in organs where a blood/tissue barrier exists, such as the central nervous system and the cortex of the thymus.

Although small hydrophilic and lipid-soluble molecules can passively diffuse across the wall of the capillary, transport of larger molecules is restricted by the endothelial cell

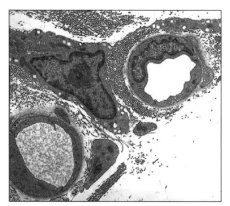

CONTINUOUS CAPILLARY
Electron Micrograph #30: Continuous Capillary; rat.

Higher magnification image:
  • caveolae

wall. The endothelium of the continuous capillary is dominated by caveolae. Caveolae typically shuttle materials across the wall by both receptor–mediated and nonspecific means. In thin regions of the endothelium two caveolae may fuse, creating a patent channel across the wall. The endothelial intercellular junction is a tight junction, termed a fascia occludens. These tight junctions are usually leaky, not perfectly tight or occluding.

Physiologists have postulated the existence of pores of two sizes in the capillary walls: small pores with a diameter of 9–11 nm and larger pores with a diameter of 50–70 nm. The intercellular junction is believed to be the morphological counterpart of the small pore and the fenestrations and caveolae are believed to be the morphological counterpart of the large pore system.

Under normal circumstances, white blood cells leave the blood and enter the tissue by crossing the walls of postcapillary venules, passing between the endothelial cells. This means of exit is termed diapedesis (*dia-*, through + *pedesis*, a leaping). Under unusual conditions, such as the inflammatory process, pharmacologically active substances like histamine and bradykinin can loosen the tight junctions of capillaries and increase vascular permeability, thereby allowing cells and increased volumes of fluid to escape into the tissue.

DISCONTINUOUS CAPILLARY. The third major category of capillary is the discontinuous type. These capillaries are also called sinusoids because architecturally they are tortuous endothelium–lined, relatively large channels passing through the parenchyma of organs like the liver. The endothelial lining is discontinuous, with gaps between the endothelial cells, and the basal lamina may be absent. Some endothelial cells lining the sinusoid are also fenestrated. Sinusoids are located in organs where the blood plasma comes into direct contact with the parenchymal cells and the blood flows slowly, allowing for maximum interaction between the parenchymal cells and the blood. Sinusoids occur in the liver, as in this electron micrograph, and in endocrine organs such as the anterior pituitary and cortex of the adrenal gland.

In light microscope tissue sections it is not possible to distinguish between continuous and fenestrated capillaries, other than reasoning which are which based on their locations. The sinusoids, because of their large size and the fact that they usually form large endothelium–lined channels through tissues rather than tubules, are clearly recognizable in light microscope tissue preparations.

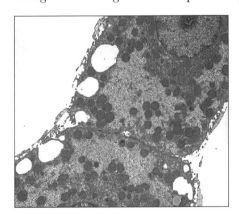

DISCONTINUOUS CAPILLARY
Electron Micrograph #21: Sinusoids; rat liver.

Higher magnification image:
• endothelium

LYMPHATIC VESSELS

Most well-vascularized tissues are well–drained by the lymphatic vessels. Lymphatic capillaries are relatively large diameter vessels with an irregular (often angular) lumen profile and very thin walls that usually appear to be no more than a single thin endothelial cell thick. Sometimes lymphatic capillaries appear to be little more than an endothelium–lined crack in the tissue section. The lumen is typically held open by small extracellular fibers called anchoring filaments, serving much like guy wires holding up a tent. These filaments cannot be visualized in a standard light microscope preparation. Electron microscopy reveals that the contiguous endothelial cells making up the wall overlap but typically do not have intercellular junctions. Because intercellular junctions are usually absent it is possible for large molecules and cells to gain access to the lymphatic system of vessels. When tissue fluid pressure exceeds the pressure within the lymphatic capillary, the interendothelial cell interface is pushed open and material flows unimpeded into the lymphatic vessel. Bicuspid valves are more frequent in lymphatic vessels than in veins, and so are more commonly observed in tissue sections. The larger lymphatic vessels have a thicker wall than the lymphatic capillaries, but the wall is thinner and of looser construction than that of veins of similar caliber. Since the lymphatic vessels are part of a blind–ending system that flows one-way toward the heart, they are typically not cleared by the vascular perfusion of fixatives. As a result, some lymphatic vessels are seen to contain lymphocytes or homogenous, pale eosinophilic lymph. Red blood cells are not normally present within lymphatic vessels.

Table 11.2 Comparison of Capillaries, Sinusoids. and Lymphatic Capillaries

	CONTINUOUS CAPILLARY	FESESTRATED CAPILLARY	DISCONTINUOUS CAPILLARY	LYMPHATIC CAPILLARY
common name	somatic capillary	visceral capillary	sinusoidal capillary	lymphatic
typical location	CNS, lung, striated muscle, many connective tissues	glomerulus of kidney, endocrine glands, most viscera	liver, spleen, bone marrow	most tissues except: brain, bone, cartilage, placenta
endothelial continuity	continuous	continuous	discontinuous	continuous
fenestrations	none (caveolae present)	present in patches, or entire endothelial cell	may be present	only in lacteals
lumen diameter and profile	small (5–12 microns), smooth profile	small (5–12 microns), smooth profile	large (30–50 microns), lines tissue channels	10–50 microns, angular profile
basement membrane	well-developed, continuous	well-developed, continuous	scanty or absent	scanty or absent
intercellular spaces	none	none	present, gaps up to 0.5 microns	usually absent
intercellular junctions	fascia occludens (tight or leaky)	fascia occludens (leaky)	absent, except in spleen	usually absent, cells overlap
pericytes	may be present	may be present	absent (macrophages may be present)	absent

12. LYMPHOID TISSUES AND ORGANS

The purpose of this chapter is to examine the lymphoid organs and tissues in the body and to recognize how they are structurally organized to perform their specific functions. As with most organ systems, the key to understanding the morphology lies in understanding the function. To this end, the lymphoid system is a series of tissues and organs established to protect the body against potentially harmful invading macromolecules. Protection is largely accomplished by cellular (cytotoxic) and humoral (antibody) defense mechanisms that together constitute the immune response. Both of these mechanisms of response involve the production of large clones of cells that include cells that carry out the immediate immune response (effector cells), and cells that are retained in the body in readiness for subsequent exposures (memory cells). A functionally key feature of the immune system — a feature that cannot be seen in tissue sections and therefore may be overlooked in the examination of static tissue sections — is circulation: lymphocytes move freely throughout the body, scouting and patrolling, and optimizing their chances of encountering the macromolecule to which they are preprogrammed to respond. Lymphocytes use the cardiovascular system and the system of lymphatic vessels for transport around the body. Lymphocytes are the only cells that typically leave and re-enter these vascular transport systems.

The lymphoid organs and the tissues may be categorized in one of two basic classes: those that produce immunocompetent cells by random proliferation, differentiation, and maturation in the absence of antigenic stimulation (the primary or central organs) and those that produce immunocompetent cells in response to antigenic stimulation (the secondary or peripheral organs). Below is a diagrammatic overview of the functional relationships among the components of the lymphoid system examined in this chapter.

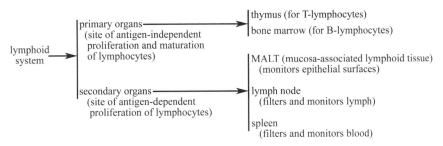

There is a hierarchy in the levels of morphological organization among the organs and tissues of the lymphoid system. The circulating lymphocytes in peripheral blood represent the simplest level of morphological organization. The second level of complexity is represented by the diffuse aggregations of lymphocytes that populate the lamina propria, dermis, and tissue surrounding ducts of glands. The third level of morphological organization is represented by the organized aggregations of lymphocytes and lymphoid follicles in the lamina propria principally of the digestive, respiratory, and urinary systems. Several of these organized aggregations are so predictably present in the body, they are named. At the highest level of morphological complexity are the organs, which are highly organized, encapsulated, and named structures. The latter category includes the lymph nodes and thymus.

The key parenchymal cells of the lymphoid system are the lymphocytes and a class of special antigen–presenting cells. There are two basic functional categories of lymphocytes: B-lymphocytes are involved in the humoral immune response, and T-lymphocytes are involved in cell-mediated immunity as well as various regulatory functions. There are additional classes of lymphocytes, but for the purpose of this exercise, which is concerned with morphology of the tissues, details of immunology are left to comprehensive texts. Antigen–presenting cells are a broad class of cells that includes some macrophages, Langerhans cells of the skin and several mucous membranes, and follicular dendritic cells. The following names refer to specific lymphocytes and other cells of the immune system, each with its own function and location. The word root peculiar to this system is the Latin word *lympha*, meaning clear spring water, reflecting the transparent, slightly opalescent watery nature of lymph.

> lymphocyte; B-lymphocyte, T-lymphocyte (*lympha*, spring water + *-cyte*, cell; B and T refer to the respective sites of precursor proliferation and maturation)
> thymocyte (*thymos*, thymus gland)
> epithelioreticular cell (epithelium + *reticulum*, a small net)
> intraepithelial lymphocyte (*intra-*, within + epithelium)
> antigen-presenting cell (APC)
> M-cell (M stands for microfold, an apical surface feature of this cell)

The following functionally important structures are common to more than one of the lymphoid organs or tissues illustrated in this exercise. A cortex (*cortex*, bark), medulla (*medulla*, marrow), and *hilum* (hilum, a small pit) characterize many other organs of the body in addition to these lymphoid organs.

> lymphoid nodules or lymphoid follicles (*nodulus*, a small knot; *folliculus*, a small sac)
> germinal center (*germen*, a sprout or bud)
> high endothelial venules (HEV)

REFERENCE DIAGRAM FOR SLIDE LOCATIONS

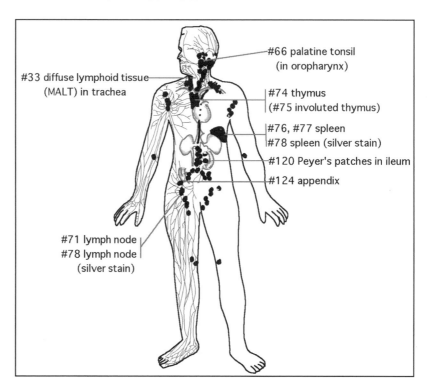

#66 palatine tonsil (in oropharynx)

#33 diffuse lymphoid tissue (MALT) in trachea

#74 thymus (#75 involuted thymus)

#76, #77 spleen
#78 spleen (silver stain)
#120 Peyer's patches in ileum
#124 appendix

#71 lymph node
#78 lymph node (silver stain)

PRIMARY LYMPHOID ORGAN: THYMUS

The following structures are specific to the functional morphology of the thymus and illustrated in this exercise.

> intralobular trabecula or septum (*intra-*, within + *lobulus*, a small lobe; *trabecula*, a small beam; *saeptum*, a partition)
> Hassall's corpuscles (after A. Hassall, a 19th century British physician)
> cytoreticulum (*cyt-*, cell + *reticulum*, a small net)

The thymus is a primary lymphoid organ, also called a central lymphoid organ. As such, it is a site of antigen–independent proliferation of lymphocytes, specifically T-lymphocytes. Several functional classes of T-lymphocytes differentiate from T-lymphocyte precursors in this organ. Mature immunocompetent lymphocytes with the appropriate "correctness of response" are released into circulation for eventual residence in secondary lymphoid tissues and organs.

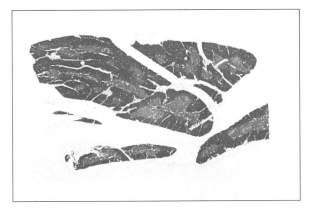

THYMUS
Slide #74: Thymus; hematoxylin & toluidine blue–phloxinate stain; 3 µm methacrylate plastic section; nonhuman primate.

Higher magnification images:
- (medium) medulla and cortex
- (medium high) intralobular septum
- (high) epithelioreticular cells
- (high) cortical vessels
- (high) macrophage and thymocytes
- (high) Hassall's corpuscle

The thymus is a bilobed organ that is of greatest size in the early years of life, i.e., before puberty. The lobes of the thymus are subdivided into lobules. Each lobule has a cortex of densely packed cells capping a less densely packed medulla. The pale-staining medulla is continuous between the lobules. A thin capsule of connective tissue envelops the lobules and thin intralobular trabeculae (or septa) of connective tissue penetrate the cortex, bringing blood vessels to the corticomedullary junction.

Thymocytes (maturing T-cells) comprise the parenchyma of the young thymus. Progenitor lymphocytes enter the thymus by crossing the walls of capillaries at the corticomedullary junction; they migrate to the outer cortex where they begin to proliferate. In the thymus cortex, mitotic figures reflect the thymocyte proliferation, whereas dark pyknotic nuclei are evidence of thymocyte death and subsequent fragmentation. The cortex is the site of a process of random proliferation and differentiation by which the successful thymocytes are those with the ability to recognize foreign antigens and the body's own cells. Approximately 95% of the thymocytes produced by this random differentiation do not have this combined ability and are destroyed. In the medulla, the thymocytes are mature and larger; they will leave the thymus via fenestrated capillaries.

The thymus is unique among all the lymphoid organs in that its stroma is a cytoreticulum of stellate–shaped epithelioreticular cells. These stromal cells are derived embryologically from epithelial cells in the developing oral cavity. The cytoplasmic processes of the epithelioreticular cells are attached to each other with desmosomes and this cellular network serves as a spongelike scaffolding within which the thymocytes develop. Several additional functional classes of epithelioreticular cells are present in the thymus. Some are distributed through the cortex and medulla and serve a variety of metabolically supportive roles. In addition, epithelioreticular cells provide barrier protection for the developing thymocytes, maintaining a special microenvironment in which they develop. The blood–thymus barrier is formed in part by epithelioreticular cells that envelop the continuous capillaries within the cortex and epithelioreticular cells that form a continuous layer underlying the capsule of the thymus. Morphologically, the various epithelioreticular cells are recognized by their large pale nuclei and relatively voluminous cytoplasm, two features that set them apart from the small, packed thymocytes with their heterochromatic nuclei. Hassall's corpuscles are structures derived from epithelioreticular cells and are unique to the thymus. They are small layered spheres of epithelioid cells that are restricted to the medulla. Some of the clustered cells of Hassall's corpuscles become filled with keratohyalin granules and keratin filaments, reflecting the stromal cells' embryologic origins from epithelial tissue. No reticular fibers contribute to the stroma of the thymus. Macrophages in the thymus can be identified on the basis of phagolysosomes present in their cytoplasm.

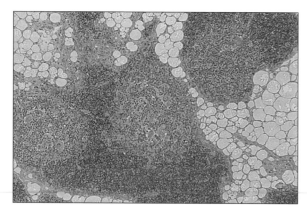

INVOLUTED THYMUS
Slide #75: Involuted Thymus; H&E stain; 3 μm plastic section; nonhuman primate.

Higher magnification image:
- (medium) medulla and cortex

By the time of puberty, the thymus has reached its greatest size; thereafter it regresses and both the stroma and the parenchyma progressively become replaced by fat cells and fibrous tissue. Contrast the involuted thymus of an adult with the previous tissue section. Note the extensive replacement of the thymocytes and epithelioreticular cells by adipocytes. In cases of severe involution, sometimes the only identifying feature is the presence of Hassall's corpuscles.

SECONDARY LYMPHOID TISSUES AND ORGANS

This group, sometimes termed peripheral lymphoid organs and tissues, includes those organs and tissues in the body populated by the fully differentiated immunocompetent T-cells and B-cells. The mature lymphocytes can undergo antigen–dependent proliferation after encountering the antigenic epitope it is specifically programmed to recognize. This lymphocyte proliferation, unlike that which occurs in the thymus, produces clones of effector and memory cells.

MUCOSA ASSOCIATED LYMPHOID TISSUE

DIFFUSE LYMPHOID TISSUE. Diffuse lymphoid tissue is the least organized of the lymphoid tissues: it is an unencapsulated concentration of lymphocytes in a connective tissue. One such concentrated infiltration of lymphocytes is illustrated in the lamina propria of the trachea. Of those lymphocytes, some traverse the overlying epithelium and enter the lumen where they can encounter and disable potentially dangerous infective agents before these agents can enter the tissues of the body. Lymphocytes observed within the epithelium are termed intraepithelial lymphocytes. In the event the epithelial barrier is breached, the lymphocytes and antigen–presenting cells mount an aggressive defense.

Lymphoid tissue located in the lamina propria of a mucous membrane is referred to with the general acronym MALT (mucosa–associated lymphoid tissue). This diffuse tissue represents an enormous total mass of lymphoid tissue in the body. The more specific acronym GALT (gut–associated lymphoid tissue) refers to the accumulations located specifically in the gut and BALT (bronchial–associated lymphoid tissue) refers to the accumulations located in the trachea and bronchi. Diffuse accumulations of

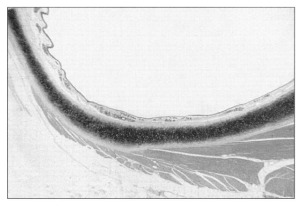

DIFFUSE LYMPHOID TISSUE
Slide #33: Trachea; eosin and toluidine blue stain; 3 μm plastic section; nonhuman primate.

Higher magnification images:
- (medium) MALT
- (medium high) MALT
- (high) MALT and intraepithelial lymphocytes

lymphocytes in these locations often occur around the ducts and secretory units of glands and add antibodies to the secretions. SALT (skin–associated lymphoid tissue) is located in the papillary layer of the dermis underlying the epidermis. Technically, SALT is not a category of MALT, since the skin is not a mucosa.

ORGANIZED LYMPHOID TISSUE. The organized forms of mucosa–associated lymphoid tissue share several common features: (*1*) They are associated with an epithelium. (*2*) They contain proliferating T-cells in interfollicular lymphoid tissue and proliferating B-cells in germinal centers. (*3*) They have efferent but no afferent lymphatic capillaries. (*4*) They contain special high endothelial venules for the directed homing of systemic lymphocytes to the tissue. (*5*) They do not have a distinct connective tissue capsule.The following structures are specific to the functional morphology of organized mucosa–associated lymphoid tissue and are illustrated in this exercise.

> reticulated epithelium (*reticulum*, a small net)
> tonsillar crypts (*tonsilla*, a stake; *crypta*, hidden)
> Peyer's patches (after J. Peyer, a 17th century Swiss anatomist)

Lymphoid nodules (or follicles) are dense aggregations of lymphoid tissue arranged in spherical masses, consisting primarily of B-lymphocytes. They are commonly embedded in diffuse internodular lymphoid tissue, comprised primarily of T-lymphocytes. The lymphoid nodule has a pale-staining center termed the germinal center; this center contains activated, proliferating, and maturing B-cells surrounded by a darker staining mantle zone (also known as the corona or cortex), consisting mostly of small lymphocytes. The dark periphery often shows a localized crescent-shaped cap at one pole, where memory cells tend to collect. Such nodules with germinal centers have been called secondary nodules, distinct from primary nodules that are spheroid concentrations of lymphocytes that lack germinal centers and are present prenatally and in the absence of antigens.

TONSIL. The palatine tonsils are a pair of organized lymphoid aggregates that, together with the pharyngeal and lingual tonsils, form a defensive ring of lymphoid tissue surrounding the entrance to the pharynx. The tonsillar lymphoid tissue is a constant (unless surgically removed) mucosa–associated lymphoid tissue that is composed of lymphoid nodules and internodular lymphocytes. The tonsils notably increase in volume in response to antigenic stimulation. The three types of tonsils differ morphologically in number (single or paired), epithelial covering, number of crypts or invaginations, and extent of encapsulation.

The palatine tonsil is a dense mass of both diffuse and nodular tissues covered by stratified squamous epithelium on its free side and by connective tissue that serves to attach the tonsil to the lateral wall of the oropharynx. The tonsil has 10–30 simple or branched crypts (deep invaginations of the mucosa) that are often filled with cellular

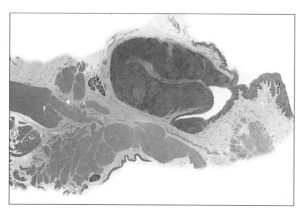

PALATINE TONSIL

Slide #66: Palatine Tonsil; hematoxylin & toluidine blue–phlloxinate stain; 3 µm plastic section; nonhuman primate.

Higher magnification images:
- (medium) nodules
- (high) reticulated epithelium

debris. The lymphoid tissue of the tonsil follows the contours of the invaginated epithelium. Lymphocyte invasion of the epithelium may be extensive, especially in the crypts. Within the overlying epithelium are patches of special modified epithelium termed reticulated epithelium. These are thinned regions of epithelium that lack the typical structure of a stratified squamous epithelium: the basal layer projects toward the free surface and the epithelial cells provide a mesh with wide spaces to accommodate infiltrating lymphocytes (intraepithelial lymphocytes) and macrophages. The basal lamina underlying this special reticulated epithelium is discontinuous to permit the passage of lymphocytes from the lamina propria across the epithelium and into the lumen of the pharynx.

PEYER'S PATCHES. The aggregation of nodules and associated diffuse lymphoid tissue in the wall of the ileum is predictably present in that location and termed Peyer's patches. A patch consists of a cluster of fewer than ten to 100's of closely associated, often confluent lymphoid nodules that typically occupy less than one half of the circumference of the ileum. A young adult may have approximately 200 such patches and the number decreases to approximately 40 with advancing age. The nodules disrupt the muscularis mucosae and invade the submucosa. The luminal portion of the lymphoid tissue is covered with a special epithelium. This epithelium is a simple columnar epithelium, like that lining the rest of the lumen, that is invaded by the lymphocytes (intraepithelial lymphocytes) and contains M-cells that are involved in the immune response. The M-cells are modified epithelial cells that capture and pass antigenic materials from the lumen of the gut to the underlying lymphocytes and antigen–presenting cells. M-cells are present in all simple epithelia that overly mucosa associated lymphoid tissue.

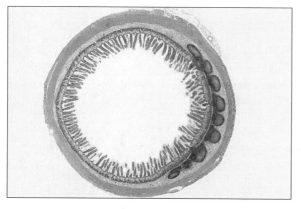

PEYER'S PATCHES

Slide #120: Ileum; H&E stain; 3 µm plastic section; cat.

Higher magnification images:
- (low) Peyer's patch
- (medium) lymphoid nodule
- (high) intraepithelial lymphocytes
- (high) lymphatic capillaries

APPENDIX. The appendix, illustrated in Slide # 128, is a small diverticulum of the alimentary canal that is characterized by the presence of dense lymphoid tissue dominating its walls. The lymphoid tissue occupies the full circumference of this blind

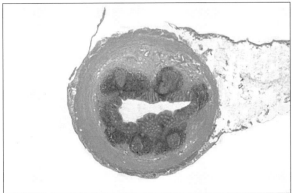

APPENDIX
Slide #124: Appendix; H&E stain; 12 µm paraffin section; human.

Higher magnification image:
 • (low) wall of appendix

tube and it obliterates the muscularis mucosae.

LYMPH NODE

The lymph node exhibits a level of organization surpassing that of the diffuse and organized lymphoid tissues. There are approximately 400 to 500 lymph nodes in the body, most of which are associated with the digestive and respiratory systems. The small bean–shaped lymph nodes are completely encapsulated. The following structures are related to the functional morphology of the lymph node and are illustrated in this part of the chapter.

paracortex of lymph node (*para-*, beside; *nodus*, a knot)
medullary sinus and cords (*sinus*, cavity or channel)
subcapsular (or marginal) sinus (*sub-*, below + *capsula*, a small chest or box; sinus, cavity)
peritrabecular (or intermediate) sinus (*peri-*, around about + *trabecula*, a small beam)
afferent and efferent lymphatic vessel (*affero*, to bring to; *effero*, to bring out)

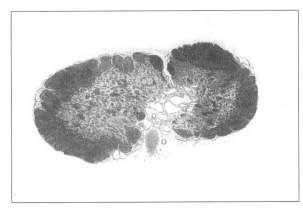

LYMPH NODE
Slide #71: Lymph Node; H&E stain; 3 µm methacrylate plastic section; nonhuman primate.

Higher magnification images:
 • (medium) medulla and cortex
 • (medium) capsule and trabecula
 • (medium) afferent lymphatic vessel
 • (high) germinal center
 • (medium) medullary cords and sinuses
 • (high) high endothelial venule

Lymph nodes are organized with an outer cortex and an inner medulla. The lymph node has a thin dense connective tissue capsule that is continuous with trabeculae that penetrate the cortex and link to the reticular fiber stroma of the lymph node. Subjacent to the capsule, and alongside the trabeculae, are sinuses supported by loose reticular networks into which the lymph flows. These spaces are called the subcapsular (or marginal) sinus and the peritrabecular (or intermediate) sinuses, respectively.

The cortex is composed predominantly of lymphoid nodules, most of which have an obvious pale germinal center and dense outer corona of smaller lymphocytes. Macrophages, some T-helper lymphocytes, and antigen–presenting cells (most are follicle dendritic cells) occur in the germinal center among the more numerous B-lymphocytes. The size and number of lymphoid nodules is directly related to the nature of the immune challenge to the lymph node. Like the tonsils, the swelling of stimulated lymph nodes is clinically remarkable. The deeper region of cortex, located between the nodules and the medulla, is the paracortex, and represents the site of T-lymphocyte concentration in the lymph node.

The medulla is divided into two compartments. Medullary cords are solid extensions of lymphoid tissue, predominantly B-cells, and medullary sinuses are the open channels coursing among the cords. Plasma cells are especially abundant in the cords; they reside in the reticular tissue and release antibodies into the percolating lymph fluid. Endothelial cells form the incomplete wall of the sinusoid.

Lymph nodes function as in–line filters for lymph: the internal sinusoidal system filters lymph and the resident cells can mount an immune response to lymph–borne alien material. Lymphatic vessels, called afferent lymphatics, approach the organ along its convex surface, penetrate the capsule, and deliver lymph to the subcapsular and peritrabecular sinuses. Lymph percolates through the cortex and paracortex toward the medulla. Efferent lymphatics arise from the medullary sinuses and carry lymph away from the node at the hilum (or hilus). Lymph nodes have a systemic blood supply that is also important to the circulation of lymphocytes: arteries carrying systemic blood enter at the hilum and form capillary beds around the lymphoid nodules and converge as veins that exit at the hilus. Special postcapillary venules, called high endothelial venules (HEV) because of their tall endothelial cells, are located in the paracortex and they are the site for special receptor-mediated egress of lymphocytes from the systemic circulation into the lymphoid tissue and circulation. Thus, the lymphocytes that leave the lymph node via the efferent lymphatic vessels either have entered by the afferent lymphatics, been generated by antigenic stimulation of the resident T-and B-lymphocytes, or have entered the node by crossing the walls of the special high endothelial venules.

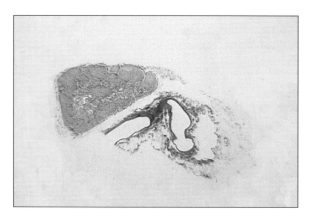

LYMPH NODE: RETICULAR STROMA
Slide #70: Lymph Node; silver stain; 15 µm paraffin section; human.

Higher magnification Images:
 • (medium) cortex and medulla
 • (high) reticular fibers

The silver-stained lymph node tissue section illustrates the reticular stroma. This supporting scaffolding is composed of reticular fibers produced by the fibroblast–like reticular cells in the cortex and medulla of the lymph node.

SPLEEN

The spleen is another encapsulated secondary lymphoid organ that contains both T-and B-lymphocytes. However, unlike other lymphoid organs, it lacks a cortex and medulla. The microscopic organization of the spleen may seem complex, but understanding this organ's dual functions helps to fathom its organization. The spleen has two basic functions, each roughly associated with its two basic components: white pulp and red pulp, named according to their appearance in the fresh spleen. The white pulp is the lymphoid tissue and represents the part where blood is filtered and an immune response to blood–borne antigens can be mounted; the red pulp is like a blood–filled sponge where the blood is cleansed of macromolecular debris and effete blood cells.

The following structures and blood vessels are related to the functional morphology of the spleen and are illustrated in this section of the exercise.

> red pulp
> white pulp
> periarterial lymphatic sheath (*peri-*, round about + artery); acronym: PALS
> marginal zone
> central artery in spleen
> radial arteriole
> penicillar arteriole (*penicillus*, a paint brush)
> trabecular artery
> trabecular vein
> cords of Billroth (after C. Billroth, 19th century Vienna surgeon)

At low power, the two compartments of the spleen are clearly illustrated. About 80% of the spleen is red pulp dominated by red blood cells. A connective tissue capsule covered with a serous membrane (peritoneum) envelops the spleen. Dense connective tissue trabeculae arise from the capsule, penetrating the mass of the organ and carrying trabecular arteries and veins into its interior. Blood vessels traveling within the trabeculae are known by their organ–specific names: they are the trabecular arteries, which are recognized by their muscular coats, and trabecular veins, which are unusual for veins because they lack a distinct tunica media.

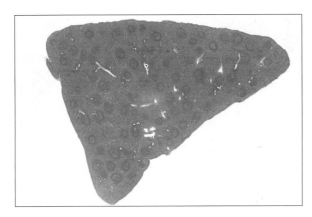

SPLEEN
Slide #77: Spleen; H&E stain; 3 mm plastic section; nonhuman primate.

Higher magnification images:
- (medium high) capsule
- (medium) red and white pulp
- (high) white pulp and marginal zone, radial artery
- (medium) central artery and trabecular vein
- (high) trabecular artery
- (high) penicillar arteries

The white pulp is the lymphoid tissue of the spleen. The trabecular artery carries blood to the white pulp by turning out of the connective tissue trabecula and becoming ensheathed by lymphocytes supported upon a stroma of reticular tissue. These lymphocyte–ensheathed arteries are termed central arteries, even though many are arterioles and they are not necessarily located in the center of the sheath of lymphocytes. The white pulp — the lymphoid tissue — surrounding the central artery has three major functional (and structural) compartments. First of these is the sleeve of lymphoid tissue surrounding the central artery, which is called the periarterial lymphatic sheath (PALS), and it is composed mostly of T-cells. Appended within the PALS is the second compartment: the splenic nodules and these are lymphoid follicles that contain mainly B-lymphocytes. The outermost region of the white pulp represents the third functional compartment: the 100-μm wide zone termed the marginal zone, which is composed of macrophages, antigen–presenting cells, plasma cells, and lymphocytes surrounding small blood sinuses. Some branches of the central artery deliver blood to the marginal zone to initiate the immune response; other branches of the central artery deliver blood to the red pulp compartment where blood is filtered. The former branches of the central artery are the radial arteries, and the latter ones are known as penicillar arterioles and sheathed capillaries.

In this tissue section, the red pulp consists of irregular, anastomosing splenic sinuses surrounded by what appear to be strips of tissue termed Billroth's cords, or splenic cords. In three dimensions, the tissue of the cords is a spongy tissue that actually surrounds the sinusoids. The tissue of the cords consists of a network of reticular fibers and the reticular cells that synthesize the stromal mesh. Macrophages also reside within the reticular tissue of the cords. When blood is delivered into the cords, the blood and its cells and other particulate matter must pass by the macrophages and the fine lattice of reticular fibers and cells in order to gain access to the splenic sinuses and out of the spleen. The sinuses are lined with special elongate endothelial cells that can shrink their width (i.e., become smaller) to widen the spaces between them, facilitating this transmural passage.

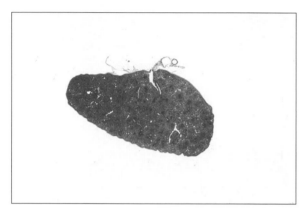

SPLEEN: RED PULP
Slide #76: Spleen; Lee's stain; 3 μm plastic section; nonhuman primate.

Higher magnification image:
• (medium) splenic cords and sinuses

Individual cords and sinuses are usually difficult to discern because of their cellular composition and tortuous architecture. In the red pulp of an unperfused spleen both cords and sinuses are filled with blood cells. The cords and sinuses are better visualized in this tissue section that has been fixed by perfusion, rendering many of the sinuses relatively free of blood cells, and leaving the cords relatively congested with blood cells. In this tissue section the occasional blood cell is seen that has been trapped traversing the wall of the sinus from the cord.

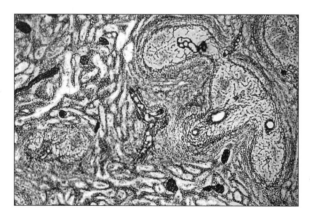

SPLEEN: RETICULAR STROMA
Slide #78: Spleen; silver stain; 12 μm paraffin section; nonhuman primate.

Higher magnification image:
• (medium) splenic sinuses

The splenic cords consist of a reticular stroma continuous with that of the white pulp and loosely formed by the cellular network of reticular cells and numerous macrophages. It is infiltrated by lymphocytes and peripheral blood cells, especially erythrocytes. The reticular stromal framework of the cords and sinuses can best be demonstrated with the silver stain, as illustrated in this tissue section. The series of zebra-like stripes are discrete bundles of reticular fibers that encircle the special fusiform endothelial cells of the sinus wall like hoops of a barrel. The discontinuity of this encircling layer facilitates the passage of blood cells from the cord into the lumen of the splenic sinuses.

SPLENIC CIRCULATION. Understanding the pattern of blood flow in the spleen helps to appreciate its dual functions. The trabecular arteries in the trabeculae give rise to the central arteries of the white pulp. Radial arterioles branch from the central artery and carry blood to the marginal zone where antigenic substances in the blood are brought into contact with the antigen-presenting cells that reside in the marginal zone. An additional set of branches from the central artery occurs within, or just beyond, the margins of the white pulp: these are the penicillar arterioles, a bundle of slender (25 μm) straight vessels that travel a short distance before some acquire a small sheath of macrophages and terminate in the red pulp. These ensheathed capillaries are called sheathed capillaries because of the encircling sheath of macrophages. Sheathed capillaries are not labeled in these tissue sections. Once the blood leaves the white pulp, by either the radial arterioles, the penicillar arterioles, or the sheathed capillaries, it enters either the cords of Billroth or the red pulp sinuses. The blood cells that pass into the cords of Billroth must be able to pass across the wall into the sinuses if they are to leave the spleen. Blood in the sinuses drains into trabecular veins and exits the spleen in the splenic artery. Thus there are two routes of circulation through the spleen: the closed circulation describes the route whereby the blood remains entirely within endothelium-lined vascular spaces, and the open circulation describes the route whereby the blood travels through the cords of Billroth before entering the sinuses. A summary of the alternate routes blood may travel through the spleen is diagrammed below.

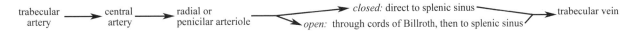

TABLE 12.1 SUMMARY OF STRUCTURAL FEATURES OF THE LYMPHOID ORGANS

	THYMUS	MALT (e.g., Peyer's patches)	TONSIL (e.g., palatine)	LYMPH NODE	SPLEEN
cortex and medulla	yes	no	no	yes	no
lymphoid nodules	no	yes	yes	yes	yes
capsule	yes	no	partial	yes	yes
cords and sinuses	no	no	no	yes	yes
lymphatic vessels	only some efferent	efferent only	efferent only	afferent and efferent	a few efferent only
high endothelial venules (HEV)	no	yes	yes	yes	no
unique characteristics	Hassall's corpuscles	located in wall of ileum	in mucosa of oropharynx	cortical nodules and subcapsular sinus	central arteries and red pulp

13. URINARY SYSTEM

The urinary system consists of the kidneys, urinary bladder, ureters, and urethra. The kidney excretes urine that is stored or carried, but not further modified, by the other urinary structures. The kidneys are impressively designed to do what they do: basically, they filter the blood and maintain the body's general fluid homeostasis. Urine is the net result of finely balanced processes of filtration, resorption, and secretion.

This chapter examines the parts of the fundamental functional unit of the kidney — the nephron — and the intimate structural and functional relationship these parts have with the microvasculature of the kidney. The task of understanding the microscopic structure of the kidney may, at first, appear daunting. However, in the case of the kidney, more than any other organ, the successful mastery of the microscopic structure is facilitated by applying three very basic principles of histology: (*1*) the inseparability of structure and function, (*2*) the significance of location, and (*3*) the relationship between numerical frequency in section and three—dimensional size. Knowledge of the architecture, structure, and ultrastructure of the nephron and its physical relationship with its blood supply will facilitate understanding how the kidney performs its vital role in the body. The intent of this chapter is to provide the morphological setting for the physiological processes carried out in the kidney, the details of which can be obtained from a comprehensive textbook of histology or physiology.

The following structures refer to specific anatomic regions of the kidney and its outflow tubes. Like many other organs, the kidney has a capsule, a cortex (*cortex*, bark), a medulla (*medulla*, marrow) and a hilum (*hilum*, a small pit). The common word root for structures related to the kidney is the Latin word *ren*, pl. *renes*, which means kidney. Many of the terms relating to the kidney use proper English words, like pyramid, ray, and column that refer to specific morphological characteristics.

> renal, or medullary, pyramid
> renal papilla (*papilla*, a nipple)
> renal column
> medullary ray
> minor calyx, pl. calyces (*calyx*, cup of a flower)
> major calyx (*calyx*, cup of a flower)
> renal pelvis (*pelvis*, a basin)
> ureter (*oureter*, urinary canal)

The following are associated with the nephron. The common word root *nephros* is the Greek word for kidney.

> nephron (*nephros*, kidney)
> renal corpuscle (*corpus*, body + *-ule*, a suffix denoting diminutive)
> glomerulus (*glomus*, a ball of yarn + *-ulus*, a suffix denoting diminutive)
> Bowman's capsule (after Sir W. Bowman, 19th century English ophthalmologist)
> podocyte (*podos*, foot + *-cyte*, cell)
> podocyte pedicels (*pediculus*, diminutive of *pes*, foot)
> filtration slit
> mesangial cell (*mes-*, middle + *angeion*, vessel)
> lacis cell or extraglomerular mesangial cell (*extra-*, outside + glomerulus)
> urinary (Bowman's) space
> proximal convoluted tubule
> distal convoluted tubule
> loop of Henle (after F. Henle, 19th century German histologist, pathologist, and anatomist)

renal interstitium (*inter-*, between + *sisto*, to stand)
thin limb of Henle's loop
thick ascending limb of Henle's loop
thick descending limb of Henle's loop
collecting tubule and duct
papillary duct of Bellini (after L. Bellini, 17th century Italian anatomist and physician)
macula densa (*macula*, spot; *densus*, thick)
juxtaglomerular cell (*juxta-*, near to + glomerulus)
renin-containing granules
juxtaglomerular apparatus

REFERENCE DIAGRAM OF SLIDE LOCATIONS

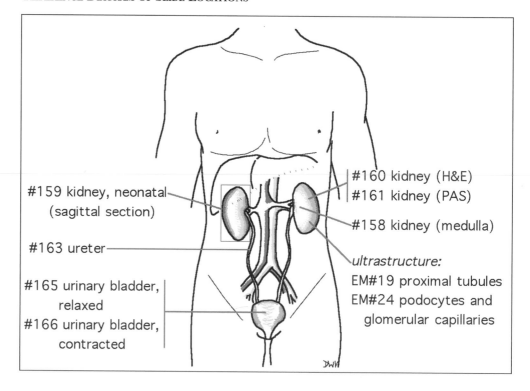

#159 kidney, neonatal (sagittal section)

#163 ureter

#165 urinary bladder, relaxed
#166 urinary bladder, contracted

#160 kidney (H&E)
#161 kidney (PAS)

#158 kidney (medulla)

ultrastructure:
EM#19 proximal tubules
EM#24 podocytes and glomerular capillaries

CD-ROM Notice: The images examined in this chapter are listed numerically on the CD-ROM by microscope slide number as they might be listed in a standard histology laboratory. Observe that some microscope slides are listed more than once because a single tissue section is used to demonstrate more than one feature, such as the parts of the nephron and the blood vessels. The labels and sets of linked images are different for each feature. To avoid confusion resulting from selecting the wrong nested series of images, read the label on the CD-ROM list carefully.

KIDNEY

Examine this sagittal section of the kidney of a neonate for the basic macroscopic morphology of the kidney. Although not fully mature (as reflected by its lobation), this kidney section clearly illustrates the dark staining cortex and paler–staining medulla. The kidney is organized into lobes. Each lobe is composed of a medullary (renal) pyramid that is conical in shape and capped by cortex. The name for the cortical substance that extends between each medullary pyramid is the renal column. The narrow zone of the cortex that parallels the interface with the medulla is known as the juxtamedullary region of cortex. The medulla is subdivided into an outer zone, near the cortical side of the pyramid, and an inner zone, toward the apex. The apex of each medullary pyramid is the renal papilla. In this tissue section a C-shaped deep pink structure caps the renal papilla. This cap of connective tissue is the wall of the minor calyx, the origin of the tubular ureters that convey urine to the urinary bladder. The minor calyx is lined with a thin, transitional epithelium. Two or more minor calyces join together to form a major calyx, and two or three major calyces in turn join to form the renal pelvis. The renal pelvis is the funnel–shaped beginning of the ureter.

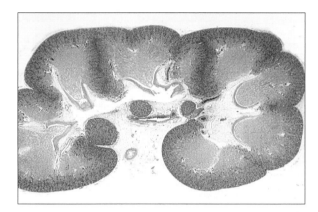

WHOLE KIDNEY: BASIC STRUCTURE
Slide #159: Neonatal Kidney; H&E stain; 10 μm paraffin section; neonatal human.

No higher magnification images

NEPHRON

The kidney is a compound tubular gland, the basic functional unit of which is the nephron. The kidneys function as excretory, regulatory, and endocrine organs, and various regions of the nephron are responsible for those functions. The nephron is an unbranched, tortuous, and tubular structure that originates with the spherical Bowman's capsule in the cortex, loops into the medulla and returns to the cortex where ultimately it empties into a collecting tubule. The collecting tubule drains into a collecting duct that travels radially to the apex of the medullary pyramid where the urine flows into the minor calyx.

Before examining the kidney with its thousands of nephrons all packed together with little intervening interstitial space, it is useful to simplify the fundamental nephron structure with an overview relating the functions of the nephron to the parts in which these functions occur. Each nephron is basically a tube of simple epithelium and it has a predictable convoluted shape that loops from its origin in the cortex into the medulla and then back into the medulla again, before emptying into the collecting duct. The geometric arrangement of the loop into the medulla, accompanied by parallel loops of capillaries, is central to the mechanism of the nephron's function. In the table below, the nephron parts are listed linearly and the paired shaded boxes indicate the typical

direction of filtrate flow	→						
nephron part	**CORPUSCLE**	**PROXIMAL CONVOLUTED TUBULE**	**DESCENDING STRAIGHT THICK LIMB**	**THIN LIMB**	**ASCENDING STRAIGHT THICK LIMB**	**DISTAL CONVOLUTED TUBULE**	**COLLECTING TUBULE AND DUCT**
			LOOP OF HENLE				
function	ultrafiltration	selective resorption		countercurrent exchange and multiplication	selective resorption and secretion		controlled water resorption
capillary bed	glomerulus	peritubular capillary plexus		vasa recta	peritubular capillary plexus		
location in kidney	cortex			medulla	cortex		medulla

location of each part within either the cortex or the medulla of the kidney. The arrow indicates the direction the filtrate flows through the nephron. Below the listed nephron parts, lined up under the appropriate region and location, are the general functions and the capillary network that participates in that function. By relating the microscopic organization of the kidney to these functions, the morphology should become understandable.

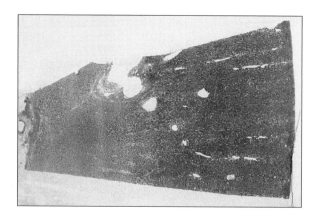

THE NEPHRON

Slide #160: Kidney, radial orientation; H&E stain; 3 μm methacrylate section; nonhuman primate.

Higher magnification images:
- (medium) cortex and medullary ray
- (high) proximal and distal tubules, cortex
- (high) poles of the corpuscle, cortex
- (higher) renal corpuscle, cortex
- (high) juxtaglomerular apparatus, cortex
- (higher) macula densa, cortex
- (high) ascending and descending thick loop of Henle, medulla
- (higher) thin loop and ascending tubule, medulla
- (higher) thin loop and vasa recta, medulla
- (high) collecting duct and ascending tubule, medulla
- (higher) collecting duct and distal tubule, medulla
- (medium) papillary ducts of Ballini, medulla

The cortex and the medulla differ distinctly in appearance. This is partly because certain structures are restricted to only one or the other of these, and partly because of the architecture of the tubules within each. In the cortical region of this tissue section, observe the renal corpuscles. Renal corpuscles occur only in the cortex. The corpuscle has two parts: a vascular tuft of capillaries, termed the glomerulus, surrounded by a double-walled epithelial sac, termed Bowman's capsule. The afferent arteriole enters the corpuscle at its vascular pole and breaks up into the glomerulus of anastomosing fenestrated capillaries. An efferent arteriole, formed from the reuniting capillary loops, exits at that same vascular pole. It is usually not possible to distinguish between the afferent and efferent arterioles in a tissue section although the afferent vessel has special modified smooth muscle cells in its wall (termed juxtaglomerular cells, described below).

Because the nephron tubules intermingle intimately with each other and are frequently convoluted, it is not possible to follow the structural changes within a single nephron in any one plane of section. The parts of the nephron are quite easily distinguished by morphology and location. Light microscope images are illustrated in this radial tissue section (Slide #160), a horizontal section through the kidney medulla (Slide #158), and a PAS-stained radial section (Slide #161). Fine structural images are provided to illustrate how the ultrastructure reflects the function.

BOWMAN'S CAPSULE AND GLOMERULUS. Bowman's capsule is composed of two layers, a parietal and a visceral layer, both of which are simple squamous epithelia. The parietal layer forms a smooth, spherical, external capsule, whereas the inner visceral layer is composed of modified cells termed podocytes. Some podocytes can be distinguished at the periphery of the glomerulus because their large, pale staining cell bodies bulge into the urinary space. A third cell type associated with the renal corpuscle is the mesangial cell. Mesangial cells have pale nuclei and are located within the base of the capillary tuft near the vascular pole.

Podocytes are highly modified cells that form the visceral layer of Bowman's capsule. They provide part of the filtration barrier in the nephron. Each podocyte has several primary processes, which give rise to multiple secondary processes called pedicels. The elongate pedicels of one podocyte interdigitate with pedicels of another podocyte and cover the outside surface of the glomerular capillaries; elongated filtration slits, approximately 25 nm wide, form between the pedicles. To visualize these pedicles and the filtration slits, place your two hands, fingers facing, flat on a table and move them together until your fingers interdigitate. A nonmembranous diaphragm spans the slit between the pedicles. The cytoplasm of the podocytes contains actin microfilaments, giving them the capacity to contract, widening the slits as needed.

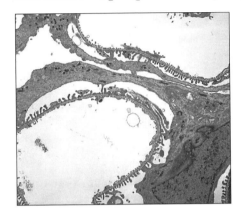

PODOCYTES
Electron Micrograph #24: Podocyte and Glomerular Capillaries; rat kidney.

Higher magnification views:
- glomerular capillary and pedicels
- filtration barrier

The endothelial cells of the glomerular capillaries are fenestrated, and the fenestrations do not have diaphragms as do most fenestrated capillaries. Between these two epithelia, the podocytes and the endothelium, a thick basement membrane forms from the fusion of the laminae densae of the podocyte layer and the endothelium. It thus consists of a central electron–dense layer, an inner lamina rara underlying the endothelium and an outer lamina rara underlying the pedicels. The basal lamina represents the filtration barrier between the blood and the urinary space.

PROXIMAL TUBULE. Return to the previous H&E stained tissue section (Slide #160) and examine the parts of the nephron that follow Bowman's capsule. There is an abrupt change in epithelium at the urinary pole of Bowman's capsule where the proximal tubule begins. The proximal convoluted tubule and the descending straight (thick) portion of Henle's loop are lined with cuboidal cells, which have large, pale, spherical nuclei, eosinophilic cytoplasm, and obscure lateral borders. The luminal surface of these cuboidal cells has a prominent brush border of long microvilli. When well fixed, the basal half of the cells exhibits vertical striations that are attributed to extensive

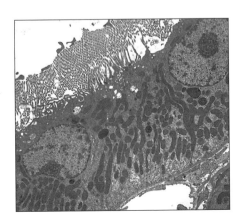

PROXIMAL TUBULE
Electron Micrograph #19: Microvilli and Basal Enfoldings, proximal tubule; kidney of the rat.

Higher magnification views:
- basal enfoldings and interdigitation
- microvilli and apical canaliculi

membrane enfolding. Proximal convoluted tubules occur only in the cortex. The descending thick portion of Henle's loop begins in the cortex and penetrates into only the outermost portion of the outer zone of the medulla. Both of these proximal regions of the nephron are actively involved in selective absorption of material from the lumen.

The epithelium of the proximal convoluted and straight tubule clearly reflects its role in absorption of materials the body retrieves from the fluid that passed into the urinary space. Abundant elongated microvilli on the luminal surface form the brush border that is visible in the light microscope. The apical cytoplasm has numerous canaliculi that open to the lumen between the bases of the microvilli and aid in absorption. Endocytic vesicles and vacuoles arise at the ends of these canaliculi, and pinocytotic vesicles form by invaginations of the apical membranes. The basal portions of these cells have elaborate membrane enfoldings and interdigitate with adjacent cells. The cytoplasm of the proximal tubule cells is dominated by mitochondria that are arrayed parallel to the membrane invaginations. This elaborate plasma membrane and mitochondria density typically characterize cells that function in active absorption activities. The proximal tubules resorb nearly 80% of the water in the ultrafiltrate and nearly all of the protein, amino acids, glucose, bicarbonate, and ascorbic acid.

THIN LIMB OF LOOP OF HENLE. Return to the light microscope images of Slide #160 to follow the next region of the nephron. The length of the thin limb of Henle's loop depends on the location of the nephron: it may be either short and only descend into the medulla or it may be long and recurved. Those nephrons whose corpuscles are in the juxtaglomerular cortex have long loops of Henle with long thin segments that extend into the apex of the medulla, whereas those nephrons whose corpuscles are located in the outer cortex have shorter loops of Henle and short thin segments. The thin portion of the loop occurs only in the medulla. The component cells of the thin segment are squamous, with a pale cytoplasm and nuclei that project slightly into the lumen. At first glance, the loop resembles a capillary, but the loop epithelium has a larger, thicker epithelial wall and more closely spaced nuclei. In this tissue section many of the capillaries have blood cells within them and so are clearly not to be confused with thin segments. The tissue space located among the tubules of the medulla is called the renal interstitium. The tonicity of the interstitium is greater in the apex of the medullary pyramids than it is in the base. This tonicity is fundamental to proper functioning of the nephron.

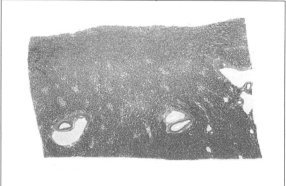

KIDNEY MEDULLA
Slide #158: Kidney Medulla; horizontal section; H&E stain; 3 μm methacrylate section; nonhuman primate.
Higher magnification images:
- (medium) vasa recta with blood
- (high) vasa recta, ducts and tubules
- (high) vasa recta and thin loops of Henle

Slide #158 has been cut in a plane oriented approximately parallel to the corticomedullary interface. The tubules and the capillaries in the medulla are sectioned transversely. This tissue was not fixed by perfusion through the vascular system and so many of the capillaries of the vasa recta and peritubular capillary plexus contain blood cells. As a result these capillaries can be distinguished from the thin-walled portion of the loop of Henle.

DISTAL TUBULE AND JUXTAGLOMERULAR APPARATUS. The next region of the nephron is the distal tubule. In contrast to the proximal tubules and the descending thick limb of Henle's loop, the ascending thick limb of Henle's loop and the distal convoluted tubule lack a brush border, have a slightly wider lumen, and are lined by somewhat smaller, less eosinophilic, cuboidal cells. Hence, in a transverse section, 5–8 nuclei may be present rather than the 3–4 in proximal tubules. For each nephron, the total length of the proximal tubule in the cortex is greater than that of the distal tubule in the cortex, so there are many more profiles of proximal tubules in a tissue section of cortex than there are of distal tubules. The distal tubules are involved in selective resorption and the collection of substances secreted from the blood into the urine.

The ascending thick limb returns to the cortex where it contacts the afferent arteriole at the vascular pole of its own renal corpuscle. At a site in its wall, at the point of contact, there is an elliptical clustering of tall columnar cells with closely packed nuclei termed the macula densa. The macula densa forms one part of a compound structure termed the juxtaglomerular apparatus. This three–part apparatus includes some extraglomerular mesangial cells and the modified smooth muscle cells in the media of the afferent arteriole. Bright pink cytoplasmic renin granules characterize the cytoplasm of the modified smooth muscle cells that are known as juxtaglomerular cells. Beyond the site of the macula densa, the distal tubule becomes convoluted. The macula densa monitors sodium levels and volume of ultrafiltrate in the lumen of the tubule.

COLLECTING TUBULES AND DUCTS. The distal tubule leads into a collecting tubule that flows into the radially oriented collecting ducts. Collecting ducts are assembled in the medullary rays of the cortex and pass into the medulla. The epithelial cells are cuboidal to tall columnar, regularly arranged, and have uniquely distinct cell boundaries; the nuclei are dark staining and basally located. There are two types of cells forming the walls of the collecting ducts: principal cells, the more numerous ones with clear pale cytoplasm and intercalated cells, the less numerous ones with darker cytoplasm attributable largely to an abundance of mitochondria. In the inner zone of the medulla, the successive union of collecting ducts results in the formation of the papillary ducts (of Bellini), many of which are seen to open into the calyx at the tip of the pyramid (renal papilla). Ducts of Bellini are straight ducts approximately 100–200 μm in diameter.

The collecting ducts travel with other straight tubules in a prominent radial structure termed a medullary ray. The medullary ray is a distinct bundle of tubules and collecting ducts that crosses the corticomedullary border from the cortex into the medulla.

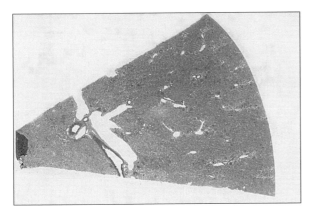

KIDNEY
Slide #161: Kidney, radial section; PAS stain; 3 μm thick methacrylate section; nonhuman primate.

Higher magnification views:
• (medium) ascending and descending tubules
• (high) brush border

The distinction between the proximal tubules, with their brush border accentuated by the PAS stain, and the other tubules of the kidney is clearly shown in this PAS-stained tissue section of kidney.

VASCULATURE

The blood vessels listed below are illustrated in this section. The blood vessels are very regularly organized in the kidney. Two sets are radially arrayed: the larger interlobar vessels, traveling radially between the medullary pyramids, and the smaller interlobular vessels that travel in the cortex, between the lobules. A lobule is defined as a roughly cylindrical region of cortex functionally associated with a medullary ray. Therefore, a medullary ray is in the middle of each lobule, and the interlobular vessels are situated between, and parallel to, the medullary rays. The arcuate arteries and veins follow the arched interface between the cortex and medulla, and connect the interlobar vessels with the interlobular vessels.

The kidney has a portal system of capillaries in the sense that two capillary beds are connected by an arteriole. The first set of capillaries is the glomerular capillaries; these capillaries collect into the efferent arteriole. The efferent arteriole, depending on the location of the corpuscle, gives rise to the second capillary bed, which is either the peritubular capillary plexus or the vasa recta. The glomeruli of the juxtaglomerular nephrons give rise to the vasa recta, the long straight loops of capillaries that descend into the medulla. These vessels participate in the countercurrent exchange process that helps to maintain the osmotic gradient in the interstitium of the medulla. The glomeruli of outer cortical nephrons give rise to the peritubular capillary plexus. This is the capillary bed that surrounds the tubules in the cortex, and collects all the substances the proximal tubules reclaim from the ultrafiltrate.

> interlobar artery and vein (*inter-*, between + *lobos*, lobe)
> arcuate artery and vein (*arcuatus*, bowed)
> interlobular artery and vein (*inter-*, between + *lobulus*, diminutive of *lobos*)
> vasa recta (*vas*, vessel; *rectus*, straight)
> peritubular capillary plexus (*peri-*, around + *tubule*, small tube; *plexus*, a braid)
> afferent arteriole (*affero*, to bring to)
> efferent arteriole (*efferro*, to bring out)

Attempt to trace the arterial supply of the kidney using the following series of tissue sections. The veins and arteries travel together up to the point of branching into the lobules of the cortex.

Interlobar arteries branch off the renal artery and pass upward between pyramids. The location of these large radially oriented interlobular vessels is illustrated in the neonatal kidney slide, illustrated below (Slide #159).

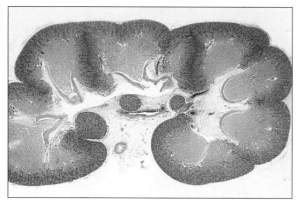

WHOLE KIDNEY: VASCULATURE
Slide #159: Neonatal Kidney; H&E stain; 10 μm paraffin section; neonatal human.

No higher magnification images

At the corticomedullary boundary, each interlobar artery bends horizontally as the arcuate artery. These arteries and their immediate branches send small, predominantly vertical (radial) branches, the interlobular arteries, into the cortex between the medullary rays. Lateral branches of the interlobular arteries, the afferent arterioles, are given off and these terminate in the glomeruli. The glomeruli give rise to the efferent arteriole that flows into the second capillary bed, as described above.

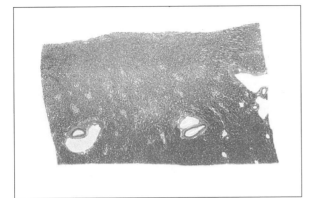

KIDNEY: VASCULATURE
Slide #158: Kidney Medulla; horizontal section; H&E stain; 3 μm methacrylate section; nonhuman primate.

Higher magnification image:
- (medium) arcuate artery and vein

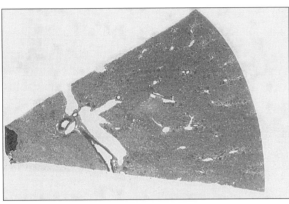

KIDNEY: VASCULATURE
Slide #161: Kidney, radial section; PAS stain; 3 μm methacrylate plastic section; nonhuman primate.

Higher magnification image:
- (medium) arcuate artery and vein

The interlobular artery and vein extend in a radial direction between the corticomedullary junction and the capsule. They travel between the renal lobules, as the name implies. The muscular wall of the artery is easily distinguished from the very thin wall of the interlobular vein. Branches of the radial interlobular artery, the intralobular arteries, are not clearly identified until they become afferent arterioles. At the vascular pole of the glomerulus, the afferent arteriole has a larger lumen than the efferent arteriole does, but unless both are in a section, it is difficult to make this comparison. The wall of the afferent arteriole contains the modified smooth myocytes termed juxtaglomerular cells whose sarcoplasm contains the prominent renin granules.

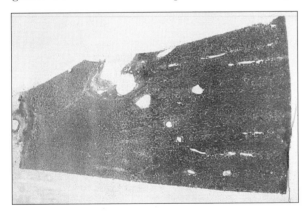

KIDNEY: CORTICAL VASCULATURE
Slide #160: Kidney, radial section; H&E stain, 3 μm methacrylate plastic section; nonhuman primate.

Higher magnification images:
- (medium) interlobular artery and vein
- (high) glomerular and peritubular capillaries
- (high) capsule and stellate veins (location)
- (high) vasa recta

Slide #158, viewed previously to demonstrate parts of the nephron, illustrates the capillaries of the vasa recta. This tissue was not fixed by perfusion through the vascular system and so many of the capillaries of the vasa recta contain blood cells. Thus these capillaries can be distinguished from the thin-walled portion of the loop of Henle. The capillaries of the vasa recta are not uniform in appearance: the descending arterial limbs of the loops (arteriolae rectae) have walls of appreciable thickness while the

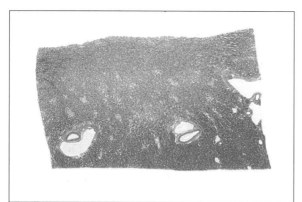

KIDNEY MEDULLA
Slide #158: Kidney Medulla; horizontal section;
H&E stain; 3 μm methacrylate section; nonhuman
primate.
Higher magnification images:
- (medium) vasa recta with blood
- (high) vasa recta, ducts and tubules
- (high) vasa recta and thin loops of Henle

ascending venous limbs (venulae rectae) are much larger, more irregular in outline and
have very thin walls.

The venous drainage of the peritubular capillary plexes in the most superficial
region of cortex includes the stellate veins that lie beneath the capsule. The stellate
veins flow into the radially oriented interlobular veins, which also receive blood from
the peritubular capillary beds of the cortex. Both the interlobular veins and the venulae
rectae (ascending vasa recta) drain into arcuate veins, which ultimately feed into the
interlobar veins coursing alongside the medullary pyramids. The interlobar veins drain
into the renal vein.

URINARY PASSAGES

The minor calyces can be seen in the tissue section of the neonatal kidney (Slide #159).
They are tapered tubes that form a cup surrounding the papilla of a pyramid. The
transitional epithelium of the minor calyx is 2–3 layers thick and continuous with the
epithelium of the papillary ducts of Bellini. Several minor calyces join to become a
major calyx, and two to three major calices form the renal pelvis. The pelvis itself is an
expansion of the beginning of the ureter.

URETER

Examine the transverse tissue section through the ureter noting the irregular pattern of
the contracted lumen. The lumen is lined by transitional epithelium of four to five cell
layers thick. The lamina propria-submucosa is a loose collagenous and elastic layer. A
muscular outer tunic consists of two or three loosely arranged and ill-defined layers of
smooth muscle bundles separated by connective tissue. The inner layer is longitudinally
arranged, the next layer circularly arranged, and the third, outermost coat, longitudinal. The third muscular layer is present only in the lower portion of the ureter.
Because the ureter is retroperitoneal, it has an adventitia.

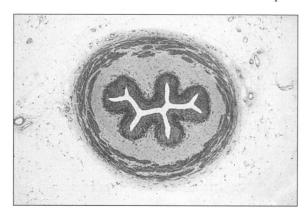

URETER
Slide #163: Ureter, transverse section; Lee's stain: 3
μm methacrylate section; nonhuman primate.

Higher magnification images:
- (medium) ureter wall
- (high) transitional epithelium

URINARY BLADDER

Examine this tissue section of relaxed (contracted) bladder illustrated below and observe that the mucosa is thrown into thick, irregular folds. In its relaxed condition, the transitional epithelium is six to eight cell layers thick. The muscular coat of the urinary bladder is well developed with many interlacing bundles of smooth muscle fibers, poorly demarcated into three layers. The urinary bladder has an adventitia, except for its superior surface, which has a serosa specifically termed a visceral peritoneum.

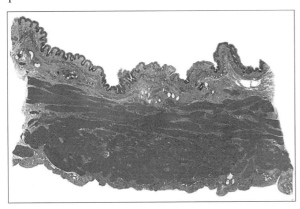

URINARY BLADDER, CONTRACTED
Slide #165: Urinary Bladder, relaxed; hematoxylin & toluidine blue–phloxinate stain; 3 μm methacrylate section; nonhuman primate.

Higher magnification Images:
- (medium) wall of bladder
- (high) transitional epithelium

The following tissue section of the entire thickness of the wall of a distended (stretched) bladder. Observe that the mucosa is comparatively thin and not folded and the transitional epithelium has been stretched to only a few layers. This low-magnification view illustrates the dispersion of the muscle fascicles in the wall of the distended bladder. When the bladder is empty, the decreased circumference of the bladder and the contraction of the myocytes condenses more muscle in the available space.

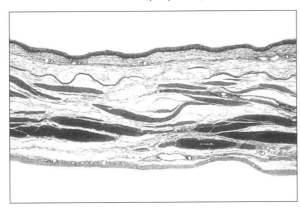

URINARY BLADDER, DISTENDED
Slide #166: Urinary Bladder, distended; Lee's stain; 3 μm methacrylate section; nonhuman primate.

Higher magnification image:
- (medium) epithelium

14. DIGESTIVE SYSTEM: ORAL CAVITY AND TEETH

The oral cavity is the physical and functional beginning of the digestive system, a specialized region where the first stages of the digestive process occur. Several structures associated with the oral cavity have an organizational pattern that is different from the basic pattern of the rest of the system, and so they are examined separately from the other components. Functionally, these structures — the lip, the tongue, the teeth, and the major salivary glands — are integral components of the digestive system.

The lip marks the transition between the outside surface of the body and the digestive system. This chapter introduces the morphological and functional characteristics of the following structures associated with the lip.

> oral mucosa
> vermilion border of lip (*vermilion*, a red pigment made from cinnabar)
> minor salivary glands

The tongue has the following specific morphological features of functional significance that are examined in this exercise.

> lingual papilla (*lingua*, tongue; *papilla*, a nipple)
> filiform papilla (*filum*, thread + *-form*, in the form of; *papilla*, a nipple)
> fungiform papilla (*fungus*, mushroom + *-form*, in the form of; *papilla*, a nipple
> circumvallate papilla (*circum-*, around; *vallum*, wall)
> von Ebner's gland (after V. von Ebner, 19th century Austrian histologist)
> taste bud
> lingual tonsil (*lingua*, tongue)

The major salivary glands associated with the oral cavity include the parotid gland, the submandibular, and the sublingual gland. Two of these are examined in this exercise. All three have the following morphological features that are illustrated in this exercise.

> parotid gland (*para-*, beside + *ot-*, ear)
> submandibular gland (*sub-*, under + *mandible*, the lower jaw)
> serous acinus, pl. acini (serous, relating to a substance, *serum*, whey, with a
>   watery consistency; *acinus*, berry)
> mucous acinus, pl. acini (mucous, relating to mucus; *acinus*, berry)
> serous demilunes (*demi-*, half + *lun*, moon)
> intercalated duct (*intercalatus*, inserted)
> striated duct (*stria*, channel, furrow; *ductus*, to lead)
> excretory duct (*excretus*, separated; *ductus*, to lead)

Teeth are unique structures. Teeth function in the very first stages of digestion, physically breaking apart the food. The complex histological structure of the tooth reveals special adaptation to the mechanical and functional demands placed upon it. The following cells and structures will be examined in this section. The development of the tooth, from its origin as an evagination of oral epithelium, is examined to facilitate the appreciation of how this complex organ evolves from a variety of developmentally interacting tissues. The word roots encountered in this portion of the chapter include the Latin word *dens* meaning tooth and the Greek word *odous* also meaning tooth.

gingiva (*gingiva*, pl. *gingivae*, the gum)

enamel (*enamelum*, enamel of teeth)

odontoblast (*odont-*, tooth + *blastos*, germ)

dentin (*dens*, tooth)

dentinal tubules

cementum (*caementum*, rough quarry stone)

anatomical crown

clinical crown

apex of the tooth (*apex*, summit or tip)

pulp cavity

periodontal ligament (*peri-*, around + *odous*, tooth)

dental lamina (*lamina*, thin plate)

Sharpey's fibers (after 19th century Scottish histologist, W. Sharpey)

inner and outer enamel epithelium

stellate reticulum (*stella*, a star; *reticulum*, a small net)

dental papillae (*dens*, tooth; *papilla*, a nipple)

ameloblast (*amel*, enamel + *blastos*, germ)

REFERENCE DIAGRAM FOR SLIDE LOCATIONS

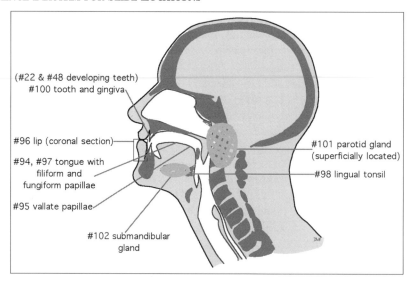

CD-ROM Notice: The images examined in this chapter are listed numerically on the CD-ROM by micro-scope slide number as they might be listed in a standard histology laboratory. Observe that some micro-scope slides — #22 and #100 — are listed more than once because, as in a real laboratory exercise, a single tissue section is used to demonstrate more than one feature. Slide #22 has more than one version, each designated with Roman numerals, and both are used for illustration in this exercise. The appro-priate lead-in images on the CD-ROM are labeled, and have the appropriate links, for the tissue or structure being illustrated. To avoid confusion arising from selecting the wrong nested series of images, read the label on the CD-ROM list carefully.

ORAL CAVITY

The oral cavity is lined by a mucosa specifically termed the oral mucosa. It is morpho-logically modified to withstand both tensile and frictional forces. In various regions of the oral cavity, the stratified squamous epithelium is either nonkeratinized with no stratum corneum, parakeratinized (*para-*, near) with a thin stratum corneum in which the keratinocytes retain their nuclei, or orthokeratinized (*ortho-*, correct) with a thin stratum corneum in which the keratinocytes have lost their nuclei.

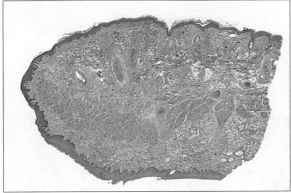

LIP

Slide #96: Lip; H&E stain; 10 µm paraffin section; nonhuman primate.

Higher magnification images:
- (medium) cutaneous portion
- (medium) vermilion border
- (medium) oral mucosa

This tissue section of the lip has been cut in the sagittal plane with respect to the body. To visualize this plane, place your open left hand with your palm facing to the right, against your nose and chin. This plane of section reveals the three parts of the lip: the outer cutaneous portion, the transitional dry red portion known as the vermilion border, and the inner mucous membrane portion. The epithelium becomes increasingly thick along the direction from the outside keratinized skin to the inside nonkeratinized oral mucosa. The vermilion (or transitional) border is thinly keratinized and appears pinkish in life because the underlying dermal papillae are tall and carry blood vessels close to the surface. It also can appear bluish when thermoregulation or poor blood oxygenation cause the red blood cells' normally scarlet oxyhemoglobin to become dark red carbaminohemoglobin. Tall dermal papillae represent a structural adaptation to strengthen the attachment of the epidermis to the underlying connective tissue. The transversely sectioned bundle of skeletal muscle fibers in this tissue section is the orbicularis oris muscle that surrounds the orifice of the oral cavity. Hair follicles and associated sebaceous glands characterize the cutaneous portion, which has all the characteristics of skin. Small mixed seromucous and mucous labial (*labium*, lip) glands lie deep in the mucus portion of the lip and secrete into the vestibule of the mouth. These glands are part of a collection of minor salivary glands that are associated with the oral cavity.

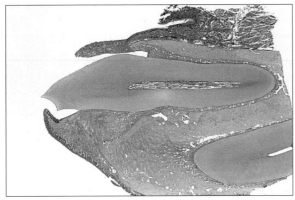

TOOTH: GINGIVA

Slide #100: Tooth; H&E stain; 12 µm paraffin section; nonhuman primate.

No higher magnification images.

The gingiva is the region of oral mucosa that surrounds the alveolar bone into which the teeth insert. Because of the considerable frictional forces to which it is subjected, the gingival epithelium is a parakeratinized or keratinized stratified squamous epithelium. The epithelial rete pegs are unusually long in the gingiva, enabling blood vessels to extend close to the surface and strengthening the connection between the epithelium and lamina propria. The lamina propria of dense irregular connective tissue in this area binds the gingiva firmly to the periosteum. The enamel of this tooth has been dissolved away in this section, leaving an artifactual gap between the surface of the tooth and the gingiva (artifact: *ars*, art + *factus*, to make). The region of epithelium that abuts the enamel of the tooth, termed the junctional epithelium, is a modified thin nonkeratinized epithelium; its superficial cells correspond to the prickle cells of skin and attach firmly with hemidesmosomes to a basal lamina associated with the tooth's enamel and cementum.

TONGUE

The tongue is a large and highly muscular organ that functions in ingestion, taste, and speech. The specific regions of the tongue include the dorsum, divided into an oral and a pharyngeal part, and an inferior surface. Each of these regions has a functionally modified mucosa. The oral part of the dorsum is covered with lingual papillae, which are numerous projections of the mucosa that increase the surface area of the tongue. The pharyngeal part of the dorsum forms the base of the tongue; its mucosa has no lingual papilla but is associated with the lingual tonsils. The inferior surface of the tongue, which is not examined in this exercise, is covered by a smooth, very thin mucosa.

In the low power images of the tongue tissue sections observe the triorthogonal (up–down, right–left, front–back) orientation of the skeletal muscle fiber groups beneath the lamina propria. These muscle fibers provide the notable flexibility of the tongue, and are functionally subdivided into two groups of muscles: the intrinsic muscle fibers that alter the shape of the tongue and the extrinsic fibers that are mostly named muscles that originate outside the tongue and move the whole tongue within the oral cavity.

The mucosa on the dorsal and lateral surfaces of the tongue forms lingual papillae, which are classified into four morphological types. Three of these are examined in the tissue sections; the fourth type, the foliate papillae, is a bilateral series of four or five vertical folds on the lateral aspect of the tongue. The most numerous of the lingual papillae are the filiform papillae. They are pointed, keratinized projections on the dorsum of the tongue. The filiform papillae function to increase the friction between the tongue and food, enabling the tongue to move particles within the oral cavity. The filiform papillae have conical or cylindrical connective tissue cores that may have

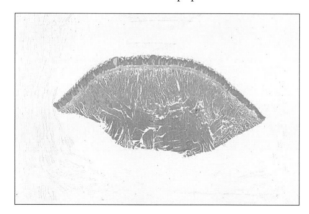

LINGUAL PAPILLAE
Slide #94: Tongue; H&E stain; 10 µm paraffin section; human.

Higher magnification image:
• (medium) fungiform papillae

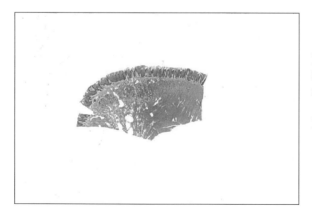

LINGUAL PAPILLAE
Slide #97: Tongue; Lee's stain; 3 µm methacrylate section; nonhuman primate.

Higher magnification images:
• (medium) filiform papillae
• (high) filiform papillae

secondary projections, giving them an irregular profile. Each apex of the connective tissue core generates a fine process of keratinized epithelium. Typically the projecting processes of stratum corneum are not well preserved and are torn away during tissue processing. The second most numerous lingual papillae are the larger mushroom–shaped fungiform papillae. They are scattered among the filiform ones. Taste buds are located on the dorsal surface of the fungiform papillae, which may be lightly keratinized.

The relatively enormous circumvallate (or vallate) papillae are arranged in a V-shaped row at the back of the oral part of the tongue. There are only 8 to 12 of these on the whole tongue. The vallate papillae differ from fungiform papillae in that they are much larger; they are encircled by a distinct sulcus and a slightly elevated wall. Numerous taste buds are located laterally on both walls of the sulcus, but not on the dorsal surface of this papilla. Taste buds are complex multicellular ovoid sensory organs that are located within the epithelium; an aperture called the taste pore opens to the surface of the tongue and provides exposure for the sensory cells of the taste bud. Von Ebner's glands, which are purely serous minor salivary glands in the tongue, empty into the sulcus of the vallate papilla.

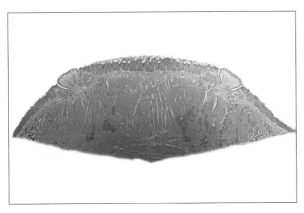

CIRCUMVALLATE PAPILLAE
Slide #95: Tongue; H&E stain; 10 µm paraffin section; nonhuman primate.

Higher magnification images:
- (medium) circumvallate (or vallate) papillae
- (medium high) circumvallate papillae
- (higher) taste bud
- (medium) von Ebner's and minor salivary glands
- (high) von Ebner's serous acini
- (high) mucous acini of minor salivary gland

The tissue section of the pharyngeal tongue illustrates some of the aggregated lymphoid nodules embedded in the submucosa of this pharyngeal region of the tongue. These nodules are some of many in this area that collectively make up the lingual tonsil. Three sets of tonsils form part of a circle of mucosa–associated lymphoid tissue at the back of the oral cavity, in the oropharyngeal cavity. The palatine tonsils, described in Chapter 12 (Lymphoid Tissues and Organs), are located in the wall of the pharynx, lateral to these lingual tonsils. The pharyngeal tonsils are located in the roof of the pharynx. These tonsils are distinguished from each other in tissue sections by the nature of epithelium that overlies the tonsil and lines the crypts: the epithelium is keratinized over the lingual tonsils, nonkeratinized stratified squamous over the palatine tonsil, and pseudostratified ciliated epithelium covers the lymphoid tissue of the pharyngeal tonsil.

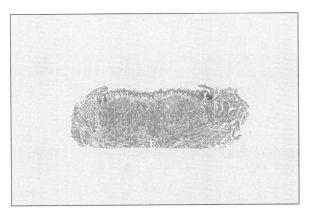

LINGUAL TONSIL
Slide #98: Tongue, Lingual Tonsil; H&E stain; 10 µm paraffin section; nonhuman primate.

Higher magnification image:
- (medium) lingual tonsil

MAJOR SALIVARY GLANDS

The submandibular gland is a compound mixed seromucous gland. Delicate connective tissue septa divide the parenchyma of the gland into lobules. Most of the secretory endpieces on this tissue section are serous acini, although mucous acini are also present. In mixed seromucous acini, serous cells are displaced away from the lumen and form a dark–staining crescent, termed the serous demilune. The serous secretions of these cells pass between the mucous cells to reach the lumen of the duct. Myoepithelial cells aid in the expulsion of the secretions. Small, low cuboidal intercalated ducts lead out of the alveoli. These initial ducts coalesce to form the more columnar columnar striated ducts. Striated ducts are named after the basal striations that are associated with the active transport of ions from the lumen. The striated ducts coalesce to form interlobular ducts, located within the connective tissue septa.

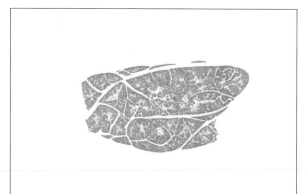

SUBMANDIBULAR GLAND
Slide #102: Submandibular Gland; H&E stain; 3 μm methacrylate section; nonhuman primate.

Higher magnification images:
- (medium) interlobular and intralobular ducts
- (medium) striated and intercalated ducts
- (high) serous demilunes

The parotid gland is also divided into lobules by connective tissue septa. The secretory alveoli are entirely serous in humans. Examine the two forms of intralobular ducts: intercalated ducts with their relatively flattened lining cells, and the larger lumen and more columnar epithelium of the striated ducts. Interlobular ducts are present between the lobes where they form the gland's excretory ducts.

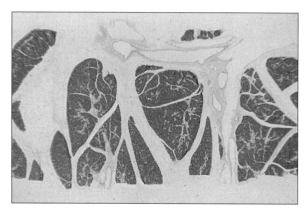

PAROTID GLAND
Slide #101: Parotid Gland; H&E stain; 3 μm methacrylate section; nonhuman primate.

Higher magnification images:
- (medium) ducts and serous acini
- (high) intercalated duct and serous acini
- (high) striated ducts

TEETH

ADULT TOOTH

The mature tooth in this tissue section is suspended in a socket in the alveolar bone. The enamel of the tooth, which normally covers the dentin deep to the gingiva and in the oral cavity, is completely lost during the demineralization process because over 96% of enamel is an inorganic calcium hydroxyapatite. The anatomic root of the tooth is the deep portion of dentin covered with cementum, whereas the anatomic crown is the portion of dentin covered with enamel. The clinical crown refers to the portion of the tooth that extends above the gingiva, the clinically observable portion. The bulk of the tooth is dentin, a tough composite material that is approximately 70% (by weight) inorganic material, a substituted hydroxyapatite. The organic matrix is mostly type I collagen with some glycosaminoglycans. Histologically, dentine has a unique regular pattern of tubules, termed dentinal tubules that are approximately 1.5 µm in diameter and extend with a slightly curved projection from the pulp cavity to the tooth surface. Each tubule contains a single process of the odontoblast, the cell responsible for synthesizing the dentin and whose cell body resides in the pulp cavity of the tooth. The tooth's pulp cavity is a cylindrical core filled with a well–vascularized loose connective tissue that is continuous with the periodontal ligament at the apex (at the root tip) of the tooth. The tooth in this tissue section is not sectioned in a plane oriented parallel to the pulp cavity, and so the full extent of the cavity is not illustrated. The odontoblast cell bodies form a pseudostratified layer upon the dentin surface within the pulp cavity. Cementum is the avascular bonelike material that covers the outer surface of the root. Its resident cells are cementocytes and they reside in lacunae interconnected by canaliculi.

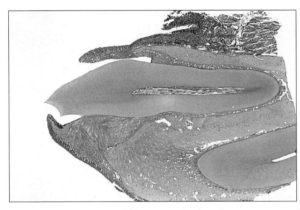

MATURE TOOTH
Slide #100: Tooth; H&E stain; 12 µm paraffin section; nonhuman primate.

Higher magnification images:
- (medium) dentin and periodontal ligament
- (high) periodontal ligament

The periodontal ligament is the dense connective tissue that anchors the tooth into its socket, connecting the cementum to the alveolar bone. It supports the tooth like a sling and provides the tooth with the ability to give under mechanical pressure. Sharpey's fibers are the collagenous attachment bundles that arise from the periodontal ligament and perforate the cementum and the alveolar bone. The small bundles of collagen that insert into the bone are considerably more coarse than the ones that insert into the cementum.

DEVELOPING TOOTH

Sequential stages of tooth development are illustrated in three tissue sections. Development of the tooth involves a series of reciprocal tissue interactions between the fetal oral ectoderm and the mesenchyme of the developing jaw. Basically — in a very simplified overview — cells residing in the mesenchyme underlying the oral ectoderm induce the formation of patches of dental epithelium in the oral ectoderm. The induced dental epithelium invaginates into the underlying primitive connective tissue and induces the underlying mesenchyme to condense into the dental papilla. The dental papilla then induces the epithelium to form the two–layered, bell–shaped enamel organ. The inner layer of the enamel organ, known as the inner enamel epithelium, next induces cells in the dental papilla to differentiate into odontoblasts. And odontoblasts from the mesenchyme induce the formation of ameloblasts from cells in the inner layer of the enamel organ. Enamel and dentin are laid down between the ameloblasts and the odontoblasts, sandwiching the two extracellular mineralizing materials between the two cell layers. The tooth thus is a composite of enamel derived from epithelial cells of the oral cavity, plus dentin and cementum derived from cells in the underlying fetal connective tissue.

The early enamel organ with its internal stellate reticulum and inner and outer enamel epithelium is connected to the oral epithelium by the dental lamina. The enamel organ plus the dental papilla is termed the tooth germ.

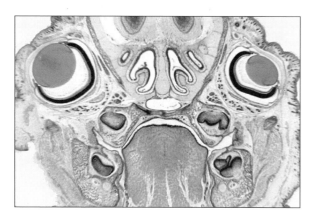

DEVELOPING TEETH
Slide #22: Embryo Head II; H&E stain; 15 μm
paraffin; rat.

Higher magnification images:
- (medium) two developing teeth
- (medium) bell stage, tooth germ
- (high) ameloblasts and odontoblasts

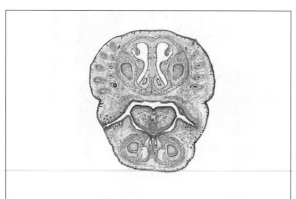

DEVELOPING TOOTH
Slide #22: Embryo Head, III; H&E stain; 15 μm
paraffin; rat.

Higher Magnification Images:
- (medium) developing tooth
- (medium high) tooth germ

In this final tissue section a developing tooth is further advanced than those observed in the fetal head. This tissue section provides a clear chronological link between the structures of the developing tooth and the mature one. In the stage of the development illustrated here, odontoblasts have produced the dentin of the growing root. Mesenchymal cells in the connective tissue surrounding the growing tooth root will differentiate into fibroblasts and cementocytes to generate the peridontal ligament and cementum, respectively. The growing dentin transforms the dental papillae into the pulp cavity of the adult tooth.

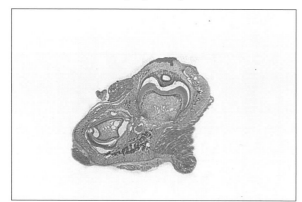

DEVELOPING TEETH
Slide #48: Developing Teeth; H&E stain; 15 μm
paraffin section; rat.

Higher Magnification Images:
- (medium) developing tooth
- (high) dentin and ameloblasts

15. Digestive System: Alimentary Canal

The alimentary canal functions in the digestion, propulsion, and absorption of food necessary to sustain the body. In an adult, this tract is a 22-foot long tube that extends from the esophagus to the anus. There is a basic organizational pattern — mucosa, submucosa, and muscularis externa — of the wall in each of the component organs and divisions. The mucosal architecture and cell populations are modified according to the function of that organ or division. Relating key morphological features to a functional role will make the histological details and differences among each region intuitive. This is a system for which understanding how the component parts function together within the context of the overall system is particularly valuable for making all the details comprehensible and retrievable.

The following diagrammatic overview illustrates relationships based on selected key morphological similarities and differences. The component parts of this system listed on the right side are those examined in this exercise. Each part has a definitive microscopic anatomy.

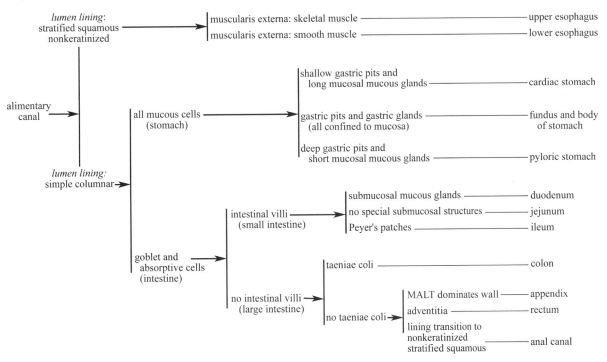

There are several different cell types associated with the mucosal epithelium and glands within the alimentary canal. Each one is morphologically distinct and has a specific function and, understandably, location. For these cells, the word roots or explanations are provided where the name itself is not adequately informative.

surface mucous cell
mucous neck cell
chief, or zymogenic, cell (-*zymo*, denoting enzymes + *genesis*, production)
parietal, or oxyntic, cell (*parieto-*, wall; *oxyno*, to make sour, acid)
stem cell
Paneth cell (after 19th century Austrian physician, J. Paneth)

goblet cell (named for its shape in histological preparations)
enterocyte, or columnar absorptive cell (*enteron*, intestine + *-cyte*, cell)
enteroendocrine cell (EEC) (*enteron*, intestine + endocrine), also APUD cell
   (for amine precursor uptake and decarboxylation)

Several glands are incorporated within the wall of the alimentary canal. Each has a distinct location and function, both of which can be understood within the context of the whole alimentary canal.

cardiac gland (*kardia*, heart)
gastric, or fundic, or oxyntic, gland (*gaster*, stomach; *fundus*, bottom; *oxyntic*, relating to acid)
pyloric gland (*pyloros*, gatekeeper)
Brunner's glands (after 17th century Swiss anatomist, J.C. Brunner)

There are several architectural modifications of the mucosa of the alimentary canal. The mucosa does not simply follow the smooth contours of the outside wall. The following structural modifications are adopted to protect the cells in the stomach or to increase the absorptive surface area of the small intestine.

rugae (*ruga*, a wrinkle)
gastric pit (*gaster*, stomach)
intestinal crypt or pit; crypts of Lieberkühn (after 18th century German anatomist, J. Lieberkühn)
villus, pl. villi (*villus*, shaggy hair)
plicae circulares (*plica*, a fold; *circulares*, circular)

The muscularis externa is modified in several regions of the alimentary tract. For example, in the upper esophagus, which is under voluntary control, the muscularis externa includes skeletal muscle fibers; whereas the lower esophagus is under involuntary control like the rest of the tube and is composed of smooth muscle. The stomach has an additional muscle layer to facilitate the mechanical churning action that is important to the stomach's digestive process. The following are named structural modifications of the external muscle layers of the alimentary canal.

pyloric sphincter (from *sphingein*, to hold tight + *-ter*, suffix denoting agent)
taeniae coli (*taenia*, band, tape; *coli*, of the colon)
internal anal sphincter
external anal sphincter

The origins of some of the component organ names are informative. The word alimentary is derived from the Latin word *alimentim* meaning nourishment. Some names correspond directly to the Greek and Latin words with the same meaning: colon from the Greek *kolon*, and anus from the Latin *anus*. Understanding the other names may assist in recalling the name and something about that part.

esophagus (*oisophagos*, from *oisein*, to carry + *phagema*, food)
duodenum (*duodeni*, twelve, based on the fact that this section of the small intestine is about 12 fingerbreadths [25 cm] in length.)
jejunum (*jejunus*, empty, based on the fact that this region of the intestine is usually found empty at autopsy)
ileum (*eileo*, to twist, referring to the coiled and twisted conformation within the abdominal cavity)
appendix (*appendix*, to hang something on)
rectum (*rectus*, straight, a straight terminal portion of the large intestine)

REFERENCE DIAGRAM FOR SLIDE LOCATIONS

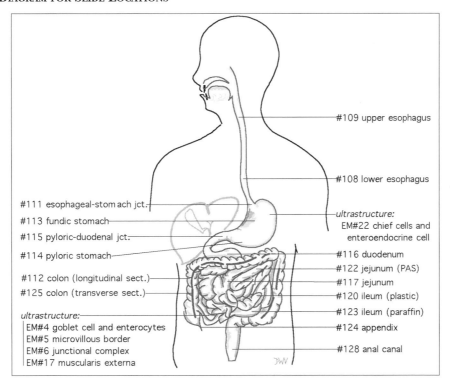

#109 upper esophagus

#108 lower esophagus

#111 esophageal-stomach jct.

#113 fundic stomach

#115 pyloric-duodenal jct.

#114 pyloric stomach

#112 colon (longitudinal sect.)

#125 colon (transverse sect.)

ultrastructure:
EM#22 chief cells and
enteroendocrine cell

ultrastructure:
EM#4 goblet cell and enterocytes
EM#5 microvillous border
EM#6 junctional complex
EM#17 muscularis externa

#116 duodenum
#122 jejunum (PAS)
#117 jejunum
#120 ileum (plastic)
#123 ileum (paraffin)
#124 appendix

#128 anal canal

CD-ROM Notice: The images examined in this chapter are listed numerically on the CD-ROM by micro-scope slide number as they might be listed in a standard histology laboratory. Observe that some micro-scope slides are listed more than once — #116, #120 — because a single tissue section is used to demon-strate more than one feature. The labels and linked images are different for each feature. Some slides have more than one version — #111, #115 — and both versions are used for illustration. To avoid confusion resulting from selecting the wrong nested series of images, read the label on the CD-ROM list carefully, and compare the images with those in this chapter.

ESOPHAGUS

This tissue section cut in the transverse plane illustrates characteristic features of the esophagus. The esophagus is the narrowest part of the alimentary canal (other than the appendix); it is normally constricted, as in this image, with deep longitudinal mucosal folds causing the near obliteration of the lumen. This part of the alimentary canal functions solely as a conduit for food: it promotes neither digestion nor absorption. The stratified squamous epithelium lining the esophagus is relatively thick, so as to withstand the friction of passing food, and this thickness persists when the esophagus distends to allow food to pass. The smooth muscle in the muscularis mucosae has a strictly longitu-dinal orientation unlike other regions of the alimentary tract in which the muscularis mucosae consists of an inner circular and outer longitudinal layer. The muscularis mucosae follows the contours of the lumen, rather than the smooth contours of the encircling muscularis externa. Submucosal mucous (mainly) glands in the submucosa are small and infrequent, and provide mucus for lubrication and a small amount of protection of the luminal surface. The muscularis externa has the usual inner circular and outer longitudinal layers. It is normally in a state of tonic contraction, and during swallowing waves of relaxation allow the bolus of food to pass. The esophagus is enveloped by an adventitia from its origin at the pharynx to the point it traverses the

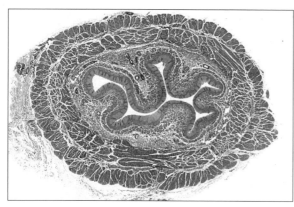

ESOPHAGUS
Slide #108: Esophagus; H&E stain; 10 μm paraffin section; human.

Higher magnification image:
• (medium) wall

diaphragm, and a serosa below the level of the diaphragm.

The second transverse tissue section is from an upper region of the esophagus. It has many of the same features as the previous section of lower esophagus, but there are some differences attributable to its location. For example, the muscularis mucosae is typically absent or present only in scattered bundles at the pharyngeal end of the esophagus. The muscularis mucosae becomes progressively thicker and more complete as the esophagus approaches the stomach, but remains a single layer of longitudinal muscle fibers. Skeletal muscle is present in the muscularis externa of the upper esophagus, and this feature also progressively changes as the esophagus approaches the stomach. The first stage of swallowing is voluntary, and in the upper quarter of the esophagus both layers of the muscularis externa are composed of skeletal muscle; the skeletal muscle is gradually replaced by smooth muscle and the bottom third of the esophagus has only smooth muscle.

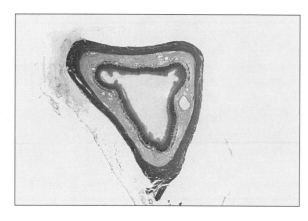

MIDDLE ESOPHAGUS
Slide #109: Esophagus, Lee's stain; 2 μm methacrylate section; nonhuman primate.

Higher magnification images:
• (medium) wall
• (high) muscularis externa

This methacrylate–embedded tissue section has been fixed by perfusion, causing most blood vessels to appear open and cleared of blood. The wall of the esophagus is very well vascularized, especially the lamina propria. Observe the capillary plexus extending into the tall connective tissue papillae that invaginate the base of the luminal epithelium.

ESOPHAGEAL–STOMACH JUNCTION

The esophagus becomes continuous with the stomach at the esophageal orifice. Both of these tissue sections have been prepared in the longitudinal plane to illustrate the histological features of this junction. In the first tissue section, the plane of section is slightly oblique to the long axis of the esophagus, and the section plane passes out of the esophageal lumen at the right side of the image. Making this image additionally challenging to interpret is the presence of one of the longitudinal folds of the esophageal mucosa within the lumen. The fold of the wall is tangentially sectioned, creating an unusual shape of the lumen. Refer to the previous transversely sectioned

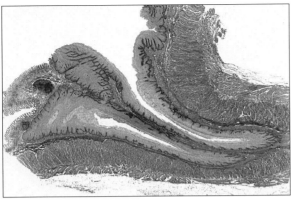

ESOPHAGEAL–STOMACH JUNCTION
Slide #111: Esophageal-Stomach Junction, I; H&E
stain; 15 μm paraffin section; nonhuman primate.

Higher magnification images:
- (medium) wall
- (high) mucosal transition

Slide #108 to help reconstruct the three dimensions that account for this image. The second section illustrates just one side of the wall with clear continuity between the esophagus and the stomach.

The bolus of swallowed food enters the stomach mixed with preliminary digestive enzymes derived from the salivary glands. The stomach is the site of substantial continued digestion facilitated by the addition of hydrochloric acid and a variety of digestive enzymes and the mechanical churning action of the stomach wall. The gastric wall consists of the same layers as elsewhere in the gut: a mucosa, submucosa, muscularis externa, and serosa. Because of the stomach's special function, these layers are modified and their morphology reflects both the digestive functions as well as the protective adaptations to keep the stomach from self–digestion. The stomach has four regions — cardiac, fundic, body, and pyloric — each with some adaptive variation in the cells and basic architecture. The cardiac and the pyloric regions, which are at the proximal and distal ends of this organ respectively, have glands that secrete mucus, whereas the fundic (the large dome-shaped portion of the stomach) and the body of the stomach have glands that secrete hydrochloric acid and digestive enzymes into the gastric pits and lumen of the stomach.

There is an abrupt transition in both the nature and architecture of the epithelium between the esophagus and the stomach. The epithelium of the stomach forms small (0.2 mm diameter), regular, tubular invaginations called gastric pits. The cells lining the entire stomach, including the gastric pits, are termed surface mucous cells and they secrete a thick protective lubricant layer of gastric mucus. The base of each gastric pit receives several tubular glands that are completely confined to the mucosa.

The narrow region of the stomach at the esophageal orifice is termed the cardiac stomach and the mucus–secreting glands that empty into the base of the pits in this region are termed cardiac glands. Cardiac glands are simple or branched tubular glands that have a smaller lumen and less prominent mucus than the pits into which they open. Similar mucus–secreting cardiac glands may occur in the lamina propria of the adjacent lower esophagus, but none are present in these tissue sections.

The second tissue section of the esophagus–stomach junction illustrates how small

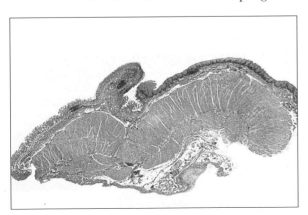

ESOPHAGEAL–STOMACH JUNCTION
Slide #111: Esophageal–Stomach Junction, II; H&E
stain; 15 μm paraffin section; nonhuman primate.

No higher magnification images.

the region of the cardiac stomach is: it is a band approximately 2 cm wide surrounding the esophageal orifice. In this second tissue section, part of the body of the stomach is present. The largest region of the stomach is termed the body of the stomach and its mucosa has relatively shallow gastric pits into which three to four long gastric or fundic glands empty. Details of these gastric glands are provided in the context the next tissue section.

There is no pronounced sphincter at the esophageal orifice, but nervous innervation maintains contraction of these muscles and generally prevents reflux of stomach contents into the esophagus. The muscularis externa in the wall of the esophagus is continuous with that of the stomach, with the addition of a third layer, a layer of oblique smooth muscle fibers on the submucosal (inner) surface of the stomach's muscularis externa. Three separate gastric muscle layers are difficult to distinguish in these tissue sections because of the plane of the cutting section. The action of the gastric muscularis externa facilitates churning and mixing the stomach's contents with secretions from the stomach's glands, producing the semi-fluid mass termed chyme (*chymos*, juice).

STOMACH

At low power three distinct layers of the fundic stomach wall are visible: the mucosa, the submucosa, and the muscularis externa. At higher power the architecture of the mucosa is apparent. Surface mucous cells cover the luminal surface and line the gastric pits. The glands of the stomach are contained within the mucosa and open into the base of the pits.

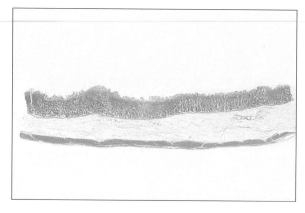

FUNDIC STOMACH
Slide #113: Fundic Stomach, H&E stain; 3 µm methacrylate section; nonhuman primate.

Higher magnification images:
- (medium) wall
- (high) gastric pits and glands
- (higher) oxyntic and parietal cells

FUNDIC AND BODY OF THE STOMACH

The fundic and body of the stomach comprise the bulk of the stomach. The glands that empty into the gastric pits are known as fundic or gastric glands. There are five functionally and morphologically distinct cells in the gastric glands of the fundic and body regions of the stomach: mucous neck cells, parietal (oxyntic) cells, chief (zymogen) cells, enteroendocrine cells, and stem cells. Proceeding from the surface toward the muscularis mucosae, the following cells can be identified. Near the opening of the gastric gland into the base of the pit are the somewhat foamy mucous neck cells that occur singly or in clusters between parietal cells. Next are the eosinophilic parietal cells, which are more frequent in the proximal than distal parts of the gland. Deeper in the gland are the numerous basophilic chief cells. Dispersed among the cells of the gland are the enteroendocrine cells, which can usually be recognized by their broad basal surface. The final cell type, difficult to identify and scattered in the neck of the glands, is the low columnar multipotential stem cell, the cell that can proliferate and differentiate into each of the cell types of the pits and glands.

With regard to the correlation between morphology and function, the oxyntic (parietal) cells produce hydrochloric acid and their pink coloration is because of a very large and complexly invaginated plasma membrane across which the chloride ions are pumped into the lumen of the gland. The zymogenic chief cells are the source of the enzymes pepsin and rennin and gastric lipase; their basophilic cytoplasm reflects their abundant rough endoplasmic reticulum. The mucous neck cells are typical mucus-secreting cells, however their mucus is different from the mucus produced by the surface mucus cells and this accounts for their slightly different morphology. Enteroendocrine cells include a variety of different cells (also known as APUD or diffuse neuroendocrine cells) that individually secrete regulatory agents such as gastrin, somatostatin, serotonin, substance P, and histamine that target relatively local cells..

The lamina propria forms a well-vascularized loose connective tissue stroma among the glands. The muscularis mucosae is relatively thin and sends strands of smooth muscle radially among the glands. Contraction of these fibers may facilitate emptying the glands. The submucosa is a layer of loose connective tissue of variable thickness. The muscularis externa has three layers of smooth muscle, and is covered by the serosa. In this tissue section, the muscularis externa appears unusually thin.

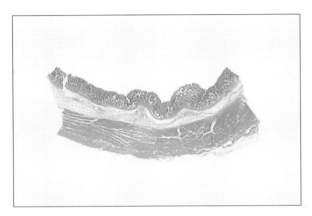

PYLORIC STOMACH
Slide #114: Pyloric Stomach, H&E stain; 3 μm methacrylate section; nonhuman primate.

Higher magnification images:
- (medium) wall
- (high) gastric pits and pyloric glands
- (higher) enteroendocrine and mucous cells

PYLORIC REGION OF THE STOMACH

The pyloric stomach is organized like the rest of the stomach. The mucosa of this tissue section illustrates the rugae, or longitudinal folds that characterize the contracted stomach, especially the pyloric region. Rugae are folds in the submucosa and overlying mucosa and they disappear when the stomach is distended. The pyloric glands are relatively short and they empty into relatively deep gastric pits The pyloric glands do not have chief cells but contain numerous mucus–secreting cells as well as enteroendocrine cells, stem cells and occasional parietal cells. The mucus–secreting cells of the glands have apical collections of mucigen granules.

The enteroendocrine cells in this tissue section have pale cytoplasm, unstained secretion granules, and usually have a broad basal side as a reflection of the direction of their secretion. Enteroendocrine cells are a diverse collection of cells that secrete endocrine or paracrine hormones to influence digestion–related activities of other cells and organs. Some enteroendocrine cells extend to the lumen and thereby can monitor the luminal contents, whereas others are confined entirely to the basal compartment of the epithelium. The granules in these EECs have an affinity for silver stains and so these cells are also collectively termed argentaffin (*argentum*, silver + *affinitas*, affinity) or argyrophilic (*argyros*, silver + -*philos*, liking) cells. The acronym APUD is also used for this collection of cells because many produce a secretion produced as a result of the uptake and decarboxylation of amine precursors.

The following PAS–stained tissue section of the pyloric stomach clearly illustrates the surface mucous cells of the surface and gastric pits and the mucus–secreting cells of the pyloric glands; the mucinogen droplets stain bright magenta. The surface mucous cells produce a thick protective layer of mucus that has been largely washed from the surface of the stomach in this tissue section. Bicarbonate ions are picked up by the surface mucous cells from the lamina propria and subsequently incorporated into this protective mucous layer. The source of the bicarbonate is the oxyntic cells in the gastric glands that produce it as a biproduct of the hydrogen ions generated for the

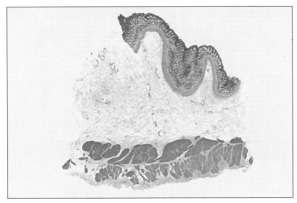

PYLORIC STOMACH
Slide #118: Pyloric Stomach, PAS and lead hematoxylin stain; 3 μm methacrylate section; nonhuman primate.

Higher magnification images:
- (medium) mucosa
- (high) gastric pits and pyloric glands
- (higher) surface mucous cells

hydrochloric acid.

The gastric pits provide a ready supply of fresh cells to replenish damaged cells that directly line the lumen. Following destruction of the surface cells, as from consuming excess alcohol or aspirin, the destroyed surface cells are rapidly replaced by existing surface mucous cells residing within the protected pits. Replacement cells quickly migrate up toward the surface along the intact basal lamina to cover the bare luminal surface. Replacement by cell regeneration takes somewhat longer and is accomplished by the mitotic division of the multipotential stem cells located principally in the neck of the glands.

The mucus–secreting cells within the pyloric glands are largely mucous neck cells and they secrete lysozyme (*lysis*, a dissolution + *zyme*, leaven), a bactericidal enzyme into the lumen.

Observe the gastric pits and pyloric glands in obliquely sectioned regions of the mucosa. It is possible to differentiate between the transversely sectioned pits and glands because of differences in the numerical density of the profiles in the mucosa. Since several branched glands empty into each pit, there are more glands packed into the deep mucosa than there are pits in the superficial half of the mucosa. In oblique section, this translates into a clear difference in the numerical frequency of profiles.

The fine granules of the enteroendocrine cells stain black with the lead hematoxylin stain. The enteroendocrine cells are discussed subsequently in this exercise.

SMALL INTESTINE

PYLORIC–DUODENAL JUNCTION

These following two tissue images are longitudinal sections of the junction between the pyloric stomach and the duodenum. In both of these tissue sections the most striking feature of the low power view is the change in the thickness of the muscularis externa and the hypertrophied inner circular layer of the muscularis externa that forms the pyloric sphincter. The pyloric sphincter controls the volume of chyme that leaves the stomach: the sphincter contracts with each peristaltic wave in the stomach, allowing only

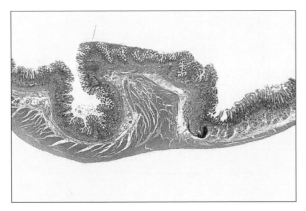

PYLORIC–DUODENAL JUNCTION
Slide #115: Pyloric–Duodenal Junction, I: H&E stain; 3 μm methacrylate section; nonhuman primate.

Higher magnification images:
- (medium) pyloric sphincter
- (medium) mucosa transition
- (medium) duodenum

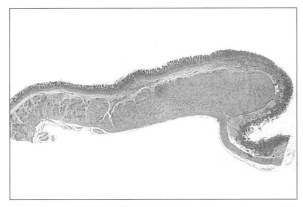

PYLORIC–DUODENAL JUNCTION
Slide #115: Pyloric-Duodenal Junction, II; H&E stain; 3 µm methacrylate section; nonhuman primate.
Higher magnification images:
- (medium) pyloric sphincter
- (medium) duodenum

the fluid and smallest particles to pass, retaining the larger particles for further digestion. In this longitudinal section it is easy to trace the relatively thick muscularis externa of pyloric stomach (three layers) through to the relatively thin muscularis externa of the duodenum (two layers).

At higher magnification, it is particularly instructive to follow the muscularis mucosae from the pyloric region into the duodenum and note its position relative to population of mucus–secreting glands. The stomach's pyloric glands are restricted to the mucosa whereas Brunner's glands of the duodenum occupy the submucosa. Considering the caustic chemical nature of the chyme that is delivered to the small intestine, the presence at this location of a major accessory gland that secretes a protective alkaline mucus is understandable.

Trace the mucosa from pyloric stomach into the duodenum and note the change in both its epithelium and architecture. The histology of the duodenal epithelium reflects one of its principal functions: absorption of nutrients. With regard to the transition in epithelium, it changes from the protective surface mucus cells of the stomach to the columnar absorptive cells (enterocytes) and goblet cells of the small intestine. With respect to architecture, the simple gastric pits of the stomach are replaced by branched invaginating tubular glands called intestinal crypts of Lieberkühn (or intestinal glands). In the duodenum leaf-like evaginations known as intestinal villi project into the lumen from the mucosal surface, increasing the surface area available for absorption.

SMALL INTESTINE: GENERAL HISTOLOGICAL FEATURES

Before illustrating the region–specific characteristics of the three divisions of the small intestine — the duodenum, jejunum, and ileum —some of the general features of the small intestine are demonstrated in several tissue sections These general features include the intestinal villi and plicae circulares, which both occur only in the small intestine, and the crypts of Lieberkühn or intestinal glands that occur in both the large and small intestine. Cells that populate the epithelium are also described in this section.

INTESTINAL VILLI AND CRYPTS. The intestinal villi are evaginations of the epithelium and lamina propria that project into the lumen and provide a nearly 10-fold amplification of the luminal surface area. Fascicles of smooth muscle derived from the muscularis mucosae extend up the core of the villi; these are thought to allow a very mild pumping in and out of the villi. Intestinal villi are not all the same size and shape: they are large and numerous in the duodenum and become smaller and shorter in the ileum; also they change from broad plate-like ridges in the duodenum to narrower finger-like projections in the ileum. These differences can be appreciated by carefully examining the various tissue sections in this exercise.

The crypts of Lieberkühn are branched tubular invaginations of the surface epithelium of the small intestine. These crypts occupy the lamina propria and open into the intestinal lumen around the base of the villi. Because the crypts are tubular structures, not folds, profiles of the crypts often appear as isolated islands of cells within the

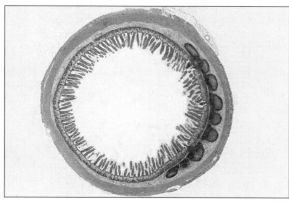

VILLI AND CRYPTS OF LIEBERKÜHN
Slide #120: Ileum, H&E stain; 3 μm methacrylate
section; cat.

Higher magnification images:
- (medium) wall
- (medium) intestinal villi and crypts

lamina propria. Like the gastric pits, they function as a source of replacement epithelial cells. Like the intestinal villi, they tend to be larger and more numerous at the proximal end of the small intestine, becoming shorter and less numerous in the ileum.

Multipotential stem cells are concentrated in a zone in the middle region of the crypts. These stem cells are among the most rapidly proliferating cells in the body. They divide mitotically and differentiate to replace the goblet, absorptive, enteroendocrine, and Paneth cells of the epithelium. Goblet cells and enterocytes migrate up the sides of the villi and are shed from the apex of the villi.

CENTRAL LACTEALS. This tissue section, Slide #117, illustrates special lymphatic vessels, termed the central lacteals, which are located in the lamina propria within the intestinal villi. The lacteals are unusually distended and easy to visualize in this tissue section; more typically they are collapsed and difficult to see. The central lacteal begins as a blind–ending dilated tube near the apex of the villus and drains into a lymphatic plexus in the lamina propria. Lacteals transport to the systemic circulation large lipoprotein droplets called chylomicra (*chylo-*, juice, chyle + *micros*, small) that are generated by the absorptive enterocytes. The loose connective tissue in the core of the intestinal villi also contains loops of fenestrated capillaries. Water, amino acids, ions, and simple sugars that are absorbed from the intestinal contents by the enterocytes and released basally into the lamina propria are carried to the liver by capillaries in this capillary bed.

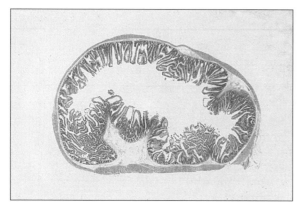

CENTRAL LACTEALS AND MUCOSAL EPITHELIUM
Slide #117: Jejunum, H&E stain; 3 μm methacrylate
section; nonhuman primate.

Higher magnification images:
- (medium) wall
- (medium high) intestinal villi and lacteals
- (high) luminal epithelium

ENTEROCYTES AND GOBLET CELLS. The luminal epithelium illustrated in Slide #117 consists principally of columnar absorptive cells (enterocytes) and goblet cells. The absorptive enterocytes bear hundreds of microvilli on their apical surface where they provide a 20-fold amplification of the absorptive surface area of these cells. These microvilli are collectively visible in the light microscope as the striated border. Because of the junctional complexes between the epithelial cells, the luminal epithelium provides an important selective barrier; materials that pass into the lamina propria must do so by passing through, not between, these cells. The goblet cells are named because the swollen accumulation of mucinogen droplets in their apical cytoplasm gives the cells a goblet shape. The secreted mucus provides protection and lubrication of the luminal surface. Goblet cells become more numerous in the distal direction along the length of the small and large intestine.

PANETH CELLS AND ENTEROENDOCRINE CELLS. Paneth cells are distinct exocrine cells clustered specifically in the base of the intestinal crypts, adjacent to the muscularis mucosae. They are particularly numerous in the duodenum and well illustrated in Slide #116. The apically located large bright eosinophilic granules in the Paneth cells contain lysozyme, an antibacterial agent. Compare the Paneth cells with the goblet cells whose apical mucinogen granules have been largely washed out during this tissue preparation.

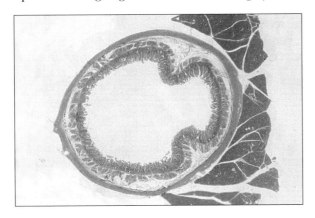

PANETH CELLS AND ENTEROENDOCRINE CELLS
Slide #116: Duodenum, H&E stain; 3 μm methacrylate section; nonhuman primate.

Higher magnification images:
- (medium) base of crypt
- (high) three cell types
- (high) Paneth and enteroendocrine cells

Enteroendocrine cells (EEC) are scattered throughout the columnar epithelium, both in the crypts and, to a smaller extent, along the walls of the villi. In this tissue section, stained with H&E, the EEC also contain eosinophilic cytoplasmic granules, but unlike the apical granules of the Paneth cells, those of the enteroendocrine cells are basally located, slightly finer and of a somewhat different hue. There are several different functional types of enteroendocrine cells distributed in the epithelium of the small intestine where they secrete bioactive amines and peptides into the lamina propria. The standard stains of light microscopy do not distinguish among the various classes of secreted substances. This diverse group of cells goes by several names including diffuse neuroendocrine or APUD cells.

The following tissue section has been stained with PAS and lead hematoxylin, which highlights the preserved PAS–positive mucinogen in the goblet cells and the glycoproteins of the glycocalyx that coats the microvilli. The glycocalyx, composed largely of the glycosylated terminals of membrane proteins, is particularly thick over the surface of the striated border. It serves as a protective coat for the epithelium, resistant to protease digestion. The glycocalyx also holds digestive enzymes so that digestion occurs close to the surface across which the products of digestion are absorbed.

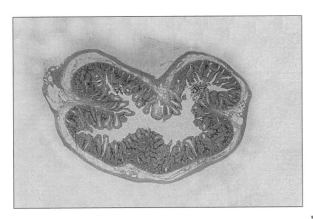

GLYCOCALYX; GOBLET AND ENTEROENDOCRINE CELLS
Slide #122: Jejunum;PAS and lead hematoxylin stain; 3 μm methacrylate plastic section; nonhuman primate.

Higher magnification image:
- (high) three cell types

The enteroendocrine cells are scattered throughout the columnar epithelium of the villi and the crypts. The lead hematoxylin stains their secretion granules black, and so these cells are recognized by the dark staining granules located basally, next to the basement membrane and the underlying lamina propria where their secreted product can pass into fenestrated capillaries.

PLICAE CIRCULARES. Infoldings of the intestinal wall that incorporate both the mucosa and submucosa are termed plicae circulares, or valves of Kerkring. These folds are oriented circumferentially around half or more of the lumen (perpendicular to the long axis of the tube) in the small intestine and provide a 2- to 3-fold amplification of the mucosal surface. Visualize the geometry of these folds by gently scrunching your shirt sleeve into horizontal folds. The plicae are particularly numerous and close together in the duodenum and proximal jejunum, but diminish in frequency to the point of being completely absent in the distal ileum. Unlike rugae, which disappear when the lumen distends, the plicae circulares remain when the lumen of the small intestine distends. These structural modifications of the lining not only amplify the surface area, but also slow the passage of intestinal contents.

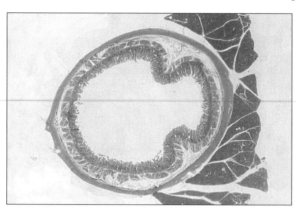

PLICAE CIRCULARES
Slide #116: Duodenum, H&E stain; 3 μm methacrylate section; nonhuman primate.

Higher magnification images:
• (medium) plicae circulares
• (high) Brunner's glands

SMALL INTESTINE: SPECIAL CHARACTERISTICS OF THE DUODENUM, JEJUNUM, ILEUM

DUODENUM. The mucus–secreting Brunner's glands illustrated in Slide #116 are located in the duodenal submucosa. Brunner's glands are diagnostic of the duodenum. The secretions are a bicarbonate–rich fluid that aids in neutralizing the chyme, which arrives in the duodenum from the stomach. The ducts of the branched compound tubuloacinar Brunner's gland open into the base of the crypts in the same way that cardiac, gastric, and pyloric glands opened into the bases of the gastric pits. In the proximal duodenum, Brunner's glands occupy the entire encircling submucosa, but they become smaller and less frequent until they are absent at the duodenal–jejunum junction.

The duodenum has the usual basic histologic features of the small intestine. The intestinal villi are tall, broad, and closely packed and the absorptive enterocytes are the most numerous cell type in the epithelium of the villi. Its histology reflects its role in absorption, although the digestive processes that began in the stomach continue, and are supplemented with the addition of enzymes from the exocrine pancreas.

ILEUM. The aggregation of lymphoid nodules in the wall of the ileum is known as Peyer's patches. Each oval mass or patch consists of a cluster of from five to hundreds of lymphoid follicles. A young adult may have more than 200 such patches, but the number declines to approximately 40 in the mature adult. Peyer's patches are most numerous in the distal ileum.

Peyer's patches represent a predictable location of mucosa–associated lymphoid tissue, specifically GALT. The lymphoid tissue extends from the mucosa deep into the

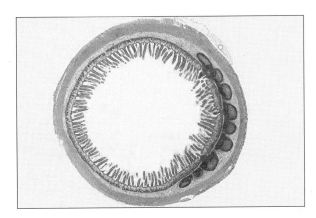

ILEUM: PEYER'S PATCHES
Slide #120: Ileum, I; H&E stain; 3 µm methacrylate section; cat.

Higher magnification images:
- (medium) Peyer's patches
- (high) intraepithelial lymphocytes

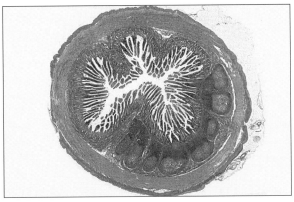

ILEUM
Slide #123: Ileum, II, H&E stain; 15 µm paraffin section; nonhuman primate.

Higher magnification image:
- (medium) lymphoid nodules

submucosa, disrupting the muscularis mucosae. Intraepithelial lymphocytes are present within the epithelium where they have migrated from the underlying lymphoid tissue for release into the ileum lumen. Specialized flattened epithelial cells, called M-cells (for microfold cells) are present in the epithelium overlying the lymphoid tissue. The M-cells transport antigenic material from the lumen to the cells of the underlying lymphoid tissue. M-cells are not identified in these standard tissue sections. Although Peyer's patches are a diagnostic feature of the ileum, the M-cells, intraepithelial lymphocytes and solitary lymphoid follicles and tissue are found dispersed throughout the intestines.

JEJUNUM. The jejunum has the usual structural and cellular features of the small intestine, but has neither Brunner's glands nor Peyer's patches in its submucosa. Its villi are slightly smaller and less numerous than those of the duodenum, although relatively broad and foliate-shaped. Its crypts are slightly shorter and less numerous than those of the duodenum, and in comparison to their numbers in the duodenum, goblet cells are slightly more numerous in the epithelium of the intestinal villi.

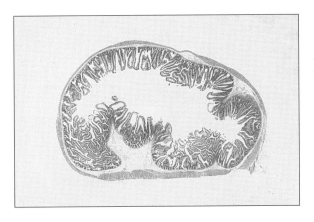

JEJUNUM
Slide #117: Jejunum, H&E stain; 3 µm methacrylate section; nonhuman primate.

Higher magnification images:
- (medium) wall
- (medium high) intestinal villi and lacteals
- (high) luminal epithelium

LARGE INTESTINE

The large intestine is most notably different from the small intestine because of its larger lumen, absence of intestinal villi and plicae circulares, and no Paneth cells. Its regions include the blind-ending caecum (which is histologically similar to the colon), the colon, the rectum, and the anus. The role of this region of the alimentary canal is one of absorption, largely water and ions, compaction of chyme into feces and short-term storage of the feces.

APPENDIX

The appendix is a narrow diverticulum of the large intestine that is located approximately at the junction of the small and large intestine. Its organization is similar to that of the large intestine (no intestinal villi) but it is specifically characterized by the dominant presence of the lymphoid tissue in the lamina propria and the submucosa. In the regions heavily infiltrated with lymphocytes and lymphoid nodules the intestinal crypts are few and the muscularis mucosae is obliterated. The luminal epithelium consists of enterocytes and goblet cells, as well as the antigen-transporting M–cells.

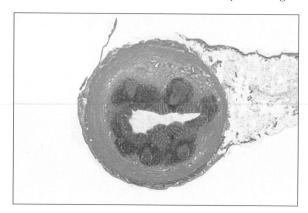

APPENDIX
Slide #124: Appendix, H&E stain; 12 μm paraffin section; human.

Higher magnification image:
* (low) wall

COLON

The layers in the wall of the large intestine resemble those of the small intestine. The surface is smooth to the extent that villi and plicae circulares are absent. Simple tubular crypts of Lieberkühn are longer in length and closer together than in the small intestine. The most numerous cells in the surface epithelium and lining the crypts are the columnar absorptive cells that are largely responsible for ion exchange and water resorption. In addition to the absorptive cells, the mucosal epithelium includes goblet cells that are like those in the small intestine, stem cells located near the bases of the intestinal crypts from where they provide replacement cells, and enteroendocrine cells. M-cells are present in the epithelium overlying solitary lymph nodules in the lamina

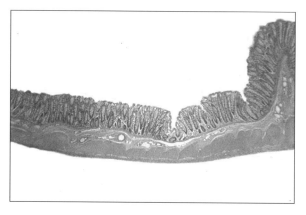

COLON: LONGITUDINAL SECTION
Slide #112: Colon, longitudinal section; H&E stain; 3 μm methacrylate section; nonhuman primate.

Higher magnification images:
* (high) intestinal crypts
* (higher) luminal epithelium

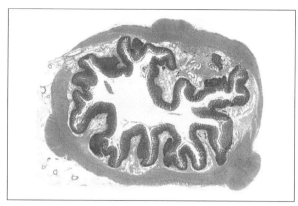

COLON: TRANSVERSE SECTION
Slide #125: Colon, H&E stain; 3 μm methacrylate section; nonhuman primate.

Higher magnification image:
- (medium) taenia coli

propria. The relative proportion of goblet cells increases in the distal direction as the lubricant properties of the mucus become more important.

The transverse tissue section of colon (Slide #125) illustrates the prominent thickenings of the longitudinal muscle in the muscularis externa: the taenia coli. These three evenly spaced longitudinal bands are shorter than the other layers of the colon wall and as a result produce tucks and pouches, or sacculations, along the length of the colon. The longitudinal folds of the mucosa and submucosa flatten when the lumen is distended.

RECTUM AND ANAL CANAL

The rectum is the short dilated terminal portion of the large intestine. The rectum is continuous with the anal canal, which is itself the last 3–4 cm of the gastrointestinal tract. The anal canal encompasses the transition from the mucosa of the alimentary canal to skin. There is an abrupt transition from simple columnar epithelium to a stratified squamous nonkeratinized, then keratinized epithelium. This transition from simple to stratified epithelium occurs at the pectinate line (*pecten*, a comb), which marks the site of the embryonic anal membrane.

The rectum is approximately 12 cm long and differs from the colon by having no taenia coli and no mesentery; the crypts (intestinal glands) are slightly deeper and fewer per unit area, and the goblet cells are even more numerous.

The mucosa of the proximal zone of the anal canal has shorter and fewer crypts and forms six to eight longitudinal ridges called anal folds (or columns of Morgagni). These anal folds terminate in crescent-shaped folds called anal valves that are situated along the pectinate line. Neither the anal columns nor the anal valves are readily identifiable in this longitudinal histological section.

The submucosa contains two plexuses of large veins that often become distended and varicose and may protrude from the anus as hemorrhoids. The internal hemorrhoidal plexus occurs above the pectinate line and the external hemorrhoidal plexus occurs at the junction of the anal canal and the anus. The anus is the external opening of the anal canal.

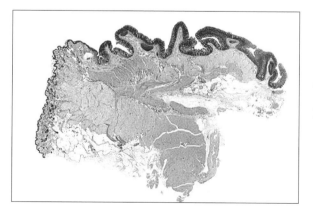

LARGE INTESTINE: RECTUM AND ANAL CANAL
Slide #128: Anal Canal, H&E stain; 12 μm paraffin section; nonhuman primate.

Higher magnification images:
- (medium) mucosa
- (medium) anal junction
- (medium) internal and external anal sphincters

The internal anal sphincter is derived from the circular layer of smooth muscle of the muscularis externa and it encloses the upper 30 mm of the anal canal. The outer longitudinal layer of the muscularis externa becomes a fibromuscular layer that attaches to the body wall. The external anal sphincter is a circumferential tube of skeletal muscle that encircles the entire anal canal external to the muscularis externa.

TABLE 15.1 SUMMARY OF MORPHOLOGICAL FEATURES OF REGIONS OF THE ALIMENTARY CANAL

Organ	ESOPHAGUS		STOMACH			SMALL INTESTINE			LARGE INTESTINE			
Division	Upper Esophagus	Lower Esophagus	Cardiac	Fundic/ Gastric	Pyloric	Duodenum	Jejunum	Ileum	Appendix	Colon	Rectum	Anal Canal
Mucosal Architecture	rugae		gastric pits (and rugae when contracted)			villi, intestinal crypts, and plicae circulares			intestinal crypts			anal columns
epithelium	stratified squamous nonkeratinized		simple columnar									transition to stratified squamous
			surface mucous cells			enterocytes, goblet, stem enteroendocrine, and Paneth cells			enterocytes, goblet, stem, and enteroendocrine cells			
lamina propria			cardiac glands	gastric glands	pyloric glands			Peyer's patches	abundant GALT	occasional GALT (gut-associated lymphoid tissue)		
			mucous neck, stem, enteroendocrine, and some parietal cells									
				parietal and zymogenic cells								
muscularis mucosae	scant, only longitudinal	only longitudinal	approximately three layers			inner circular, outer longitudinal						
submucosa	scattered submucosal glands					Brunner's glands		Peyer's patches	abundant GALT			
muscularis externa	inner circular, outer longitudinal		inner oblique, middle circular, outer longitudinal			inner circular and outer longitudinal						internal anal sphincter
	skeletal muscle	smooth muscle			pyloric sphincter					taeniae coli		
serosa or adventitia	adventitia		serosa			serosa and adventitia	serosa			serosa and adventitia	adventitia	
Organ	ESOPHAGUS		STOMACH			SMALL INTESTINE			LARGE INTESTINE			

16. Liver, Gall Bladder, and Pancreas

The liver is the largest organ in the body and it performs numerous metabolic activities that are essential to life. The functions of the liver are broadly categorized as nutrition, homeostasis, and defense. Its parenchymal cells, known as hepatocytes, are bathed in slowly moving blood, thus enabling them to remove, modify, or add substances to the blood. The key to comprehending the liver's microscopic structure lies in understanding (*1*) the source and flow of blood through the liver and (*2*) the liver's dual role as both an exocrine organ and an absorptive organ. Knowledge of the liver's microscopic and fine structure provides the morphological framework with which to understand normal hepatic physiology and patterns of liver pathology.

The gall bladder and pancreas are accessory digestive organs that function in bile storage and the production of digestive enzymes, respectively. The architecture of the gall bladder clearly reflects its function as a concentrator and storage site for bile. The pancreas is a gland with both exocrine and endocrine roles. In the context of this chapter, only the exocrine pancreas is examined. Visualization of the pancreas microstructure facilitates appreciation of the susceptibility of this multifunction organ to injury and pathology.

The following structures associated with the liver are illustrated in this exercise. The word liver arises from the Anglo-Saxon *lifer*. The word roots related to this system are portal from the Latin *portalis*, pertaining to a gate (portal), and hepatic from the Greek word *hepar*, meaning liver.

> hepatocytes (*hepar*, liver + -*cyte*, cell)
> Kupffer cell (after K. von Kupffer, 19th century German anatomist and
>   histologist)
> portal canal or portal triad (*portalis*, gate; *trias*, three)
> hepatic lobule or classic lobule (*lobus*, lobe + -*ule*, suffix denoting diminutive)
> portal lobule (*portalis*, gate; *lobus*, lobe + -*ule*, suffix denoting diminutive)
> liver acinus or hepatic acinus (*hepar*, liver + *acinus*, berry)

The named blood vessels and the structures associated with the vasculature in the liver are as follows.

> hepatic artery
> perisinusoidal (Disse's) space (*peri-*, around + *sinus*, channel + -*oid*,
>   resemblance; after J. Disse,19th–20th century German anatomist)
> portal vein
> central vein

Structures related to the secretion, concentration and storage of bile in the liver include the following.

> bile canaliculus (*bilis*, bile; *canaliculus*, diminutive of *canalis*, canal)
> canal of Hering (after K.E.K. Hering, 19th–20th century German physiologist)
> bile duct

The following functionally significant structures are illustrated in the pancreas. The name pancreas comes from the Greek word *pankreas* meaning the sweetbread.

pancreatic acinar cells (*acinus*, berry)
zymogen granules (*zyme*, leaven + *-gen*, producing)
centroacinar cells (*kentron*, center + *acinus*, berry)

REFERENCE DIAGRAM OF SLIDE LOCATIONS

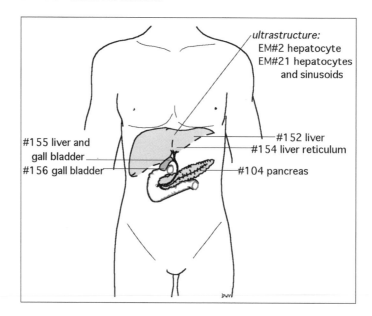

LIVER

Two light microscope tissue sections illustrate the cellular organization of the liver. Use both of these linked series of images for the initial study of the organization of the liver.

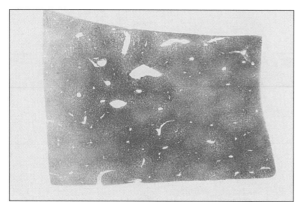

LIVER
Slide #152: Liver; H&E stain; 3 μm thick methacrylate section; nonhuman primate.

Higher magnification images:
- (medium) classic lobule
- (high) portal triad
- (higher) central vein
- (higher) sinusoids and Kupffer cells
- (high) bile canaliculus
- (high) bile canaliculus

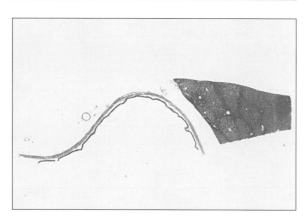

LIVER AND GALL BLADDER
Slide #155: Liver and Gall Bladder; Lee's stain; 3 μm thick methacrylate section; nonhuman primate.

Higher magnification images:
- (medium) liver and gall bladder
- (medium high) capsule and lobules
- (medium high) classic lobule
- (high) small portal triad
- (medium) large portal triad
- (high) central vein
- (higher) Kupffer cell and sinusoid

Slide #155 is a section of liver that includes part of the wall of the gall bladder. The liver is surrounded by a fibroelastic capsule called Glisson's capsule. Since most of the liver is covered by peritoneal reflections, it has a serosa. However, where the liver shares a wall with the gall bladder, its capsule is thin and the liver is covered by an adventitia.

At low power, observe that the liver parenchyma is divided into small lobules that consist of plates of liver cells (hepatocytes) and intervening hepatic sinusoids. The branching and anastomosing plates are usually one-cell thick, and radiate spoke-like from the hub of the central vein. The individual hepatocytes are large and polyhedral; the nucleus is prominent and has one or more nucleoli. Occasional polyploid cells have either very large or multiple nuclei.

The hepatic sinusoids are blood sinusoids that surround the plates of hepatocytes. The blood supplied to the sinusoids is from the interlobular branches of the portal vein as well as small terminal branches of the hepatic artery. The portal vein carries poorly oxygenated blood from the intestines. These portal veins are the intervening vessels in a portal system, a system in which the first capillary bed is located in the lamina propria of the intestines and the second capillary bed, specifically the sinusoids, is in the liver. The hepatocytes are the first cells in the body to "see" both the healthy and the potentially harmful material absorbed from the alimentary canal and their function includes dealing appropriately with these substances. The much smaller hepatic artery carries well–oxygenated blood from the general circulation and contributes approximately 25% to the total blood in the sinusoids. The sinusoid is lined by endothelial cells, which lie close to the hepatocytes but are separated from them by the narrow perisinusoidal space of Disse. They have dark, flattened nuclei and attenuated cytoplasm. Within the sinusoids are large, irregularly shaped phagocytes, called Kupffer cells, which are the resident macrophages of the liver. Kupffer cells are part of the diffuse mononuclear phagocyte system derived from blood monocytes.

The small, roughly triangular area of connective tissue and vessels is termed the portal triad (or portal canal) and it carries the blood vessels that supply the sinusoids. The largest caliber vessel in a portal triad is the portal vein, which has very thin walls and few, if any, encircling muscle fibers. The artery, or arteriole, is the hepatic artery and it has a well-developed tunica media and internal elastic lamina. A third standard component of the portal triad is the bile duct, which is recognized by its cuboidal to low columnar epithelium. Because of the branching of these three structures, multiple profiles of each may appear together in a single portal canal. A fourth standard component of the portal canal is a lymphatic vessel. Lymphatic vessels appear as irregularly shaped endothelium–lined spaces in the connective tissue of the portal canal. Occasionally nerves are observed in the largest portal canals.

The direction of blood flow in the sinusoids is toward the central vein. The central veins empty into sublobular veins and the sublobular veins converge into collecting veins and then into the hepatic vein to exit the liver. It is not difficult to distinguish between the veins that carry blood away from the central veins and those that carry blood to the sinusoids because the veins into which the central veins flow are not accompanied by arteries or bile ducts.

HEPATOCYTE ULTRASTRUCTURE

The hepatocyte cytoplasm typically includes a variety of organelles to support this cell's multiple functions as an absorptive and secretory cell. This electron microscope image shows multiple phagocytic vacuoles that are involved in the hepatocytes' internalization of blood-borne substances. The pronounced smooth endoplasmic reticulum is involved in the deactivation and detoxification of a variety of substances carried in the blood. This electron micrograph also illustrates the extent of exposure the hepatocytes have to the blood. There are large gaps between the endothelial cells and because of the large sinusoidal channels, the blood moves slowly. The endothelial cells are loosely applied to the walls of the sinusoid and there is no basement membrane. Many of the endothelial cells have fenestrations. Beneath the endothelial cells is the narrow extracellular space of Disse into which the stubby hepatocyte microvilli project.

A small channel, the bile canaliculus, is formed between the opposed faces of hepatocytes. The canaliculi are the first portions of the excretory bile duct system. The hepatocyte plasma membrane forms the lining of this tiny channel (1–2 μm), tight junctions seal it off from the extracellular space, and a small number of microvilli project into their interiors.

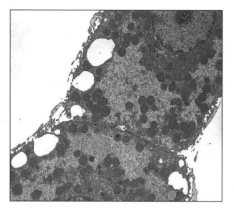

HEPATOCYTES

Electron Micrograph #21: Hepatocytes and Sinusoids; prepared from rat liver.

Higher magnification views:
- bile canaliculus
- space of Disse

The canaliculi form a network within the plates of hepatocytes. The bile canaliculi can be seen in the light microscope in the H&E stained tissue section of Slide #152, examined previously. Bile canaliculi appear as small circles located in the center of a plate of hepatocytes in transverse section, and as elongated channels in the center of a plate of hepatocytes in longitudinal section. At the periphery of the hepatic lobules, the bile canaliculi empty into tributaries of the bile duct, called canals of Hering. These ductules are not illustrated in this material.

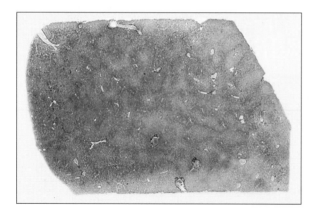

RETICULAR STROMA OF THE LIVER

Slide #154: Liver, reticulum; Silver stain; 12 μm thick paraffin section; dog.

Higher magnification images:
- (medium) central veins and portal canals
- ((high) hepatic plates and sinusoids

Examine the stromal framework of the liver in the silver–stained preparation and observe the delicate network of reticular fibers supporting the plates of hepatocytes. At the periphery of each hepatic lobule loose connective tissue supports the portal canals.

LIVER LOBULES

Return to the H&E stained tissue sections of the liver to examine the liver's lobular organization. There are three structural entities described that are based on various organizations of the components just described: the classic liver lobule, the portal lobule and the liver acinus. In these tissue sections the plates of hepatocytes are seen to be radiating around the central vein with the portal canals, or portal triads, marking the corners of each lobule. This structural arrangement, with the central vein it the center, represents the hepatic or classic lobule. There are two other lobular arrangements of the hepatocytes, both based on functional considerations: the liver's excretory function and its absorptive function. The portal lobule is centered on the bile ducts in the portal areas and includes the draining parts of three adjacent hepatic lobules. The liver acinus is formed from parts of two adjacent hepatic lobules centered on the terminal portal veins that travel in the periphery of the classic hepatic lobule, and drain into the sinusoids.

GALL BLADDER

The gall bladder functions to store bile, concentrate bile and, when stimulated, to eject bile into the lumen of the duodenum. Its microscopic anatomy reflects all those functions. Examine the tissue sections of gall bladder on the H&E–stained slide examined for liver microstructure (Slide #155) and this following tissue section, noting its general structure. Bile is continuously produced by the hepatocytes, delivered to the gall bladder, and stored until a meal is ingested. The mucosa is highly folded and the folds flatten as the gall bladder fills. The epithelium consists of tall, very narrow, columnar cells, with basally positioned nuclei. These cells absorb water and ions from the bile, thereby concentrating the organic components of bile. The lamina propria is a vascularized loose connective tissue, with a dense capillary plexus to take up and return the resorbed substances to circulation. There is no muscularis mucosae so a submucosa as such is absent. External to the lamina propria is a muscularis layer containing bundles of smooth muscle, mostly circularly arranged. These muscle cells are stimulated to contract by the hormone cholecystokinin, which is released by enteroendocrine cells in the luminal epithelium of the duodenum and jejunum. Beyond the muscle layer, a thick, very loose layer of areolar connective tissue, the subserosal connective tissue, provides room for the expansion of the gall bladder as it accumulates bile. A serosa covers the surface of the gall bladder that faces the peritoneal cavity and an adventitia covers the wall shared with the liver.

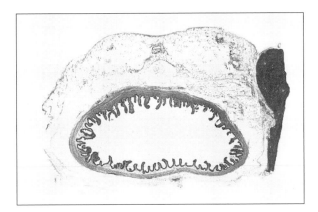

GALL BLADDER
Slide #156: Gall bladder, serosa and adventitia; 3 μm methacrylate section, H&E stain; nonhuman primate.

Higher magnification views;
- (medium) wall
- (high) luminal epithelium

PANCREAS

This compound tubulo-acinar gland is both exocrine and endocrine in nature. The endocrine portion of the pancreas consists of scattered groups of pale cells referred to as the islets of Langerhans, and they are examined in Chapter 17: Endocrine System.

The exocrine portion of the pancreas consists of the serous acini, which produce an enzyme–rich secretion, and the duct system that produces an enzyme-poor secretion. The acini are clusters of secretory cells containing eosinophilic zymogen granules within their apical cytoplasm. These granules contain a large number of digestive enzymes and proenzymes, as well as a trypsin inhibitor, which protects the cells from accidental activation of the trypsin. Pale–staining centroacinar cells appear in the center of serous acini and are diagnostic of the exocrine pancreas. These small polygonal cells are the beginning of the duct system and grade into the intercalated ducts. They and the cells of the intercalated ducts produce a bicarbonate–rich alkaline serous fluid that neutralizes and buffers the chyme that comes from the stomach into the duodenum. The ducts are composed of low cuboidal epithelial cells, have a small lumen, no prominent connective tissue sheath, and join with other ducts to form the larger intralobular ducts. Intralobular ducts join to form the interlobular ducts, identified by their location and prominent connective tissue sheath. The interlobular ducts eventually join to form the main pancreatic duct. The pancreatic duct may share a common opening into the duodenum with the common bile duct.

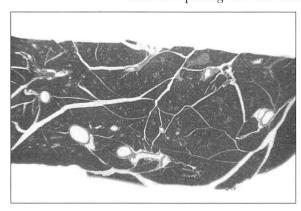

PANCREAS
Slide #104: Pancreas; eosin and toluidine blue stain; 3 μm methacrylate section; nonhuman primate.

Higher magnification views:
- (medium) endocrine and exocrine
- (high) acini and ducts
- (high) centroacinar cells

17. Endocrine System

This chapter examines organs and cells of the endocrine system. The role of this system is to respond to and regulate many metabolic activities of the body by means of secreted chemical messages, known as hormones, that target specific cells. The chemical messages are secreted into and transported by capillaries, so the hallmark feature of endocrine tissues is an extensive capillary bed. Unlike most histological structures in which the morphology provides a great deal of information about function, the histology of endocrine cells is minimally informative. Specific endocrine cells can be identified by unique location and morphology, but beyond that, the secreted products, targets, and effect have to be remembered.

Endocrine organs and cells are clearly distinguishable from exocrine ones. Exocrine secretion occurs from the apical side of the cell onto a free surface or into a duct, whereas endocrine secretion usually occurs from the basal side of the cell (if it has clear polarity) into the underlying tissue where the secreted agent either acts locally or is transported by the systemic circulation to its targets. If stored intracellularly in a polarized cell, exocrine secretion granules are located apically and endocrine secretion granules are stored basally.

As a class of cells, endocrine cells secrete a variety of specific hormones that require special stains or immunocytochemistry to differentiate among the specific ones. Hormones are classified biochemically as either steroids, peptides/proteins or amines. It is possible to distinguish morphologically between cells that produce steroids and the cells that produce peptides/proteins or amines. The steroid–producing cell has an elaborate smooth endoplasmic reticulum and stores its lipid substrate, giving the cell's cytoplasm a foamy appearance in standard histological preparations. The protein/peptide–producing cell typically has basophilic cytoplasm that is rich with rough endoplasmic reticulum. The amine-producing cell also has polyribosomes for protein production, but not for producing the secreted product, rather the ribosomes are for synthesizing the enzymes required to produce the amine hormones. Also, cells that produce steroids cannot store their products, whereas peptide producing cells and amine-producing cells often visibly store granules.

A diagrammatic overview of the principal components of the endocrine system, based on morphological features, follows. Most of the various endocrine cells and tissues are not isolated in single-function organs, rather many exist in combination with other

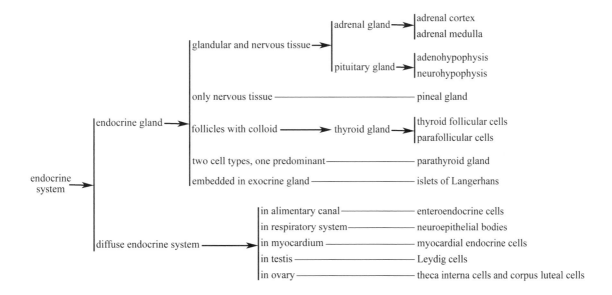

tissues. Several endocrine organs combine separate endocrine tissues that independently respond to and influence very different metabolic events; in some instances, the separate endocrine tissues in an organ are of different embryological origins.

REFERENCE DIAGRAM FOR SLIDE LOCATIONS

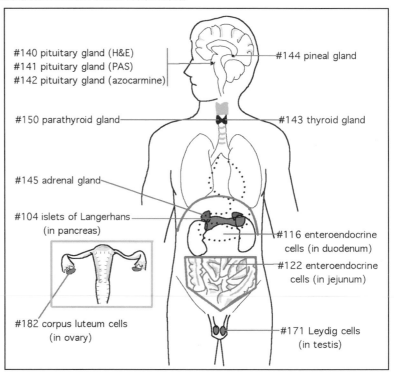

#140 pituitary gland (H&E)
#141 pituitary gland (PAS)
#142 pituitary gland (azocarmine)

#144 pineal gland

#150 parathyroid gland

#143 thyroid gland

#145 adrenal gland

#104 islets of Langerhans
(in pancreas)

#116 enteroendocrine
cells (in duodenum)

#122 enteroendocrine
cells (in jejunum)

#182 corpus luteum cells
(in ovary)

#171 Leydig cells
(in testis)

PITUITARY GLAND

The pituitary gland is also called the hypophysis (*hypo-*, under + *physo*, to grow) because of its anatomical position below the diencephalon of the brain. The cells and structural components of the pituitary gland are listed below with their word roots. The three common systems of nomenclature applied to the subdivisions of the pituitary gland — anterior/posterior, adeno-/neuro- and distalis/intermedia/nervosa — are based on anatomical, tissue and embryological considerations, respectively.

infundibular stalk (*infundibulum*, funnel)
posterior pituitary (*pituita*, phlegm)
anterior pituitary (*pituita*, phlegm)
neurohypophysis (*neuron*, nerve + *hypo-*, under + *physo*, to grow)
adenohypophysis (*adeno-*, gland + *hypo-*, under + *physo*, to grow)
pars distalis (*pars*, a part; *distalis*, situated away from the center)
pars nervosa (*pars*, a part; *nervus*, nerve)
pars intermedia (*pars*, a part; *intermedia*, in the middle)
acidophils, basophils, and chromophobes (*chroma*, color + *phobos*, fear)
Herring bodies (after P. Herring, 19th century English physiologist)
pituicyte (pituitary + *-cyte*, cell)

Examine this tissue section of a pituitary gland and identify the divisions of the pituitary: the pars distalis (anterior pituitary), pars nervosa (posterior pituitary), and pars intermedia. This material was fixed by perfusion through the vascular system and so the cleared capillaries and sinusoids reveal the rich blood supply in all of the regions of this compound endocrine gland, but especially in the pars distalis.

The secretory cells in the anterior pituitary are arranged as branching cords separated by vascular sinusoids. The H&E stain reveals differences among the cells with respect to the content and nature of the granules. The distinction between the chromophobes and the acidophils and basophils (the latter two are known as chromophils) is not particularly obvious. Chromophobes constitute the majority of the anterior pituitary cells but they are not conspicuous because of their small size and poor staining. There are five different anterior pituitary chromophil cells, classified according to their secretory products, but specific immunocytochemical methods are necessary to differentiate among them.

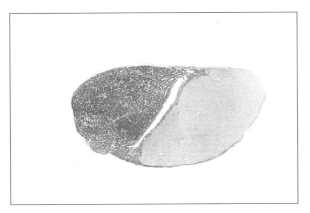

PITUITARY GLAND
Slide #140: Pituitary Gland; H&E stain; 2 μm methacrylate section; nonhuman primate.

Higher magnification image:
• (high) anterior pituitary
• (high) posterior pituitary
• (higher) neurohypophysis

The posterior pituitary has a comparatively nonglandular appearance. The resident pituicytes are neuroglial cells. The hormones secreted by the pars nervosa are actually synthesized in cells residing in the hypothalamus of the brain. The tract of axons, termed the hypothalamohypophyseal tract, delivers the hormones to the capillaries for release. The axons of this tract constitute most of the volume of the pars nervosa.

The narrow band of adenohypophysis cells situated between the pars distalis and pars nervosa is the pars intermedia. It contains scattered cords of basophilic cells that secrete a melanocyte–stimulating hormone. This region may contain Rathke's cysts that are remnants of the lumen of a structure termed Rathke's pouch. Rathke's pouch is the embryological evagination of the oral cavity from which the adenohypophysis originates.

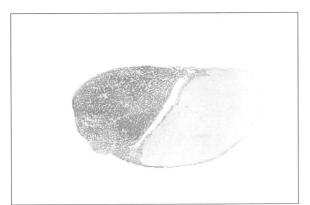

PITUITARY GLAND
Slide #142: Pituitary Gland; azocarmine stain; 2 μm methacrylate section; nonhuman primate.

Higher magnification image:
• (medium) anterior pituitary

This tissue section, Slide # 142, is stained with azocarmine, which stains the granules of the acidophils, which typically outnumber basophils in the pars distalis. There are two varieties of acidophils. Somatotrophs are the more numerous cells and they tend to be located laterally in the pituitary, frequently in clusters. Their granules are numerous and relatively small. Mammotrophs are smaller cells, usually situated individually, with relatively large secretory granules.

This tissue in this third section of pituitary, Slide #141, has been stained with PAS- –lead hematoxylin to reveal two of the three varieties of basophils. The thyrotrophs and gonadotrophs both have glycoprotein secretion granules (thyroid-stimulating hormone and follicle-stimulating hormone plus luteinizing hormone, respectively) that are PAS-positive. Thyrotrophs have smaller, darker granules, tend to be located away from the sinusoids, and are concentrated centrally and anteriorly in the anterior pituitary. Gonadotrophs have slightly larger granules and they are scattered uniformly throughout the gland, generally situated adjacent to the blood sinusoids. The granules of the third variety of basophil, the corticotroph, contain ACTH (adrenocorticotropic hormone), which is a polypeptide that is not PAS–positive.

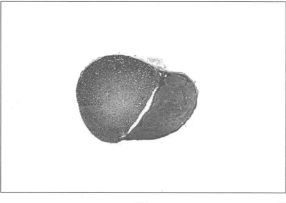

PITUITARY GLAND
Slide #141: Pituitary Gland; PAS–lead hematoxylin stain; 2 μm methacrylate section; nonhuman primate.

Higher magnification images:
- (medium) anterior pituitary
- (high) basophils
- (medium) posterior pituitary
- (medium high) posterior pituitary
- (high) Herring bodies and pituicytes

There are no secretory cells in the neurohypophysis. The cells whose nuclei appear in the posterior pituitary are neuroglial-like supporting cells called pituicytes, and they occupy nearly one-quarter of the volume of the posterior pituitary. The large PAS-positive structures are Herring bodies. Herring body is the light microscope term for the stored accumulation of neurosecretory granules located within the course and termination of axons whose cell bodies are located in the hypothalamus. Some axons store oxytocin whereas others store vasopressin, and stimulation of the parent neurons results in the release of the hormone into the vicinity of the numerous fenestrated capillaries.

PINEAL GLAND

The cells and structural components of the pineal gland (*pineus*, relating to a pine cone) illustrated in this exercise are listed below. The pineal gland, or pineal body, is also known as the epiphysis cerebri (*epi-*, on + *physo*, to grow; *cerebri*, of the cerebrum) because of its location in the central nervous system. This small gland is an elongated oval structure attached to the diencephalon, anatomically located beneath the overlying cerebral hemispheres.

brain sand or corpora arenacea (*corpus*, body; *arena*, sand)
pinealocytes or pineal chief cells (*pineus*, pine cone + *-cyte*, cell)

The pineal gland is an outgrowth of the brain. A thin capsule derived from the pia

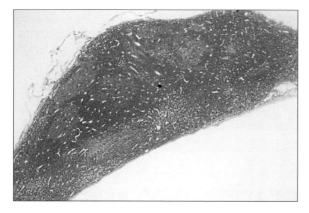

PINEAL GLAND
Slide #144: Pineal Gland; Lee's stain; 3 μm methacrylate section; nonhuman primate.

Higher magnification images:
- (medium) pinealocytes and glia
- (medium) brain sand

mater, the thin collagenous layer that covers the entire central nervous system, envelopes the gland. Septa (trabeculae) of neuroglial cells extend through the pineal gland, separating it into incomplete lobules. Blood vessels give rise to a rich blood supply comprised primarily of fenestrated capillaries. This perfused tissue section illustrates the density of the capillary bed in this gland.

The parenchymal cells of the pineal gland are pinealocytes, which are modified neurons that have large, round-to-oval nuclei with prominent nucleoli. Their cell bodies are arranged in clusters and their highly branched processes intertwine with other process in the pale surrounding neuropil. The second cell population is the neuroglial cells. There are fewer of these supporting cells than there are pinealocytes. The glial cells have smaller, darker nuclei and are dispersed between the clusters of pinealocytes.

Deposits of calcified organic matrix, called corpora arenacea, or brain sand, are characteristic of the pineal gland. These irregular basophilic extracellular bodies consist of concentric layers of calcium and magnesium phosphate in an organic matrix. The number and size of brain sand particles increase with advancing age.

ADRENAL GLAND

This gland is also termed the suprarenal gland (*supra-*, above + *ren*, kidney). The cells and structural components of the adrenal (*ad-*, to + *ren*, kidney) gland are as follows. The names of the regions are based on architectural features. The morphology of the cells reflects the general nature of the hormones they secrete.

> cortex (*cortex*, a bark)
> medulla (*medulla*, marrow)
> zona glomerulosa (*zona*, a girdle, or zone; *glomerulus*, a small ball)
> zona fasciculata (*zona*, a girdle, or zone; *fasciculus*, a small bundle)
> zona reticularis (*zona*, a girdle, or zone; *reticulum*, a small net)
> chromaffin cells (*chroma*, color + *affinis*, affinity)

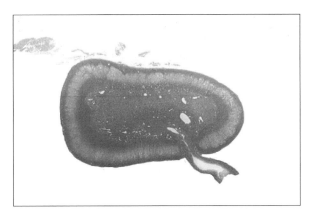

ADRENAL GLAND
Slide #145: Adrenal Gland; H&E stain; 3 μm methacrylate section; nonhuman primate.

Higher magnification images:
- (medium) cortex and medulla
- (medium high) outer cortex
- (high) zona glomerulosa
- (high) zona fasciculata
- (high) zona reticularis
- (medium) cortex/medulla junction
- (high) chromaffin cells
- (medium) medullary and suprarenal veins

Beginning with the low magnification image, observe the overall structure of the adrenal gland in this tissue section. Identify the capsule, cortex, and medulla and the three distinct zones in the cortex. The outermost zona glomerulosa of the cortex is a thin subcapsular zone composed of small compact cells arranged in spherical clumps. The middle zona fasciculata occupies most of the cortex and is composed of large rectangular cells with finely vacuolated cytoplasm as a result of accumulated lipid droplets; the cords of cells are arranged in vertical columns separated by capillaries. The zona reticularis contains cells with eosinophilic cytoplasm arranged in a branching network of clumps and columns surrounding a prominent capillary network.

Examine the centrally located medulla. The adrenal medullary cells, called chromaffin cells, have large, pale-staining nuclei and their cytoplasms are usually finely granular and relatively basophilic. These cells are usually arranged in clumps or cords and are surrounded by a rich network of capillaries. There are two types of chromaffin cells: one produces epinephrine and the other produces norepinephrine and they can be distinguished from each other with special histological stains. These chromaffin cells are actually neurons without their dendrites and axon; they are modified postganglionic cells of the sympathetic division of the autonomic nervous system.

The vascular system in the cortex of the adrenal gland is an anastomosing network of capillary sinusoids supplied by branches of a subcapsular capillary plexus. The sinusoids travel between the cords of secretory cells in the zona fasciculata and converge upon the central vein of the medulla. The medulla is additionally supplied by small arterioles that pass directly through the cortex into the medulla; in the medulla they form a dense capillary network. The large central medullary vein drains the medullary capillaries into the suprarenal vein. Contraction of the longitudinal bundles of smooth muscle in the wall of the large suprarenal vein may regulate blood flow through the cortex and medulla.

THYROID GLAND

The cells and structural components of the thyroid gland are as follows. The architecture of this organ reflects its unique means to provide its hormone quickly when needed.

> thyroid follicle (*thyreos*, an oblong shield + *-oid*, shaped like)
> colloid (*kolla*, glue + *-oid*, shaped like)
> follicular cell (*folliculus*, a small sac)
> parafollicular cell (*para-*, beside + *folliculus*, a small sac)

The thyroid parenchyma consists of large numbers of glandular follicles of varying sizes. The height of the follicular cells decreases with decreasing activity. In this tissue section, the follicular cells appear quite active. Highly vascularized strands of reticular connective tissue separate the follicles and a large number of capillaries form an extensive network among the follicles. The PAS–positive colloid within the follicles shows different staining intensities, reflecting different concentrations of the large glycoprotein thyroglobulin. Thyroglobulin binds the stored thyroid hormone within the follicles. Examine the epithelium lining the thyroid follicles and observe the colloid, not only within the follicles proper but also as small magenta–stained phagosomes within the apical portions of the follicular cells themselves. The thyroid hormones are cleaved from the thyroglobulin by lysosomes within the follicular cell and released to the surrounding capillaries.

Parafollicular or C-cells occur as single or grouped clusters in the walls of the follicles and intrafollicular spaces. These cells are enclosed within the basement membrane of the follicles but do not extend to the lumen. The basally localized granules contain calcitonin and are visible with the lead-hematoxylin stain.

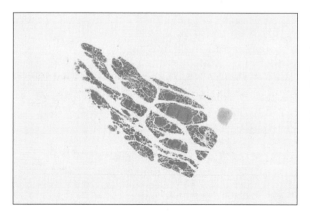

THYROID GLAND
Slide #143: Thyroid Gland; PAS–lead hematoxylin stain; 2 μm methacrylate plastic section; cat.

Higher magnification images:
- (medium) thyroid follicles
- (medium high) thyroid follicles and capillaries
- (high) parafollicular cells

PARATHYROID GLAND

The cells of the parathyroid (*para-*, beside + thyroid) gland are as follows.

chief cell
oxyphil cell (*oxys*, acid + *philos*, liking)

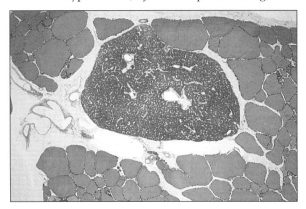

PARATHYROID GLAND
Slide #150: Parathyroid Gland; H&E stain; 2 μm methacrylate section; nonhuman primate.

Higher magnification image:
• (high) chief and oxyphil cells

The parathyroid glands are small lightly encapsulated glands embedded in the posterior surface of the thyroid gland. The follicles of the thyroid gland are visible in this low power image. Arterial vessels enter the parathyroid and then break up into a network of fenestrated capillaries supported by the reticular interstitial stroma. There are two parenchymal cell types in the parathyroid gland: chief cells and oxyphil cells. The chief cells predominate and are characterized by a relatively large nucleus with an open chromatin network and by a nearly agranular cytoplasm. The oxyphil cells are much less numerous and occur singly or in groups scattered throughout the gland. Oxyphil cells are larger than the chief cells; they have small, dark nuclei and a highly eosinophilic cytoplasm that is filled with an extraordinary number of mitochondria. The oxyphil cells secrete parathyroid hormone, while the oxyphil cell is generally believed to be an inactive phase of the former.

ISLETS OF LANGERHANS

Spherical clumps of endocrine tissue known as islets of Langerhans, or simply the endocrine pancreas, occur within the pancreas, which itself is a major exocrine gland. The islets vary in size and make up only 1%–2% of the volume of the pancreas; most are located in the tail of the pancreas. Each islet is a compact mass of epithelial cells supported by a fine reticular network containing numerous fenestrated capillaries. There are four types of cells in the islets, each secreting a different hormone. In H&E –stained preparations it is not possible to distinguish among the cells that secrete the different hormones. Immunocytochemical procedures enable differentiation among the cells and show that the type A (α) cells secrete glucagon; they are the second most numerous and located peripherally in the islets. The type B (β) cells secrete insulin;

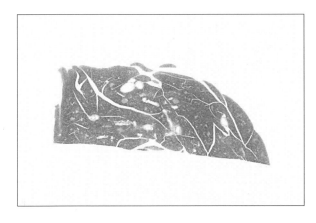

PANCREAS
Slide #104: Pancreas; eosin and toluidine blue stain; 3 μm methacrylate section; nonhuman primate.

Higher magnification images:
• (medium) lobules
• (high) islets of Langerhans

they are the most numerous cell type and tend to be centrally located. The third cell type, the D(δ) cells secrete somatostatin; they represents about 5% of the cells and are located in the periphery of the islet among the glucagon-secreting A cells. A fourth cell type represents less than 1% of the islet cells and is scattered among the others; it is the F or PP cell and it secretes pancreatic polypeptide.

ENTEROENDOCRINE CELLS

Enteroendocrine cells (EEC) are a diverse group of endocrine cells that are specifically located in the epithelium lining the alimentary canal. The broader class of cells, of which they are a subgroup based on their location, is also referred to as the diffuse endocrine system or diffuse neuroendocrine system. These cells are additionally referred to as APUD cells, an acronym referring to a common function as amine precursor uptake and decarboxylation cells.

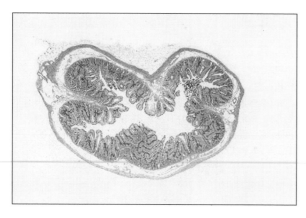

ENTEROENDOCRINE CELLS: JEJUNUM
Slide #122: Jejunum; PAS–lead hematoxylin stain; 2 µm methacrylate section; nonhuman primate.

Higher magnification images:
• (low) mucosa
• (high) endocrine and exocrine cells

Examine enteroendocrine cells in this PAS–stained tissue section of the small intestine (Slide #122) where they are scattered among the columnar cells of the mucosal epithelium. The basally located granules of the enteroendocrine cells are stained with the lead hematoxylin (not the PAS) and so the granules are stained blue–black. These endocrine cells may be located anywhere in the epithelium, from the base of glands where they tend to be more numerous, to the tips of villi. The stains used in this and the following tissue section are not specific for any hormone. A variety of hormones are produced by the variety of enteroendocrine cells, although each cell generally produces only one type. The apically located mucinogen granules of the nascent goblet cells are PAS–positive and distinguish these cells as exocrine.

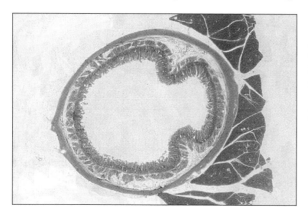

ENTEROENDOCRINE CELLS: DUODENUM
Slide #116: Duodenum; H&E stain; 2 µm methacrylate section; nonhuman primate.

Higher magnification images:
• (medium) wall
• (high) endocrine and exocrine cells

In this tissue section (Slide #116) the granules of the enteroendocrine cells stain a red color, as do the granules of a second type of cell, the Paneth cell. Differentiate between the exocrine Paneth cells and the endocrine APUD cells in two ways: the location of the cell in the epithelium (base of crypt: Paneth cell vs. anywhere in epithelium: EEC) and the location of the granules within the cells (apical: Paneth cell vs. basal: EEC). The granules in the Paneth cells are larger and of a slightly different red coloration than the granules of the enteroendocrine cells, but this morphological distinction is not particularly functionally significant beyond indicating that they are different granules.

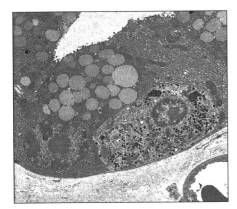

ENTEROENDOCRINE CELL
Electron Micrograph #22: Enteroendocrine Cell; rat stomach.

Higher magnification images:
- (high) exocrine and endocrine cell cytoplasm
- (high) basal secretion

This electron micrograph illustrates an enteroendocrine cell adjacent to zymogenic cells in the mucosal epithelium of the rat stomach. It should be easy to appreciate the continuum between the fine structure of this image and the light microscope images of the previous two tissue sections. The apical accumulation of the secretion granules in the zymogen cell, which releases its product into the lumen of the gastric gland, contrasts with the basal accumulation of the granules in the enteroendocrine cell. The closely associated capillary in the lamina propria can transport the released hormone to target cells. The organelles of these two secretory cell types also reveal a difference in the process by which the respective secretory products are produced. The zymogenic cell cytoplasm is rich in rough endoplasmic reticulum, which synthesizes the protein product for release. In contrast, the cytoplasm of the APUD cell indicates the cell is not synthesizing proteins for secretion since there is little rough endoplasmic reticulum. The large number of cytoplasmic free ribosomes reflects the synthesis of cytosolic proteins involved in this endocrine cell's production of amines.

ENDOCRINE CELLS OF THE REPRODUCTIVE SYSTEMS
Hormone-producing cells and tissues in the male and female reproductive systems are examined within the context of Chapters 19 and 20, the Male and Female Reproductive Systems, respectively. The endocrine tissues include the Leydig cells in the testis and the theca interna cells and the cells of the corpus luteum in the ovary.

18. RESPIRATORY SYSTEM

The respiratory system functions to oxygenate the blood, conducting air from the atmosphere into the lungs where atmospheric oxygen is exchanged for carbon dioxide in the blood. Thus the components of the system are passageways that ultimately lead to the key functional site, the interface between air and blood across which gases are exchanged. Given the vital importance of oxygen to cells in the body, the interface between the air and the blood in the lung ideally should have maximal surface area and minimal separation between blood and air. The conducting airways, in addition to being conduits of respired air, have the ability to trap and dispose of inhaled debris and other potentially harmful material that invariably enters the lungs from the external environment.

This chapter examines the parts of the respiratory tree that conduct air into the site of gas exchange and describes the functional significance of the cellular composition and architecture of the layers in the walls of these conduits. The exercise examines the composition and the functional significance of the blood–air barrier. Finally, this exercise explains the relationship between, and differences in, the distribution of branches of the vascular systems that (*1*) deliver the blood for gas exchange and (*2*) provide systemic circulation to the respiratory tissues.

An overview of the hierarchical relationships among the identified components of the respiratory system follows. The structures listed to the far right are arranged from top to bottom in the direction of the flow of air from the outside to the site of gas exchange. This exercise does not examine tissue from the nasal cavity, nasopharynx or larynx, but they are included in this diagram for the sake of completeness.

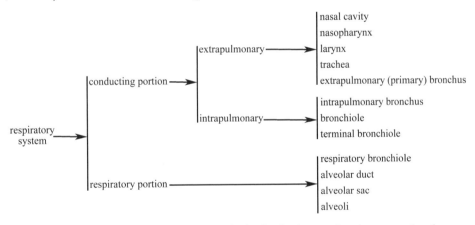

The word roots common to this system include the Latin word *pulmo*, meaning lung, the Greek word *bronchos*, meaning windpipe, and the Greek word *pneumonos*, meaning lung. The following cells are associated with the airways. Each has a specific structure, distribution, and function.

> ciliated cell (*cilium*, eyelid)
> mucus secreting cell
> basal cell
> neuroendocrine (APUD) cell
> Clara cell (after M. Clara, a 20th century Austrian anatomist)
> great alveolar cell or type II pneumocyte (*alveolus*, a small cavity; *pneumonos*, lung + -*cyte*, cell)
> squamous alveolar cell or type I pneumocyte (*alveolus*, a small cavity; *pneumonos*, lung + -*cyte*, cell)

alveolar macrophage, also dust cell or pulmonary macrophage (*macro-*, large + *phagein*, to eat)

The pulmonary circulation consists of the arteries and veins that carry blood to the lungs for gas exchange. Pulmonary arteries transport deoxygenated blood; pulmonary veins transport oxygenated blood. Branches of the pulmonary arteries travel in parallel with the branches of the respiratory tree, tracing the branches from the hilum of the lung all the way to the capillaries in the interalveolar (*inter-*, between + *alveolus*, little cavity) septa. The postcapillary venules travel toward interlobular (*inter-*, between + *lobulus*, little lobe) septa and form veins that travel between the lobules, not rejoining the path of the arteries before reaching the level of the larger intrapulmonary bronchi. The bronchial circulation, in contrast, represents the systemic system that provides metabolic support to the tissues of the lung. Unlike the large diameter vessels of the pulmonary system that transport large volumes of blood at low pressure, the vessels of the bronchial system are relatively small, and typical of systemic blood vessels in any organ. The bronchial capillary beds flow some into the pulmonary postcapillary veins and some into bronchial postcapillary veins and small veins, which eventually flow into the pulmonary veins. The pulmonary veins transport all blood away from the lungs.

REFERENCE DIAGRAM FOR SLIDE LOCATIONS

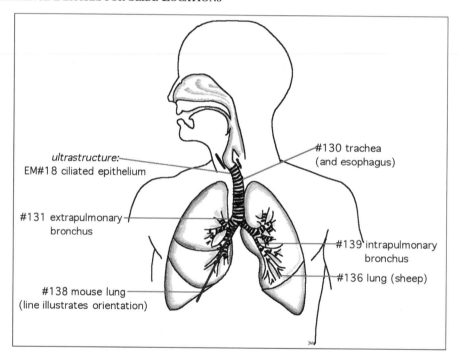

TRACHEA AND EXTRAPULMONARY BRONCHUS

The trachea is a mucosa-lined, cartilage and fibromuscular tube that extends from the larynx to the bifurcation of the two primary bronchi. It is approximately 10 cm in length in an adult. In this low–power tissue section note the organization of the tracheal wall into concentric layers: mucosa, submucosa, and adventitia. The posterior wall of the trachea contacts the anterior wall of the esophagus. The mucosa of the trachea consists of a thick pseudostratified columnar epithelium and underlying lamina propria. A layer of elastic fibers, which is difficult to discern in this H&E–stained tissue, separates the mucosa from the submucosa. Submucosal seromucous glands reside in the submucosa.

The tracheal rings are located in the adventitia of the trachea. These rings of hyaline cartilage are actually a series of incomplete rings located within the anterior and lateral walls of the trachea; the rings are not continuous in the posterior wall of the

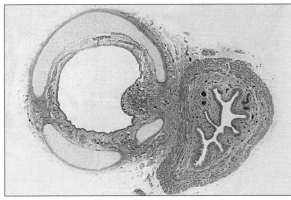

TRACHEA
Slide #130: Trachea; H&E stain; 12 mm, paraffin
section; human infant.

Higher magnification images:
- (medium) wall
- (medium) seromucous glands

trachea. A comparison of the lumen of the trachea with that of the esophagus clearly illustrates the role of the tracheal cartilages in keeping the tracheal lumen open. In this tissue section, the cartilaginous ring appears incomplete because the tissue block has been cut at an angle, catching the fibrous adventitia between adjacent rings (at approximately 8 o'clock and 5 o'clock, if this lumen were a clock face) and including part of the adjacent ring (at 6 to 7 o'clock). The connective tissue adventitia between the rings provides the trachea with flexibility and the ability to alter its length, as it must during deep inspiration. The muscularis in the trachea is represented by bands of smooth muscle (the trachealis muscle) joining the open ends of the cartilage, as well as by a few deeper longitudinal fibers. Contraction of these muscles reduces the cross-sectional area of the lumen. The bulging mucosa overlying the region of the trachealis muscle in this tissue section indicates the muscle is contracted.

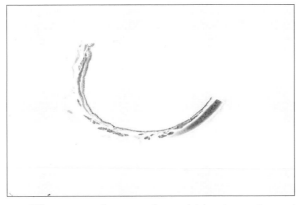

EXTRAPULMONARY BRONCHUS
Slide #131: Extrapulmonary Bronchus; PAS–lead
hematoxylin stain; 3 µm methacrylate section;
nonhuman primate.

Higher magnification image:
- (medium) bronchial wall
- (medium high) bronchial gland

The extrapulmonary bronchi begin at the point of the bifurcation of the trachea and they become intrapulmonary bronchi when they enter the substance of the lung. They are smaller than the trachea but similar in structure. The cartilage in the adventitia loses its regular circumferential arrangement and has the form of irregular plates; scattered spiraling bundles of smooth muscle form a muscularis layer inside the adventitial layer, rather than being restricted to the gap at the posterior wall. The seromucous glands in the submucosa are called bronchial glands. They are invaginations of the epithelial lining, with serous and mucous cells intermixed in tubular and acinar secretory units. The PAS stain accentuates the mucus secreting cells in this tissue section. Details of the epithelium are to be examined later in this chapter.

THE LUNG

This tissue section from a sheep lung has been fixed by immersion. Although its cellular preservation is not ideal, the multiple generations of the branching intrapulmonary bronchi and bronchioles can be identified because of the characteristic arrangement of tissues comprising their walls.

The body has two lungs, and each lobed lung resides in a pleural cavity. The pleural cavity is lined by a smooth, moist serosal layer termed the pleura. The part of the pleura enveloping the lung is called the visceral pleura, whereas the pleura lining the inside of the pleural cavity is called the parietal pleura. The visceral pleura is an integral part of the lung; it consists of a mesothelium under which a loose connective tissue carries arteries and veins that are part of the bronchial circulation, lymphatic vessels that join those of the lung, and nerves of the autonomic nervous system.

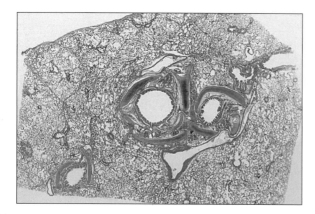

LUNG

Slide #136: Lung; H&E stain; 12 μm thick paraffin section; sheep.

Higher magnification images:
- (medium) intrapulmonary bronchus
- (medium high) bronchus wall
- (medium) lung lobule
- (high) bronchiole
- (high) respiratory bronchiole
- (high) alveolar duct

This tissue section (Slide #136) illustrates several generations of intrapulmonary bronchi, each smaller than the one from which it arose. Intrapulmonary bronchi are recognized by the prominent cartilaginous plates encircling the lumen and the bundles of spiraling smooth muscle fascicles in the muscularis. Like the larger extrapulmonary bronchi, these passageways are lined by pseudostratified epithelium and have numerous seromucous bronchial glands in the submucosal space.

The large blood vessels that accompany the airway are pulmonary arteries. Pulmonary arteries branch with every branch of the bronchial tree following the conducting airway and the respiratory airway all the way to the alveolus. At the alveolus the pulmonary artery gives rise to continuous capillaries that entwine the interalveolar septa, beneath the thin walls of the alveoli.

Returning to the bronchial tree: after a series of dichotomous branchings a small bronchus eventually leads to its own lobule of lung. This lobule is separated from other lobules by connective tissue. As the bronchi become smaller the epithelium becomes simple columnar, the cartilage becomes less prominent, and the glands diminish until both cartilage and glands disappear from the wall. As the airway becomes progressively smaller, the trend is for the relative amount of smooth muscle and elastic tissue to increase. Eventually, small airways called bronchioles (*bronchos*, windpipe + *-iole*, suffix denoting diminutive) are reached and there is a transition in the epithelium. Ciliated cells and an occasional mucus-secreting cell line the larger bronchioles along with a new cell, the Clara cell. With decreasing diameter of the bronchioles the epithelium becomes increasingly cuboidal, the mucous–secreting cells disappear and the Clara cells increase proportionally. After several generations of bronchioles, a terminal bronchiole is reached and the terminal bronchioles branch into airways called respiratory bronchioles. Respiratory bronchioles mark the beginning of the respiratory portion of the airway. The respiratory bronchiole is characterized by a wall that is interrupted by small pulmonary alveoli. The numbers of alveoli in the wall increase with distal progression. When the alveoli occupy most of the area of the wall the structure is called an alveolar duct. Beyond the alveolar ducts, the airway branches into 2–6 alveolar sacs, which are grapelike clusters of alveoli.

Many of the structures described in the previous tissue section can be seen in the following tissue section of mouse lung (Slide # 138). This mouse preparation is useful for following the transition from large airway to alveolar sacs, and for examining the pulmonary circulation that follows the bronchial tree. The branching of the bronchial tree is always an unequal dichotomy, that is, from the trachea to the alveolar ducts, each

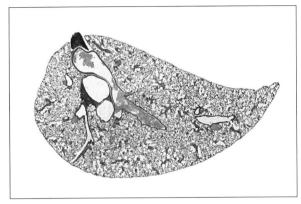

LUNG (MOUSE)
Slide #138: Lung; lead hematoxylin and resorcin–fuchsin stain; 2 μm methacrylate section; mouse.

Higher magnification images:
- (medium) bronchial tree
- (high) respiratory epithelium
- (medium) bronchiole
- (high) Clara cells and pulmonary artery

branch point forms two branches of unequal diameter. It is not until the alveolar sacs that the airway branches into more than two paths.

Because the mouse is a very small animal, the bronchial tree of the mouse is greatly telescoped into a very small package relative to the larger human lung, and there are many fewer than the 20+ generations of branching airway typical of the human lung. Also, there is no cartilage associated with the intrapulmonary airways in the mouse lung, so the airways are recognized principally by the lining epithelium. This tissue was fixed by perfusion through the airways and so the blood vessels appear engorged with blood and the airway epithelium is particularly well fixed.

In this tissue section elastic fibers are stained reddish-purple by the resorcin-fuchsin stain. There is a predominantly longitudinal elastic fiber network along the bronchial tree that continues all the way to the elastin networks of the interalveolar septa. This stromal framework in the lung provides important elastic recoil during expiration and therefore is vital to the proper function of the lung.

The mouse lung tissue section is valuable for observing the bronchioles. In these small airways the predominant cell is the tall, nonciliated bronchiolar (or Clara) cell. In human lungs, the bronchiolar cells are restricted mainly to the terminal and respiratory bronchioles. The Clara cell is a cuboidal, nonciliated cell whose apical surface bulges prominently into the airway lumen. It is generally believed that the Clara cell functions to degrade inhaled toxins, to produce a surfactant that helps maintain the patency of these small airways, and to serve as a stem cell to replace other epithelial cells as needed. Note also the bronchial lymphoid tissue (BALT). These lymphocytes are involved with immune surveillance and the destruction of virus-infected cells.

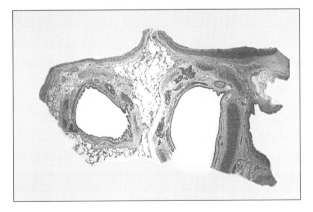

LUNG (HUMAN)
Slide #139: Intrapulmonary Bronchus; PAS–lead hematoxylin; 2 μm methacrylate section; human.

Higher magnification images:
- (high) respiratory epithelium
- (medium) bronchial artery and vein
- (medium) alveoli
- (high) type I and type II pneumocytes
- (high) alveolar macrophages

Slide #130 is a tissue section of human intrapulmonary bronchus. The pseudo-stratified ciliated epithelium lining the bronchus and the trachea is termed a respiratory epithelium because it is unique to the respiratory system. Its mucous cells and ciliated cells constitute the mucociliary apparatus that is responsible for clearing the larger airways of inhaled debris: particulate debris clings to the thick, sticky, luminal carpet of mucus and the cilia, beating within a layer of serous fluid that underlies the lighter mucus layer, sweep the carpet of mucus up the airway into the pharynx where it is coughed out or swallowed.

Several cell types are present in this epithelium. Ciliated cells are the most numerous cells in proximal parts of the airway, becoming less frequent in the terminal and respiratory bronchioles. Single mucous cells and short (or basal) cells are present and represent the cycling stem cells of this region. This epithelium also contains small-granule cells (termed neuroepithelial cells or APUD cells) that are located mainly in the basal part of the epithelium and have bluish staining granules in their basal cytoplasm. These small granule cells are quite rare; innervated groups of these cells form structures termed neuroepithelial bodies in the human bronchial and bronchiolar epithelium. The small granule cells may function in detecting hypoxia and the regulation of bronchial secretion and smooth muscle contraction; in fetal lungs they play an important role in pulmonary development. The basement membrane underlying the respiratory epithelium is typically quite thick; ultrastructurally it is composed of a normal basal lamina with an unusually thick lamina reticularis. Beneath the epithelium are rather delicate bundles of smooth muscle cells and a network of elastic fibers.

Clusters of secretory acini of the seromucous bronchial glands occur in the submucosa and adventitia; their ducts empty into the bronchial lumen. The plates of hyaline cartilage lie deep to the submucosa and form part of the adventitia. The small vessels in the bronchial wall are bronchial arteries and bronchial veins belonging to the systemic circuit of the cardiovascular system. These bronchial arteries give rise to capillary beds in the region, which in turn collect into a venous plexus and thence into bronchopulmonary veins. Bronchopulmonary veins flow into the pulmonary veins.

There is a small amount of respiratory (alveolar) tissue to one side of the bronchus in this tissue section. The alveoli are the thin walled cavities that provide the surface for gas exchange. The thin connective tissue wall between the backs of two abutting alveoli is termed the interalveolar septum, and the capillaries for gas exchange entwine that septum. Examine the structure of the interalveolar wall; it is made up of the capillaries covered by an epithelium consisting of the squamous alveolar epithelial cells (type 1 pneumocytes) and the great alveolar cells (type II pneumocytes). The barrier between the air and the blood within the capillaries may be as thin as 0.2 μm. Where the blood–air barrier is thinnest, the attenuated cytoplasm of the squamous type I pneumocyte overlies a thin basal lamina that may be fused with the basal lamina of the underlying attenuated wall of the continuous capillaries. The vacuolated cytoplasm of the rounded type II great alveolar cells contains multilamellar bodies that contain the precursors for alveolar surfactant.

Many rounded alveolar macrophages with large PAS positive heterolysosomes are artifactually free in the alveolar space; they normally crawl along the surface and clear the alveoli of small inhaled particles. These macrophages can migrate up the airways to the bronchioles where they are swept out of the lungs by the mucociliary apparatus or they migrate into the connective tissue and enter the lymphatic vessels. These lung-specific cells are part of the mononuclear phagocyte system derived from blood monocytes; they are also termed dust cells.

The table on the following page summarizes the structural features of the elements of the respiratory tract.

TABLE 18.1 SUMMARY OF STRUCTURAL FEATURES IN THE RESPIRATORY SYSTEM

function	region	epithelium	principal epithelial cells	mucous cells in epithelium	submucosal glands	cartilage	elastic fibers	smooth muscle
CONDUCTING PORTION								
	TRACHEA	pseudostratified	ciliated, mucous,* and basal cells*	present	seromucous ++++	C-shaped rings	present	spans open ends of C-rings
	LARGE BRONCHUS				seromucous +++	irregular open rings	abundant	spiral bundles
	SMALL BRONCHUS				seromucous +	irregular plates		
	BRONCHIOLE	transition to simple columnar	ciliated and Clara cells*	few-to-none	none	none	very abundant	wide-spread spiral bundles
RESPIRATORY PORTION								
	RESPIRATORY BRONCHIOLE	simple columnar and alveoli	ciliated, Clara,* and type I and II* pneumocytes	absent				sparse bundles
	ALVEOLAR DUCT	alveoli and simple columnar	type I and type II* pneumocytes					minimal bundles
	ALVEOLAR SAC	simple alveolar epithelium						none
	ALVEOLUS							

Notes: The + signs under seromucous glands indicate the relative amounts of glandular material, with multiple +++ indicating more glands.
The * denotes a cycling stem cell in the epithelium.

19. MALE REPRODUCTIVE SYSTEM

The male reproductive system functions to generate and deliver the male germ cells (spermatozoa) and it is the source of the hormone testosterone. To this end, the system consists of a series of ducts and tubules that not only generate and transport spermatozoa, but also modify, absorb, and supplement the secretions that accompany the spermatozoa from their origin to their excretion. This exercise examines the functional significance of variations in the wall structure of the ducts within which the spermatozoa travel from the origin to the end of the excretory pathway. The morphology of the tubes becomes understandable after considering the overall function of the system, and what must be subtracted from and added to the initial product to produce the final product.

A diagrammatic overview of the structural relationships among the components of the system appears below. The components of this system listed on the right are those examined in this chapter and their descending order corresponds to the direction the spermatozoa travel from genesis to exit. Each of these components is structurally and functionally different from the others. In man, pairs of each component are arranged in a bilaterally symmetric manner, beginning with the testis through to the level of the prostate gland. Within the prostate gland, the bilaterally symmetric ejaculatory ducts (the name of the portion of the ductus deferens that continues beyond the confluence with the seminal vesicle lumen) join the prostatic portion of the urethra. The urethra continues as a single tube into the penis.

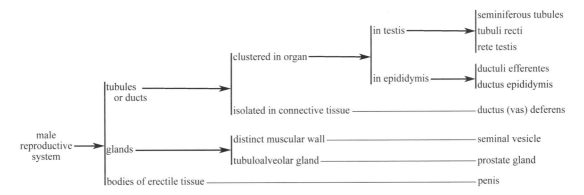

The names of the various organs and glands of the male reproductive system, listed above, are Latin words or are derived from Latin or Greek words. The commonly used word semen is the Latin word *semen*, meaning seed, and the word sperm is derived from the Greek word *sperma*, also meaning seed. Recognizing the translation of many of these frequently used words and word roots assists in relating the name to the function, morphology, or location. Translations or derivations of the parts listed in the diagram above are as follows:

> testis, pl. testes (*testis*, testicle)
> seminiferous tubule (*semen*, seed + *fero*, to carry; *tubule*, diminutive of tube)
> tubulus rectus, pl. tubuli recti (*tubule*, diminutive of tube; *rectus*, straight)
> rete testis (*rete*, a net; *testis*, of the testis)
> ductulus efferentes, pl. ductuli efferentes (*ductulus*, diminutive of duct; *efferens*, bringing out)
> ductus epididymis (*epi-*, upon + *-didymos*, twin)

187

ductus (or vas) deferens (*deferens*, carrying away; *vas*, vessel)
seminal vesicle (relating to *semen*, seed)
prostate (*prostates*, standing before)
penis (*penis*, a tail)

The testes are ovoid organs that produce spermatozoa and testosterone. Understand the relationship between the name, the structure, and the function of the following resident cells and component parts of the testis.

tunica albuginea of testis (*tunica*, a coat; *albugo*, a white spot)
septum, pl. septa, of testis (*septum*, a partition)
mediastinum testis (*mediastinum*, a middle septum; *testis*, of the testis)
Sertoli cell (after the 19th century Italian histologist)
spermatogonium (*spermat-*, seed + *-gon-*, generation)
spermatocyte (primary and secondary) (*spermat-*, seed + *-cyte*, cell)
spermatid (early and late) (*spermat-*, seed + *-id*, ending indicating small or young)
spermatozoon, pl. spermatozoa (*spermat-*, seed + *-zoon*, animal)
Leydig (or interstitial) cell (after the 19th century German anatomist; *inter-*, between + *-sisto-*, to stand)

REFERENCE DIAGRAM FOR SLIDE LOCATIONS

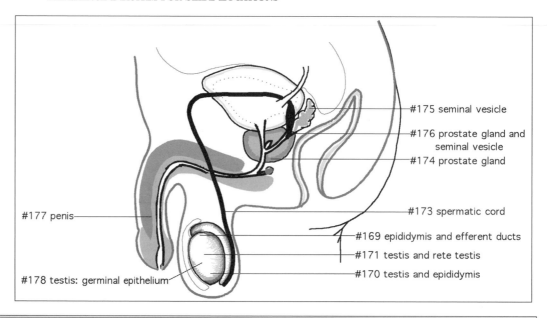

#175 seminal vesicle
#176 prostate gland and seminal vesicle
#174 prostate gland
#173 spermatic cord
#169 epididymis and efferent ducts
#171 testis and rete testis
#170 testis and epididymis
#177 penis
#178 testis: germinal epithelium

CD-ROM Notice: The images examined in this chapter are listed numerically on the CD-ROM by microscope slide number as they might be listed in a standard histology laboratory. Observe that some microscope slides — #169, #171 — are listed more than once because a single tissue section is used to demonstrate more than one feature. The labels and series of linked images are different for each feature. To avoid confusion resulting from selecting the wrong nested series of images, read the label on the CD-ROM list carefully.

TESTIS

The testis functions as both an exocrine gland and an endocrine gland. The germinal epithelium of the seminiferous tubules generates the male germ cells (spermatozoa) and the interstitial cells of Leydig that reside among the seminiferous tubules produce the male sex hormone, testosterone.

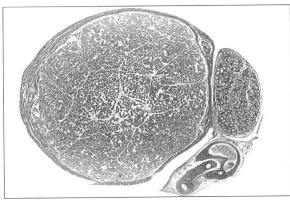

TESTIS AND EPIDIDYMIS
Slide #170: Testis and Epididymis; H&E stain; 12 μm paraffin section, dog.

No higher magnification images.

For orientation, examine the horizontal (in terms of the upright human body: parallel to the floor) tissue section of testis and epididymis in this low magnification view. This horizontal plane of section corresponds to the level of the leader for Slide #170 in the diagram on the previous page. Distinguish the encapsulated lobulated testis with its seminiferous tubules from the attached epididymis. The epididymis is a body that caps the posterior aspect of each testis and its main component is a very long (approximately 16 feet in length) tightly packed tortuous canal, the ductus epididymis. The epididymis is divided roughly into three parts: the caput (*caput*, head), corpus (*corpus*, body), and cauda (*cauda*, tail). The ductus epididymis begins in the head of the epididymis and becomes continuous with the ductus deferens in the tail of the epididymis. Within the scrotum (*scrotum*, the sac containing the testis), the anterior and lateral surfaces of the combined testis and epididymis are covered by the visceral layer of the serosal tunica vaginalis. The tunica vaginalis is a peritoneal outpocketing that lines the scrotal cavity. The testis, but not the epididymis, is enveloped by a dense connective tissue capsule beneath the serous membrane, termed the tunica albuginea.

Posteriorly, the tunica albuginea of the testis is thickened into a larger septum, the mediastinum testis (not present in this tissue section, but to be examined later, in slide #171) that projects into the interior of the gland. Ducts, blood vessels, lymphatics, and nerves enter or leave the testis through the mediastinum. Radiating from the mediastinum to the capsule are the delicate septa of the testis that subdivide the testis into 200–300 lobules. The lobules differ in size, being largest in the central region. Each of these lobules contains one to three or more long highly coiled loops of seminiferous tubule that open at each end into short tubules termed tubuli recti. Each testis has 400–600 seminiferous tubules, each 70–80 cm in length. Therefore, each testis may contain approximately 375 meters of seminiferous tubules. The septa and lobules are evident in this tissue section.

SEMINIFEROUS TUBULES
The microscopic structure of the seminiferous tubule is best observed in the methacrylate tissue section of the human testis. The tubules are lined with a specialized,

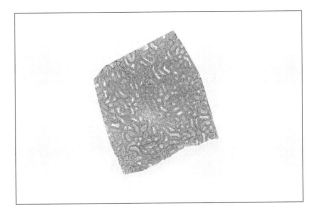

TESTIS, SEMINIFEROUS TUBULES
Slide #178: Testis; H&E stain; 1.5 μm methacrylate section, human.

Higher magnification images:
- (medium) seminiferous tubules
- (medium high) seminiferous tubules
- (high) germinal epithelium, early spermatids
- (high) germinal epithelium, late spermatids
- (high) Sertoli cell

complex stratified epithelium, called germinal or seminiferous epithelium, which contains two populations of cells: spermatogenic cells and supportive cells. The germinal epithelium rests on a distinct basement membrane and the tubule itself has a thin encircling connective tissue layer. The interstitial space among the tubules is a loose well-vascularized elastic connective tissue containing fibroblasts and the interstitial cells of Leydig, which will be examined subsequently.

The cells of the epithelium lining the tubules form a dynamic population, undergoing the process of proliferation and differentiation from spermatogonia to spermatozoa, a process that involves both mitosis and meiosis. The duration of spermatogenesis takes approximately 64 days in man, and in different regions in the seminiferous tubule the spermatogenic cells are at different stages of the spermatogenic cycle. Thus, the whole circumference of one segment of the tubule may be at one stage of the cycle, whereas adjoining regions are at preceding or succeeding stages, resulting in waves of spermatogenesis passing along the length of tubules. The following cells can be identified in the germinal epithelium.

SERTOLI CELLS. The nongerminal cells in the epithelium are known as Sertoli cells or sustentacular cells (*sustento*, to hold upright). They are solitary, columnar cells, radially oriented, with their bases on the basement membrane of the tubule and their apices bearing recesses into which spermatids and spermatozoa are inserted until the latter are released into the lumen. The nucleus lies some distance from the base of the cell; it is large, elongated and irregularly indented, often oriented radially, pale staining, and has a pronounced nucleolus. Sertoli cells have lateral cytoplasmic projections that extend among the germ cells, at a level that separates the spermatogonia from the primary spermatocytes. Tight junctions join these Sertoli cell processes creating a permeability barrier between the basal (abluminal) compartment and the luminal (adluminal) compartment. This barrier constitutes the blood–testis barrier, and isolates developing germ cells from the connective tissue compartment below.

SPERMATOGONIA. Also in contact with the tubule's basement membrane are spermatogonia, the diploid stem cells of the seminiferous tubule. Their rounded nuclei are circumferentially disposed at the periphery of the tubule. The nuclei of these stem cells vary in staining density depending upon whether they are active or inactive. Thus, functionally and morphologically there are three types: dark type A, pale type A, and type B. The dark type A spermatogonia are small cells with relatively inactive–appearing heterochromatic nuclei; they are the true stem cells that divide infrequently to maintain the reserve supply of type A spermatogonia. Pale type A spermatogonia, distinguished from the previous ones by a more euchromatic nucleus, proliferate mitotically and give rise to both type A and type B spermatogonia. Type B spermatogonia look like the pale type As except the euchromatic nuclei are larger, and they divide mitotically for several generations, eventually giving rise to primary spermatocytes. To summarize: of the actively proliferating cells, type As give rise to both As and Bs, and type Bs are all committed to generating haploid germ cells.

SPERMATOCYTES. The largest germ cells, known as primary spermatocytes, have a diploid chromosome complement and undergo two meiotic divisions to produce spermatids that have a haploid chromosome complement. The nuclei of the primary spermatocytes are prominent and usually exhibit chromatin organizing into chromosomes as the cells enter the final stages of meiosis I. Most of the spermatocytes in the germinal epithelium are in the first meiotic prophase, which is a slow process extending over many days. Fewer secondary spermatocytes are evident in these tissue sections because the second meiotic division (the division that gives rise to spermatids) progresses much more rapidly than the first meiotic division. Spermatids mark the end stage of spermatocytogenesis, i.e., the proliferation of germ cells.

SPERMATIDS. They do not divide, but mature into spermatozoa by a series of nuclear and cytoplasmic modifications. Thus, early (spheroid) spermatids can be distinguished from late (elongate) spermatids. The early spermatids begin as round cells approximately 9 μm in diameter; they occur in clusters, and are located near the lumen of the seminiferous tubule. The nuclei of these early spermatids are small, densely stained, and spherical. The late spermatids have radially elongated, dark–staining nuclei that are embedded in the apical cytoplasm of the Sertoli cells. The late spermatids are completing spermiogenesis. Spermiogenesis is the name of the complex differentiation process that involves elaboration of the acrosome (*acro*, extremity + *soma*, body), elongation of the nucleus, formation of the motile flagellum, and discarding the early spermatid cytoplasm that is no longer needed. Scattered among the late spermatids are residual bodies, which are spherical structures containing the cytoplasmic residue derived from the differentiating spermatids. These residual bodies are either phagocytosed by the Sertoli cells or they escape into the lumen.

SPERMATOZOA. Independent germ cells with pear-shaped heads (acrosome and nucleus) and long, slender tails are known as spermatozoa. The late spermatid becomes a spermatozoon after its head is actively extruded from the invaginated Sertoli cell cytoplasm. This final releasing phase is called spermiation. The released spermatozoa are not yet motile, and are carried out of the tubules by the fluid generated across the wall of the germinal epithelium.

A single type B spermatogonium can divide and give rise to very large numbers of spermatozoa during the active reproductive life of a male. Spermatogonia undergo four to seven mitotic divisions before the first meiotic division. Unlike most proliferative processes that produce physically independent daughter cells, the proliferation of type B spermatogonia produces a progeny of cells interconnected by cytoplasmic bridges. This occurs because the nuclear division of spermatocytogenesis is followed by incomplete cytokinesis, producing a syncytium (*syn-*, together + *-cyte*, cell; a multinucleated

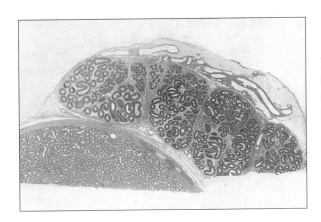

EPIDIDYMIS, LEYDIG CELLS
Slide #169: Epididymis, Ductuli Efferentes; H&E stain; 3 μm methacrylate section; nonhuman primate.

Higher magnification image:
• (high) Leydig cell

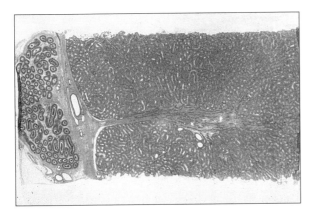

TESTIS, LEYDIG CELL
Slide #171: Rete Testis; H&E stain; 3 μm methacrylate section; nonhuman primate.

Higher magnification image:
• (high) Leydig cells

protoplasmic mass). The cytoplasmic connections cannot be seen in the light microscope, but account for the synchronized development evident in the seminiferous tubules.

LEYDIG CELLS. These cells are illustrated in Slides # 169 and 171, illustrated on the previous page. The endocrine interstitial cells of Leydig constitute a major endocrine component of the body. These cells synthesize and secrete androgens. They are large, ovoid eosinophilic cells with frothy cytoplasm. This frothy appearance is attributable to the content of lipid droplets typical of steroid-producing cells. They can be best seen in the angular spaces between the profiles of the seminiferous tubules, isolated or clustered among the vessels and nerves and connective tissue cells.

TUBULI RECTI AND RETE TESTIS

Observe the mediastinum testis in this next tissue section, Slide #171. At the apex of each lobule of the testis, the seminiferous tubule becomes the short tubulus rectus. Tubuli recti are lined only by Sertoli cells, with no germinal elements, and they end with the transition to the simple epithelium of the rete testis. The rete testis consists of a series of irregularly interconnected chambers embedded in the well-vascularized mediastinum. Simple cuboidal cells, the apical surfaces of which bear short microvilli and an occasional single flagellum, line the walls of the rete testis. Many lymphatic vessels are present in the mediastinum.

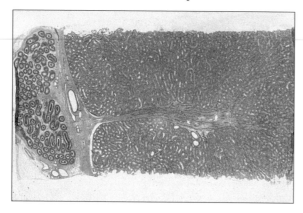

TESTIS, TUBULI RECTI, AND RETE TESTIS
Slide #171: Rete Testis; H&E stain; 3 μm
methacrylate section; nonhuman primate.

Higher magnification images:
* (medium) rete testis
* (medium) tubuli recti

EPIDIDYMIS AND DUCTUS DEFERENS

DUCTULI EFFERENTES

The ductuli efferentes (efferent ductules) are clustered within the head of the epididymis in this tissue section, Slide #169. Twelve or more efferent ductules arise from the rete testis and eventually unite to form the single coiled duct of the epididymis. The individual coiled ductules are embedded in the connective tissue of the epididymis; each ductule is surrounded by a thin layer of circularly arranged smooth muscle. The

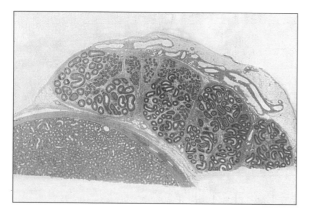

EPIDIDYMIS, EFFERENT DUCTS
Slide #169: Epididymis, Ductuli Efferentes; H&E
stain; 3 μm methacrylate section, nonhuman
primate.

Higher magnification images:
* (medium) epididymis
* (high) ductuli efferentes
* (high) ductus epididymis

epithelium of the efferent ductules is basically simple columnar but its luminal pattern appears scalloped because of the presence of patches of shorter, pale, clear cells interspersed between the more frequent tall, eosinophilic, obscurely granulated cells. Typically the columnar cells are ciliated and the shorter ones bear numerous microvilli. The cilia beat in the direction of the epididymis and assist in the movement of the spermatozoa; the microvilli absorb most of the fluid produced in the seminiferous tubules.

DUCTUS EPIDIDYMIS

Examine the ductus epididymis on the previous tissue section as well as on this next one, slide #171. The ductus epididymis is the principal component of the epididymis, the body that caps the testis. This single, highly coiled duct arises from the confluent ductuli efferentes. It differs from them by having a larger lumen and a distinctly more uniform and thicker epithelium. Typically, the lumen may contain a coagulum of spermatozoa, as well as some cells that have escaped from the seminiferous tubules and residual bodies generated by the process of spermiogenesis. The epithelium is pseudostratified, with two cell types: principal cells and basal cells. The former are abundant, tall, columnar cells that reach the lumen; they have a prominent Golgi apparatus in their apical cytoplasm and long, nonmotile stereocilia. These cells continue the process of resorption of the luminal fluid and remove remnants of the residual bodies not disposed of by the Sertoli cells. Also, various secretions of the epididymal cells facilitate the motility of the spermatozoa and inhibit their capacitation (*capacitas*, capable of; the process through which spermatozoa acquire the ability to fertilize ova). The basal cells are rounded cells scattered along the basement membrane and may be stem cells. The epididymal duct is surrounded by a layer of smooth muscle. The muscle layer is thin over most of its length but it thickens markedly in the tail region of the epididymis near the ductus deferens. Peristalsis of this muscle moves the spermatozoa on to the ductus deferens.

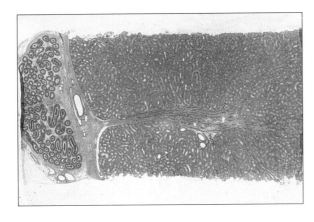

TESTIS, EPIDIDYMIS

Slide #171: Rete Testis; H&E stain; 3 μm methacrylate section; nonhuman primate.

Higher magnification image:
• (high) ductus epididymis

DUCTUS DEFERENS

The epididymal duct in the tail of the epididymis eventually enlarges to form the ductus deferens. This duct retains the pseudostratified epithelium but the principal cells are shorter and the stereocilia have shortened to become just long microvilli. The mucosa is thrown into three to six longitudinal folds, giving the lumen a stellate outline. The thin, dense lamina propria contains many elastic fibers. Unlike the epididymal duct, the muscular coat of the ductus deferens is very thick, approximately 1 mm in thickness, and it is arranged in three layers: a thin inner layer of longitudinal fibers, an extremely thick middle layer of primarily circular smooth muscle fibers, and a thick outer layer of longitudinal fibers. A fibroelastic connective tissue forms an adventitial layer.

The ductus deferens originates at the tail of the epididymis and ascends along the posterior aspect of the testis. It ascends toward the body cavity as part of the spermatic cord. Upon entering the peritoneal cavity the ductus deferens takes an indirect route

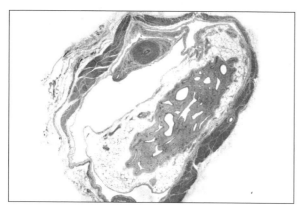

SPERMATIC CORD WITH DUCTUS DEFERENS
Slide #173: Spermatic Cord; H&E stain; 2 μm methacrylate section, rat. (The linked images are not from this tissue section, but from Lee's stained human material.)

Higher magnification images:
- (medium) ductus deferens; human
- (high) lumen of ductus deferens
- (low) pampiniform plexus
- (medium) pampiniform vein; testicular artery

toward the body's midline and the base of the urinary bladder. Near its termination the ductus deferens becomes dilated and tortuous and this segment is known as the ampulla. The ampulla then becomes confluent with the duct of the seminal vesicle after which it becomes diminished in caliber again. This segment of the duct following the seminal vesicle is known as the ejaculatory duct. The ejaculatory duct marks the end of the bilaterally paired structures of the male reproductive system. The ejaculatory ducts flow into the midline urethra where the urethra traverses the prostate gland.

This tissue section of the ductus deferens is from the spermatic cord, so it includes the pampiniform (*pampinus*, a tendril + *forma*, form) plexus of veins, as well as arteries, lymph vessels, and nerves of the testis and epididymis. The veins of the plexus have unusually thick muscular walls. Examine the walls of the vessels carefully and note the diagnostic presence of bundles of smooth muscle in the adventitia of the veins. The testicular artery tends to be coiled so there are multiple profiles of the artery among the vessels.

ACCESSORY GLANDS

PROSTATE AND SEMINAL VESICLE

SEMINAL VESICLE. The low–power view of this methacrylate–embedded specimen (Slide #176) enables a direct comparison of the architecture of the prostate and seminal vesicle. The seminal vesicle is technically not a gland, rather it is a hollow organ that arises as a very convoluted glandular diverticulum of the ductus deferens. This fact is reflected by the presence of a well-defined muscle coat surrounding the lumen of the seminal vesicle. The prominent outer wall consists of smooth muscle arranged into inner circular and outer longitudinal layers. The mucosal lining resembles a honeycomb of branching chambers. The elaborately folded mucosa has a secretory epithelium of pseudostratified columnar cells. Secretory granules and lipid droplets give the cells a frothy appearance. The seminal vesicles contribute approximately 70% of the seminal fluid. Their secretory products include water, potassium ions, fructose, and other agents concerned with modifications of sperm activity.

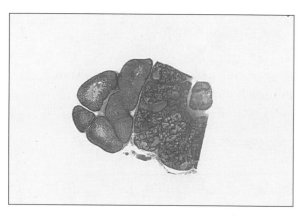

PROSTATE AND SEMINAL VESICLE
Slide #176: Prostate and Seminal Vesicle; Lee's stain; 4 μm methacrylate section; nonhuman primate.

Higher magnification images:
- (medium) seminal vesicle
- (high) seminal vesicle wall
- (medium) prostate gland
- (high) prostate gland parenchyma
- (higher) prostate gland epithelium

PROSTATE GLAND. The prostate gland is a collection of up to 50 individual compound tubuloalveolar glands. The fibromuscular stroma, dense with collagen and irregularly arranged smooth muscle is continuous with the capsule. The secretory nature of its epithelium is apparent; it is a simple columnar or pseudostratified epithelium with basal, excretory (including mucus-producing cells), and diffuse endocrine cells. Under the influence of testosterone, the glandular component of the prostate increases and the stromal component diminishes. After puberty, the prostate secretory units are large and generally referred to as follicles, as they become expanded by accumulated secretory product. Folds, or papillae of acinar epithelium multiply the glandular epithelium of the follicles. The secretory cells of the prostate produce a white serous fluid containing a number of products including acid phosphatase, fibrinolysin, proteolytic enzymes, and citric acid.

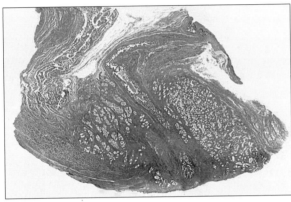

PROSTATE AND SEMINAL VESICLE
Slide #175: Prostate and Seminal Vesicle; H&E stain; 12 μm paraffin section; human.

Higher magnification image:
• (high) secretory epithelia

The tissue section illustrated above (Slide #175) also includes portions of the seminal vesicle and prostate gland and provides a different view for the comparison between the respective architectures: the seminal vesicle is a diverticulum with a distinct lumen, and the prostate is a compound tubuloalveolar gland. The prostate gland is the largest of the accessory glands of the male reproductive system and surrounds the urethra as it leaves the bladder. It is an aggregate of many glands that empty by 12 to 20 ducts into the prostatic urethra. The wall of the seminal vesicle, in contrast, is composed primarily of smooth muscle. When the seminal vesicle is sectioned through its center, it reveals a prominent central lumen; when the lumen of the seminal vesicle is cut parasagittally, it displays small round profiles that can be mistaken for the follicles of the prostate.

PROSTATIC CONCRETIONS. With advancing age, the epithelial folding of the follicles tends to diminish and the follicular outlines become more regular. Unique ovoid or spherical bodies frequently occur in the glandular follicles of the prostate, especially in the prostate gland of older men. These bodies are the prostatic concretions, or corpora amylacea (*amyl-*, starch). They are lamellar structures composed of acidophilic glycoprotein that may become calcified.

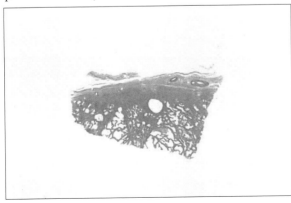

PROSTATE GLAND, PROSTATIC CONCRETIONS
Slide #174: Prostate Gland; H&E stain; 10 μm paraffin section, human.

Higher magnification images:
• (medium) concretions
• (high) concretion

PENIS

The penis is an organ that functions as a copulatory organ in addition to functioning as an excretory organ. Understand how the following component parts of the penis contribute to its functions.

septum penis (*septum*, a partition; *penis*, of the penis)
penile urethra (*urethra*, urethra, from *uron*, urine)
urethral gland of Littré (after the 17th century Paris anatomist)
corpus cavernosum penis, pl. corpora cavernosa penis (*corpus*, body; *cavernosa*, cavernous)
corpus cavernosum urethrae, or corpus spongiosum (*urethrae*, of the urethra; *spongi-*, sponge)
tunica albuginea of penis (*tunica*, a coat; *albuginea*, white)
helicine arteries (*helic-*, helix, spiral)

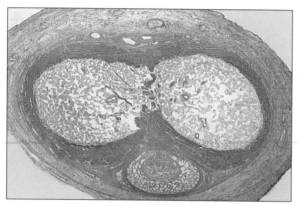

PENIS
Slide #177: Penis; H&E stain; 12 µm paraffin section; human.

Higher magnification images:
* (medium) outer surface
* (high) tunica albuginea of penis
* (medium) corpus spongiosum
* (high) erectile tissue
* (high) urethra and glands of Littré
* (higher) urethral epithelium

In the low–power view of this tissue section examine the general characteristics of a transverse section of the penis. The paired corpora cavernosa are separated by an incomplete midline septum penis. The septum is thick and complete in the proximal penis but incomplete in the distal half, as in this tissue section. The single corpus spongiosum (corpus cavernosum urethrae) is located ventrally and contains the penile urethra in its center. A fibrous tunica albuginea surrounds each cavernous body. The penis is enveloped by thin skin with tall dermal papillae; the subcutaneous layer has no fat, but does have abundant smooth muscle.

The corpora cavernosa are elongate bodies composed of erectile tissue that increase in size by filling with blood. This filling enables the penis to change from a flaccid to a rigid state. The tunica albuginea of the corpora cavernosa is very thick encapsulating tissue that consists of an outer longitudinal layer of collagen fibers and an inner circular layer of collagen fibers. The interior of these cavernous bodies is honeycombed by a network of vascular spaces that are lined with typical endothelium and bordered by trabecular walls of connective tissue and smooth muscle. In the corpora cavernosa, the central spaces are larger than the peripheral spaces, an arrangement that facilitates the retention of blood necessary for erection of the penis.

In the corpus spongiosum the encapsulating tunica albuginea is relatively thin, having elastic fibers among the collagenous ones. The trabeculae of its erectile tissue are thinner than those in the corpora cavernosa. Specialized veins within the erectile tissue have accumulations of fibroblasts and smooth muscle in the intima of their walls; these accumulations are longitudinal ridges known as posters that are believed to have a role in constricting the lumen and slowing venous outflow during erection. Unlike the corpora cavernosa, the peripheral vascular spaces in the corpus spongiosum are larger than the more central vascular spaces. This arrangement, in conjunction with the more flexible tunica albuginea, prevents the high-pressured retention of blood, and during erection preserves the patency of the urethra for ejaculation. The corpus spongiosum expands distally to form the somewhat conical glans penis.

The erectile tissues receive blood from the deep and dorsal arteries of the penis. These branch and enter the walls of the trabeculae of the erectile tissue. Among the vessels in the stroma of the trabeculae of the corpora are the coiled helicine arteries that open into the vascular spaces. Venous drainage occurs through the deep dorsal vein located on the dorsal aspect of the penis.

The penile urethra has a somewhat folded mucosa. Its epithelium is variable, being transitional near the bladder from which it arises, then pseudostratified or stratified columnar throughout most of its length, and finally stratified squamous beginning near the meatus. The mucus-secreting periurethral glands of Littré are located in the lamina propria near the urethra.

20. FEMALE REPRODUCTIVE SYSTEM AND ORGANS OF PREGNANCY

The female reproductive system functions in the production and development of the human baby. Central to this function are the ovaries, which are the site of gametogenesis and steroidogenesis. Many of the structures examined in this exercise undergo progressive or cyclic functional and histological change. Thus the dimension of time must be considered along with the usual three dimensions as these static tissue sections are examined. The histological changes within and among the ovary, oviduct, and uterus accompany hormonal changes of the menstrual cycle, and so there is a temporal coordination among the dynamic changes.

The diagrammatic overview below illustrates the basic structural relationships among some of the components of the female reproductive system. The organs of the female reproductive system have functionally significant microscopic features that are examined in this exercise and that can be related to their role in support of human reproduction. The principal word roots specific to this system are the Latin *ovum*, meaning egg, and the Greek *oon* also meaning egg.

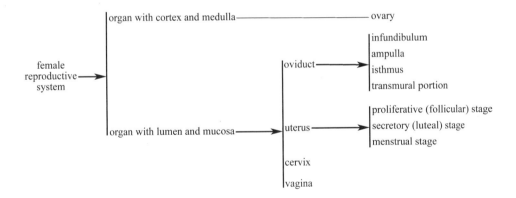

OVARY

The structures and cells associated with the ovary, and their word roots, include the following. Like many other organs of the body, the ovary has a cortex (*cortex*, bark) and medulla (*medulla*, marrow).

> germinal epithelium (*germen*, a sprout or bud)
> ovarian follicle (*folliculus*, a little sac)
> oocyte (*oon*, egg + -*cyte*, cell)
> primordial follicle (*primus*, first + *ordior*, to begin)
> primary follicle (*primus*, first)
> secondary follicle
> Graafian follicle (after R. de Graaf, 17th century Dutch histologist)
> atretic follicle (*atretos*, imperforate, having no opening)

zona pellucida (*zona*, zone; *pellucidus*, allowing the passage of light)
follicular cells
granulosa cells (*granulum*, a granule)
corona radiata (*corona*, crown; *radiata*, radiate)
cumulus oophorus (*cumulus*, a heap; *oon*, egg + *phoros*, bearing)
antrum (*antrum*, a cave)
theca folliculi (*theke*, a box; *folliculi*, of the follicle)
theca interna (*theke*, a box; *interna*, internal)
theca externa (*theke*, a box; *externa*, external)
corpus luteum (*corpus*, a body; *luteus*, saffron-yellow)
theca lutein cells (relating to the theca and corpus luteum)
granulosa lutein cells (relating to the granulosa– derived cells of the corpus luteum)
corpus albicans, pl. corpora albicantia (*corpus*, a body; *albicans*, white)

REFERENCE DIAGRAM FOR SLIDE LOCATIONS

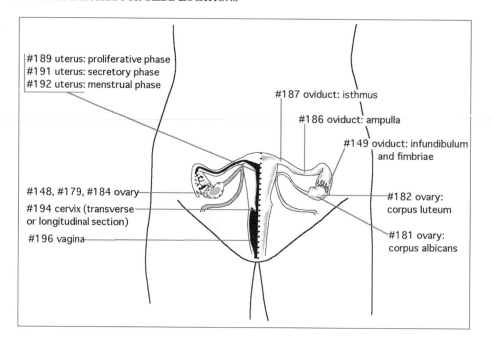

CD-ROM Notice: The images examined in this chapter are listed numerically on the CD-ROM by microscope slide number as they might be listed in a standard histology laboratory. Observe that several microscope slides have more than one version, each designated with Roman numerals or with different identifying titles. To avoid confusion resulting from selecting the wrong nested series of images, read the label on the CD-ROM list carefully.

Each ovary is an almond-shaped organ (approximately 3 x 1.5 x 1 cm in human) that has a central medulla and a peripheral cortex. The medulla is the inner zone and consists of loose connective tissue and numerous tortuous arteries and veins from which small branches reach into the cortex. There is not a clear line of demarcation between the cortex and the medulla. The cortex contains a very large number of multicellular ovarian follicles that, in the ovary postpuberty, are at different stages of development and exhibit a wide range of sizes. The small primordial follicles are peripherally situated in the cortex and are the most numerous, numbering approximately 40,000 in a young woman. Spindle-shaped cells of the stroma look like fibroblasts; many have the potential to differentiate into the steroid–secreting cells of the theca interna.

The ovary is suspended in the peritoneal cavity within a fold of peritoneum called the mesovarium. The ovary is covered by a simple cuboidal epithelium, a mesothelium derived from the peritoneum that is specifically termed the germinal epithelium. This germinal epithelium has no gametogenic properties, although it is a very dynamic epithelium that rapidly recovers the ruptures that occur with ovulation (and is a source of ovarian cancers). The dense connective tissue capsule between the germinal epithelium and the cortex is the tunica albuginea of the ovary.

A woman does not generate new oocytes in the manner that a man generates new spermatogonia. A woman is born with all the oocytes she will ever have. During a woman's own fetal development, primordial germ cells proliferate by mitotic division and when these germ cells enter prophase of the first meiotic division their progress is arrested for over a decade until after puberty. Then, over the next 40 years in a cyclic manner, selected primary oocytes resume development.

OVARIAN FOLLICLES

In the ovary, the stages in the development of the oocyte are distinguished by the histology of the ovarian follicle. The follicle consists of the oocyte and its cellular investment of epithelial and stromal cells. Most of the oocyte—containing ovarian follicles are embedded in the connective tissue of the cortex. The following follicles are identified.

The histology of the ovaries is illustrated in four tissue sections.

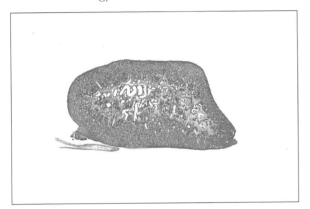

OVARY
Slide: #184: Ovary; H&E stain; 3 μm methacrylate section; nonhuman primate.

Higher magnification images:
- (medium) medulla and cortex
- (high) primordial follicles and germinal epithelium

PRIMORDIAL FOLLICLE. The small primary oocytes are relatively large cells, approximately 25 μm in diameter and in the early stages the primary oocyte is enveloped by a single layer of squamous epithelial cells. These encircling cells are called follicular cells. Being epithelial cells, they rest on a basement membrane, are capable of proliferation, and perform synthetic and barrier functions important to the development of the oocyte. This primary oocyte and its follicular cells constitute the primordial follicle. These are dormant ovarian follicles.

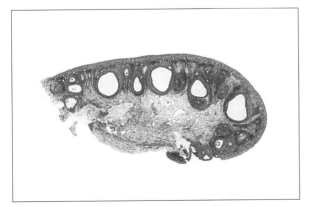

OVARY, I
Slide #148: Ovary, I; H&E stain; 3 μm methacrylate section; nonhuman primate.

There are no higher magnification images.

OVARY II
Slide #148: Ovary, II; H&E stain; 3 μm methacrylate section; nonhuman primate.

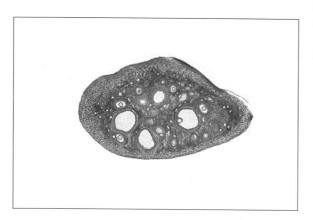

Higher magnification images:
- (medium) ovary cortex
- (medium) primordial, primary and secondary follicles
- (high) multilaminar primary follicle
- (medium) primary and secondary follicles
- (high) secondary follicles
- (high) cumulus oophorus
- (high) membrana granulosa
- (medium) normal and atretic follicle
- (high) atretic granulosa
- (medium) atretic follicle

PRIMARY FOLLICLE. In each menstrual cycle, a cohort of primordial follicles begins a phase of rapid growth in which the oocyte increases in size and the surrounding epithelium and stroma undergo change. As the activated oocyte grows, the follicular cells become cuboidal to columnar in shape, and then stratify. These epithelial cells are now called granulosa cells. The zona pellucida, which is a protective glycosaminoglycan-rich highly refractile layer, forms between the granulosa cells and the oocyte. A follicle with the single layer of cuboidal granulosa cells is known as a unilaminar primary follicle and one with a stratification of the granulosa cells is a multilaminar primary follicle. The theca folliculi forms in the stroma immediately surrounding the spheroid follicle. The theca folliculi is a poorly defined highly cellular area of stroma that develops into two circumferential zones: an internal well-vascularized layer that contains steroid–secreting cells, the theca interna, and an encircling external fibrous layer, the theca externa.

SECONDARY FOLLICLE. The ovarian follicle continues to grow and reaches a diameter of approximately 200 μm. This stage is marked by the formation of a fluid–filled space, called the antrum, within the follicle. The antral fluid (or liquor folliculi) is a transudate of blood. As the antrum increases in size, the oocyte is pushed to one side. The membrana granulosa can now be separated into two regions: the granulosa proper (membrana granulosa or mural granulosa; *murus*, wall) and the cumulus oophorus, the pedestal of granulosa cells upon which the oocyte rests. The corona radiata refers to the layer of granulosa cells that immediately surrounds the oocyte at the time of ovulation.

GRAAFIAN FOLLICLE (OR TERTIARY FOLLICLE). This is a very large dominant follicle (approximately 25 mm in diameter) that is destined to ovulate. There are no Graafian follicles present in these tissue sections. Only one such tertiary follicle, between the two ovaries, develops to this stage per menstrual cycle. Prior to ovulation, the Graafian follicle bulges above the surface of the ovary and the oocyte with its corona radiata floats free in the antrum. At this stage in its development the oocyte resumes its meiotic division within the confines of the zona pellucida and generates a tiny cell with little cytoplasm called the first polar body and the huge secondary oocyte. The secondary oocyte immediately begins the second meiotic division and is arrested in metaphase II, where it remains until its plasma membrane is penetrated by the spermatozoa.

ATRETIC FOLLICLE. Many primordial follicles begin to mature, but only a few actually develop to the tertiary stage. More than 99% of all follicles present in the ovary at the time of a woman's birth eventually degenerate. Atresia can occur at any stage in

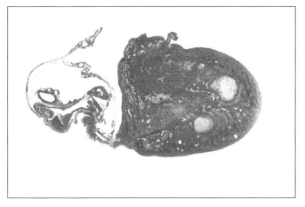

OVARY, ATRETIC FOLLICLES
Slide #179: Ovary; H&E stain; 3 mm methacrylate section; nonhuman primate.

Higher magnification image:
- (medium) pyknotic nuclei and atretic follicle

follicular development. In the first sign of atresia, the granulosa cells begin to degenerate and distinctly small, dense, pyknotic nuclei (*pyknos,* thick, dense) appear among the normal granulosa cell nuclei. The granulosa proceeds to deteriorate and eventually the remnant of the follicle is invaded by blood vessels, macrophages, and fibroblasts.

CORPUS LUTEUM

The corpus luteum is a temporary endocrine gland formed from the collapsed remnants of the Graafian follicle wall following ovulation. It is about 10 mm in diameter. The previously avascular granulosa is invaded by blood vessels and the basement membrane begins to break apart. Both the granulosa cells and the enfolded cells of the theca interna enlarge and become part of this structure. The granulosa lutein cells are large, spherical steroidogenic cells that produce progesterone and the theca lutein cells are smaller, have less cytoplasm, and secrete estrogen. If pregnancy occurs the corpus luteum increases to approximately 25 mm in diameter and persists through birth of the baby.

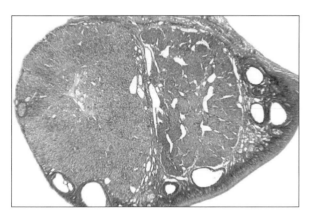

CORPUS LUTEUM, I
Slide #182: Ovary: Corpus Luteum, I; H&E stain; 12 μm paraffin section; human.

Higher magnification images:
- (medium) corpus luteum
- (medium high) corpus luteum
- (high) granulosa and theca luteum cells

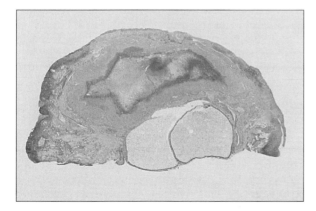

CORPUS LUTEUM, II
Slide #182: Ovary: Corpus Luteum, II; H&E stain; 12 μm paraffin section; human.

Higher magnification images:
- (medium) granulosa lutein cells
- (medium) granulosa and theca lutein cells
- (high) corpus luteum cells

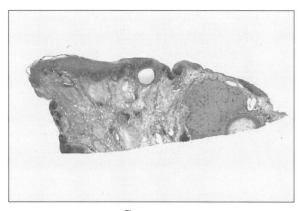

CORPUS LUTEUM, III
Slide #182: Ovary: Corpus Luteum, III; H&E stain; 12 μm paraffin section; human.

There are no higher magnification images.

CORPUS ALBICANS

A corpus albicans is the degenerated corpus luteum. It is easily recognized as a fibrous scarlike tissue that replaces the steroidogenic cells of the corpus luteum. Like the atretic follicles, it is eventually removed by macrophages.

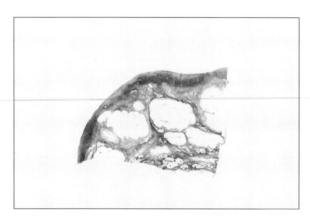

CORPUS ALBICANS
Slide #181: Ovary: Corpus Albicans; H&E stain; 12 μm paraffin section; human.

Higher magnification images:
• (medium) corpus albicans
• (medium) corpus albicans (trichrome stain)
• (high) corpus albicans

OVIDUCT

The oviduct is also known as the uterine tube or Fallopian tube (after G. Fallopius, a 16th century Italian anatomist). The divisions, component parts, and cells of the oviduct are named according to their morphological appearance.

fimbria, pl. fimbriae (*fimbria*, a fringe)
infundibulum (*infundibulum*, a funnel)
ampulla (*ampulla*, a two-handled bottle)
isthmus (*isthmus*, a narrow passage connecting two larger parts)
intramural segment (*intra-*, within + *murus*, wall)
peg cells (name based on peglike appearance in tissue section)
ciliated cells of the oviduct (*cilium*, eyelid)

There are two oviducts in the female, a bilaterally symmetric pair, that open into the peritoneal cavity at the ovarian end and extend to the uterus with which its lumen is continuous. The oviduct is supported within a mesenteric fold (the mesosalpinx; *salpinx*, trumpet, tube), which is attached to the broad ligament. Each oviduct is divided into four parts: the infundibulum, the ampulla, the isthmus, and the intramural portion. There is no tissue section in this exercise of the fourth portion, the intramural portion, which penetrates the uterine wall.

The structure of the oviduct is basically similar throughout. The mucosal folds, which begin as very tall, complex folds, decrease in height and complexity in the proximal direction, that is, from the infundibulum to the isthmus. Toward the ovarian end of this tube, in the infundibulum, the lumen is large with a labyrinthine system of narrow spaces between the elaborately branched thin mucosal folds; the muscularis is thin. Fingerlike extensions of the mucosa are termed fimbriae and they extend into the peritoneal cavity. The epithelium of the uterine tube is simple columnar, although occasional basal stem cells may occur. In the infundibulum the cells are taller than those nearer the uterus. The epithelium of the fimbriae is continuous with the serosal mesothelium of the infundibulum.

There are two types of columnar cells in the mucosal epithelium: ciliated cells whose cilia beat in the direction of the uterus, and nonciliated (peg) cells that secrete a viscous fluid containing substances believed to support the function of the spermatozoa and create an environment conducive to the development of the zygote. The relative numbers of each of these epithelial cells are influenced by the level of circulating estrogen: in the preovulatory period almost half of the cells are ciliated (to move the ovulated cell into the oviduct and toward the uterus), in late luteal period only approximately 5% of these cells are ciliated.

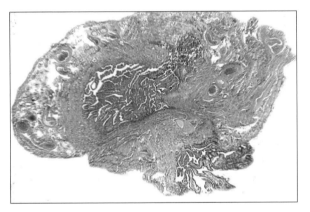

INFUNDIBULUM
Slide #149: Fimbria and Infundibulum of Oviduct; H&E stain; 12 μm paraffin section; human.

There are no higher magnification images.

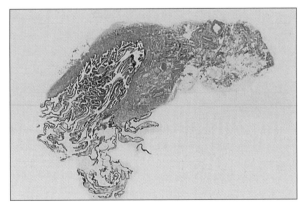

FIMBRIA AND INFUNDIBULUM
Slide #185: Fimbria and Infundibulum of Oviduct; H&E stain; 12 μm paraffin section; human.

Higher magnification images:
  • (medium) oviduct infundibulum
  • (high) epithelium and peritoneum

The lamina propria/submucosa is highly cellular with only a sparse accumulation of collagenous fibers. The tunica muscularis is composed of two somewhat intermingled layers, an inner mainly circular and an outer longitudinal layer; the circular layer becomes progressively thicker with distance from the infundibulum to the isthmus. Peristaltic (*peri-*, around + *stalsis*, contraction) contractions of the muscularis assist the cilia in moving the oocyte or zygote toward the uterus. The serosa is continuous with the broad ligament.

The progressive decrease in the height and complexity of the mucosal folds and the progressive increase in the thickness of the muscularis is apparent in the following series of tissue sections of the ampulla, the distal isthmus and the proximal isthmus, respectively. In the proximal isthmus at the uterine end, the lumen is reduced in caliber, the mucosal folds are much simpler and not much more than low ridges; and the muscularis is thickest

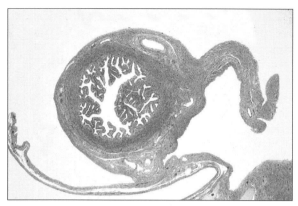

AMPULLA
Slide #186: Ampulla of Oviduct; H&E stain; 3 μm methacrylate section; nonhuman primate.

Higher magnification images:
- (medium) ampulla
- (medium high) mucosa
- (high) epithelium

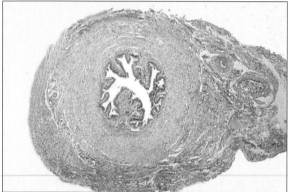

ISTHMUS, DISTAL
Slide #187: Isthmus of Oviduct; H&E stain; 12 μm paraffin section; human.

There are no higher magnification images.

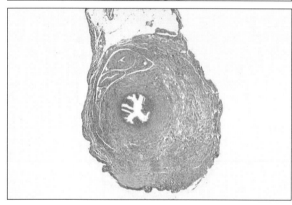

ISTHMUS, PROXIMAL
Slide #187: Isthmus of Oviduct; H&E stain; 12 μm paraffin section; human.

There are no higher magnification images.

UTERUS

The uterine wall has three layers, each with a specific name. The names of the layers have as a common root the Greek word *metra* for uterus. In women between the ages of approximately 13 and 52, the uterine mucosa (endometrium) undergoes cyclic changes under the influence of hormones. Structures in the uterus include the following:

endometrium (*endo-*, within + *metra*, uterus)
endometrial glands
stratum basalis (*stratum*, layer; *basalis*, basal)
stratum functionalis (*stratum*, layer; *functio*, performing)
endometrial spiral (or coiled) arteries
straight arteries
myometrium (*myo-*, muscle + *metra*, uterus)
perimetrium (*peri-*, around + *metra*, uterus)
uterus: proliferative (or follicular, referring to the ovarian follicle) stage
uterus: secretory (or luteal, referring to the corpus luteum) stage
uterus: menstruating stage (from *menis*, pl. *menses*, month)

There are several tissue sections of the uterine wall. The pattern of the wall is similar to that of other hollow organs, but the layers are known by organ–specific names. The endometrium corresponds to the mucosa/submucosa. The myometrium is a broad muscularis and consists of interlacing bundles of smooth muscle obscurely arrayed in three layers. These muscle cells increase in both size (hypertrophy; *hyper-*, over + *trophe*, nourishment) and in numbers (hyperplasia; *hyper-*, over + *plasis*, a molding) during pregnancy. The perimetrium is the serosa and it covers much of the outer surface of the uterus. An adventitia covers part of the anterior aspect of the uterus where it rests against the urinary bladder.

In the endometrium, a simple columnar epithelium with occasional groups of ciliated cells forms simple tubular uterine glands that extend through the thickness of the mucosa. The connective tissue surrounding the endometrial glands is called the endometrial stroma; it is quite cellular and contains reticular fibers. The endometrium is divided into two zones: the stratum functionalis and the stratum basalis, which are identified in this material primarily by location. The stratum functionalis (pars functionalis) is the superficial layer that under the influence of ovarian hormones grows cyclically and sloughs off during the menstrual cycle. The stratum basalis (pars basalis) is the deeper permanent layer that includes the basal portions of the uterine glands; it is retained during menstruation. Branches of the arcuate arteries, which are located in the myometrium, give rise to two sets of arteries that supply the endometrium: straight arteries and spiral arteries. In tissue sections it is difficult to distinguish between straight and spiral arteries except by location; both are present in the stratum basalis but only the spiral arteries extend into the functionalis.

ENDOMETRIAL PHASES

The endometrium is subject to cyclic changes throughout the potential years of parturition, from puberty until menopause. The most obvious morphological differences among the stages lie in the development of the uterine glands.

PROLIFERATIVE STAGE. This stage follows menstruation and during this stage, cells in the epithelium of the stratum basalis restore the surface epithelium of the stratum functionalis. There is a progressive elongation of the endometrial (uterine) glands. A proliferation of the stromal cells of the lamina propria accompanies this growth. Initially the glands are relatively straight and lined by a columnar epithelium. Mitotic figures are evident in the glandular epithelium and in the stroma. In the very late stages of the proliferative phase, marking the beginning of the secretory stage and the influence of the hormone progesterone, the columnar epithelial cells accumulate glycogen in their basal portions, displacing the nucleus toward the apex of the cell. This first tissue section (Slide # 189) is from the late proliferative stage, where the glands are straight but the epithelial cells have begun to accumulate glycogen.

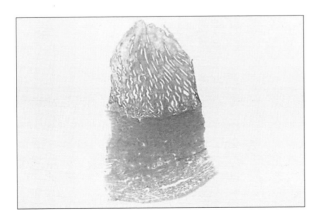

UTERUS: PROLIFERATIVE STAGE
Slide #189: Uterus: Proliferative; H&E stain; 3 μm methacrylate section; nonhuman primate.

Higher magnification images:
- (medium) uterus, proliferative stage
- (medium) endometrium, stratum functionalis
- (medium) stratum basalis
- (high) mucosa
- (high) uterine gland

SECRETORY STAGE. By this stage the endometrial glands have become irregular in shape. From day 16 to day 28 in the menstrual cycle the glands of the functionalis become more tortuous and develop lateral sacculations and the lumen of the gland enlarges. Mitotic figures are absent. The columnar epithelial cells are pale and the glycogen is now apical as these cells become a source of the glycogen– and glycoprotein–rich secretions that provide nutrition for the conceptus. The stroma is at its most vascularized stage. Near the end of this stage, the stroma becomes edematous.

The series of images linked on the CD-ROM to this lead-in image (slide #191) illustrate the progression of change from early to late secretory period. Despite the presence of linked hotspots, most of the linked images are drawn from different tissues.

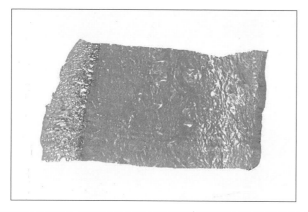

UTERUS: SECRETORY STAGE
Slide #191: Uterus: Secretory; H&E stain; 3 μm methacrylate section; nonhuman primate.

Higher magnification images:
- (medium) endometrium
- (medium) secretory endometrium
- (medium) secretory stage, early
- (medium) secretory stage, late
- (high) late secretory endometrial glands

MENSTRUAL STAGE. This stage occurs when the spiral arteries constrict and deprive the cells of the stratum functionalis of blood and oxygen. The glands no longer secrete nutritive materials and lymphocytes invade the stroma. Blood escapes from the damaged spiral arteries into the stroma and lumen. The ischemic stratum functionalis begins to degenerate and break apart. Clumps of necrotic fragments of endometrium are shed until the entire functionalis is sloughed off. The stratum basalis is spared because its straight arteries remain intact during this process. By day 5 of the menstrual cycle the basalis has begun to regenerate a new functionalis.

Blood escapes from the necrotic blood vessels in the stratum functionalis and the functional layer is shed. Under the influence of estrogen, the cycle repeats and a new functionalis develops from the stratum basalis.

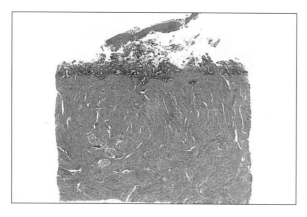

UTERUS: MENSTRUAL STAGE
Slide #192: Uterus: Menstrual; H&E stain; 3 μm methacrylate section; nonhuman primate.

Higher magnification images:
- (medium) endometrium
- (medium high) stratum functionalis

CERVIX

The cervix is the narrow distal third of the uterus and it has its own characteristic morphological features. Its mucosa does not cycle in the manner of the endometrium in the body of the uterus. The cervix (*cervix*, neck) communicates with the vagina (*vagina*, sheath), which is the female copulatory organ.

Structures associated with this part of the female reproductive system include the following:

plicae palmatae, also known as endocervical or cervical glands (*plica*, a fold; *palma*, palm)

external and internal os of the cervix (*os*, mouth)

endocervix and ectocervix (*endo-*, within and *ecto-*, outside the cervix)

portio vaginalis (*portio*, portion; *vaginalis*, of the vagina)

The cervix is the cylindrical lower portion of the uterus and its lumen is the cervical canal. The bulk of its wall is dense connective tissue. The distal end of the cervix bulges into the vaginal cavity as the portio vaginalis. The projection into the vagina creates a recess in the vaginal cavity called the fornix vaginae (*fornix*, arch). The opening of the cervical canal into the larger lumen of the uterus is termed the internal os; the aperture at the end of the canal opening into the vagina is the external os. In this longitudinal tissue section the mucosa of the cervical canal, called the endocervix, forms irregular branching folds, termed the plicae palmatae. The epithelium is a simple columnar epithelium whose cells contain apical droplets of mucus. There is an abrupt demarcation between the epithelia of the cervical canal and the stratified squamous epithelium the vagina. Typically the transition in epithelium occurs just inside the opening of the cervical canal into the vagina, at the external os.

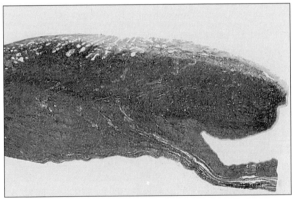

CERVIX (LONGITUDINAL SECTION)
Slide #194: Cervix, longitudinal plane; azan stain; 15 μm paraffin section; human.

Higher magnification image:
• (medium) epithelium at transition

This following tissue section is a transverse section of the cervix near the portio vaginalis. For orientation, the central lumen of this tissue section is the cervical canal and the stratified squamous epithelium on most of the outer surface is of the vagina. The mucosa lining the cervical canal is the endocervix and the mucosa of the outside surface of the portio vaginalis is the ectocervix. The epithelium of the endocervix consists of tall columnar cells with basal nuclei; some are ciliated but most are mucoid. The cervical mucosa changes only slightly during menstruation and does not slough. Very complex, deep furrows or compound clefts, called the plicae palmatae characterize

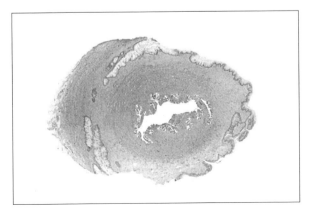

CERVIX (TRANSVERSE SECTION)
Slide #194: Cervix, transverse plane; H&E stain; 15 μm paraffin section; human.

Higher magnification image:
• (low) plicae palmatae

the endocervix. These folds are irregularly arranged and often misinterpreted to be a system of branching tubular glands, and so are also known as endocervical or cervical glands. The wall of the cervix is unlike that of the rest of the uterus in that it consists mostly of dense collagenous and elastic fibers among which are distributed a variable number of smooth muscle cells. The portio vaginalis has no smooth muscle cells.

VAGINA

The vagina is a distensible fibromuscular sheath that extends from the cervix to the external genitalia. It is lined with a mucosa that forms transverse rugae (*ruga*, wrinkle). The epithelium is a stratified squamous epithelium that is rich in glycogen, the amount of which is controlled by estrogens. Bacterial metabolism of this glycogen results in lactic acid accumulation and the vaginal lumen's typically low pH. The lamina propria has a dense papillary layer, particularly well developed on the posterior wall, and a looser vascular layer with an extensive capillary plexus. The muscularis layer consists mainly of longitudinal smooth muscle but includes some interlacing inner circular fibers. A sphincter of skeletal muscle, not present on this tissue section, encircles the lower end of the vagina.

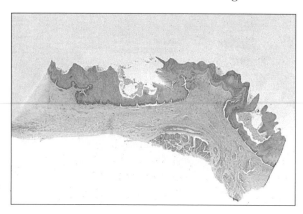

VAGINA
Slide #196: Vagina; H&E stain; 15 µm paraffin section; human.

Higher magnification image:
- (low) mucosa

ORGANS OF PREGNANCY

PLACENTA

The placenta is the site of active and passive transport of gases, ions, amino acids, and macromolecules between the fetal blood and maternal blood. In addition, the placenta is a major endocrine organ.

EARLY DEVELOPMENT. If fertilization occurs, the zygote (*zygotos*, yoked) develops into a fluid-filled hollow blastocyst that attaches to the surface of the secretory endometrium at approximately 6 days after ovulation. The uterine wall supports the development of the fetus with contributions from the extraembryonic tissues of the conceptus (*con-*, together + *capio*, to take). The embryo develops from a specific inner cell mass within the hollow blastocyst, whereas the surrounding cells of the sphere, called trophoblast cells, generate most of the placental structures. Proliferation of these trophoblast cells produces a two–layered wall consisting of an inner cytotrophoblast layer and an outer syncytiotrophoblast layer. This outer layer is a syncytium (*syn-*, together + *-cyt*, cell), that is, a multinucleate layer of protoplasm formed by the fusion of originally separate cells. The syncytiotrophoblast will eventually become the only cellular layer separating the fetal capillaries within the placental villi from the maternal blood. Although the formation of the placenta requires a precise developmental progression of the trophoblast cells, it requires as well certain developmental changes in the endometrium. During pregnancy the endometrium is known as the decidua.

With the initial growth of the trophoblast cells into the endometrium, the endometrial stromal cells develop into enlarged secretory cells. These cells are called decidual cells. At this stage in pregnancy, the uterine endometrium is properly termed the decidua; that region of the decidua specifically underlying the developing fetus will later form the maternal portion of the placenta and it is called the decidua basalis.

MORPHOLOGY: LATE PREGNANCY. Morphologically, the placenta (*placenta*, a cake) is a composite organ: the maternal contribution to this organ develops from the uterine endometrium, whereas the fetal contribution develops from the extraembryonic trophoblast and amnion. This portion of the chapter examines the full-term placenta. The following structures are part of the placenta and illustrated in the tissue sections.

decidua basalis (*deciduus*, falling off; *basalis*, basal)
decidual cells
chorionic villi, also termed floating or free or terminal villi (*chorion*, a
    membrane; *villus*, shaggy hair)
primary and secondary villus, pl. villi (*villus*, shaggy hair)
stem villus
anchoring villus
syncytial knot (*syn-*, together + *-cyt*, cell)
amnion (*amnion*, the membrane around the fetus)
chorionic plate (*chorion*, a membrane)
syncytiotrophoblast (*syncitio-*, syncytium + *tropho-*, nourishment + *-blast*, germ)
cytotrophoblast (*cyto-*, cell + *tropho-*, nourishment + *-blast*, germ)
peripheral cytotrophoblast cells

Examine the tissue section of placenta. It consists of a chorionic plate, a basal plate, and between these two, the placental villi and the intervillous spaces. The placental villi extend from the fetal chorionic plate like branches of a tree, most ending freely. Some villi are attached to the compact maternal layer that is known as the basal plate of the placenta. The free chorionic villi float in the intervillous spaces that are filled with maternal blood.

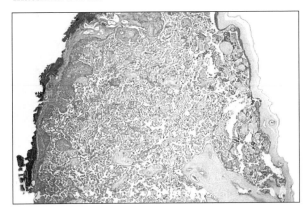

PLACENTA
Slide #199: Placenta; H&E stain; 10 μm paraffin section; human.

Higher magnification images:
 • (medium) fetal side of the placenta
 • (medium high) chorionic plate
 • (medium) basal plate
 • (high) decidual cells
 • (low) anchoring villus
 • (medium) stem villus
 • (high) placental villi

As the placenta forms, the fusiform stromal cells of the endometrium accumulate glycogen and lipid and develop into enlarged polygonal cells with lightly basophilic cytoplasm. These cells are the decidual cells and they constitute almost the entire stroma in the basal plate of this tissue section. Decidual cells produce a variety of secretory products. Fetal peripheral cytotrophoblast cells, which differ in location and morphology from the cytotrophoblast cells of the placental villi, are scattered among the decidual cells in the basal plate and recognizable because their cytoplasm is more distinctly basophilic than that of the decidual cells.

The chorionic plate is the fetal side of the placenta. In late pregnancy it is composed of the amnion and the chorion. The amnion is the membrane that surrounds the amniotic cavity within which the fetus grows; the chorion is derived from trophoblast cells. The smooth, simple cuboidal cells of the amnion rest on a thick basement membrane beneath which is an avascular extraembryonic mesenchymal layer. In the early stages of pregnancy an extraembryonic coelom exists between the amnion and the chorion, but as the fetus grows in size, the extraembryonic coelom is obliterated and the amnion and chorion fuse becoming the chorionic plate or chorio-amnion. The large villi that arise from the chorionic plate, bearing placental arteries and veins, are called stem villi. Those large villi that cross the intervillous space and fuse to the cytotrophoblast of the basal plate are called anchoring villi. The rest of the villi are variously termed placental, chorionic, floating, or tertiary villi.

The placental villi illustrated in this mature placenta consist of a core of very loose fibromuscular tissue supporting the fetal blood vessels enveloped by the syncytiotrophoblast. Resident macrophages in the villi are called Hofbaur cells. In the last half of pregnancy the internal cellular cytotrophoblast layer that characterizes the villi of the early placenta is absent; its cells have been incorporated into the syncytiotrophoblast. In the mature placenta, the blood–placenta barrier is formed of the syncytiotrophoblast, the fetal capillary epithelium and their basal laminae. Although the syncytiotrophoblast is usually thin, there are occasional regions where the nuclei are clumped together in a bulge called the syncytial knot. In mature placenta, degenerative changes result in the production of the eosinophilic fibrinoid material in the intervillous space.

MAMMARY GLAND

The mammary gland undergoes significant developmental changes during pregnancy to prepare for the nutrition of the neonate. Under the influence of the hormones of pregnancy, the exocrine ducts proliferate and generate increased numbers of secretory acini. The stroma becomes reduced as the parenchymal compartment increases. The following structures are illustrated in the tissue sections of the mammary gland and the nipple:

>mammary gland (*mamma*, breast)
>lactiferous duct and sinus (*lactis*, milk + *fero*, to bear)
>interlobular duct (*inter-*, between + *lobule*, diminutive of lobe)
>intralobular duct (*intra-*, within + *lobule*, diminutive of lobe)
>secretory acinus, pl. acini, or secretory alveolus, pl. alveoli
>nipple (diminutive of Anglo-Saxon *neb*, beak)
>areolar sebaceous gland

NIPPLE. Examine the tissue sections of the female and the male nipple. The epithelium if the nipple is thin and pigmented, and the dermis has tall papillae and bundles of smooth muscle. In the nipple, the areolar sebaceous glands are not associated with hairs. There is no morphological difference between the male and female nipple.

In the dermis of the nipple tissue section large lactiferous ducts with their simple or stratified columnar epithelium underlie the epidermis. Some of these ducts may join

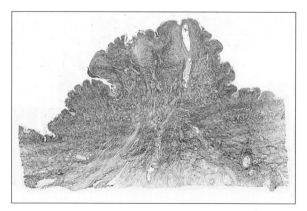

MALE NIPPLE
Slide #92: Male Nipple; H&E stain; 12 µm paraffin section; human.

There are no higher magnification images.

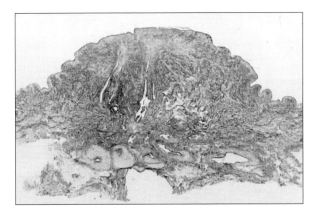

FEMALE NIPPLE
Slide #91: Female Nipple, I; H&E stain; 12 μm paraffin section; human.

There are no higher magnification images.

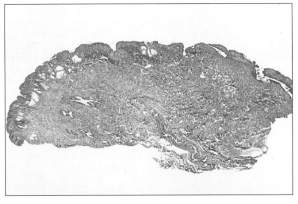

FEMALE NIPPLE: LACTIFEROUS DUCTS
Slide #91: Female Nipple, II; H&E stain; 12 μm paraffin section; human.

Higher magnification image:
- (medium) lactiferous ducts and sebaceous glands

together before emptying by pores on the nipple surface; the pores are usually lined by stratified squamous epithelium. Before terminating at the surface, the lactiferous ducts exhibit a dilatation, the lactiferous sinus, which is difficult to specifically identify in longitudinal section. Each of the lactiferous ducts drains a lobe of the mammary gland.

MAMMARY GLAND. These various sections of the mammary gland tissue illustrate differences in the relative proportions of the stroma and parenchyma in the pregnant versus the lactating gland. The mammary gland is a compound tubulo-alveolar gland consisting of 15–20 lobes, each drained by a branched lactiferous duct. The lobes are separated by dense irregular connective tissue and adipose tissue. Each lobe consists of several small lobules, which are groups of alveoli clustered around the terminal branch of a lactiferous duct. This terminal branch of the lactiferous duct is termed an intralobular duct and it connects to the small saccular alveoli.

In the mammary gland of the nonpregnant female it is difficult to distinguish alveolar ducts from alveoli in histological sections. Major changes occur in the pregnant adult mammary gland as it prepares for lactation. These changes include growth in length and branching of the duct system and proliferation of alveoli. The stroma

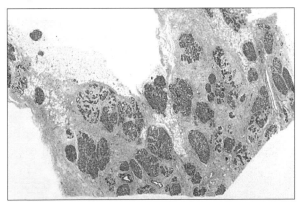

MAMMARY GLAND, PREGNANCY
Slide #90: Mammary Gland, Pregnancy; H&E stain; 10 μm paraffin section; human.

Higher magnification images:
- (medium) lobules
- (medium) lactiferous duct
- (high) alveoli and lobules

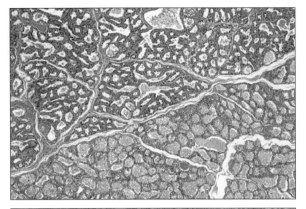

MAMMARY GLAND, LACTATING, I
Slide #90: Mammary Gland, Lactating, I; H&E stain;
10 μm paraffin section; human.

There are no higher magnification images.

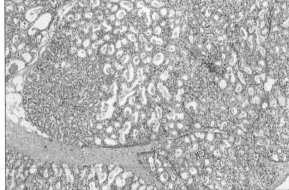

MAMMARY GLAND, LACTATING, II
Slide #90: Mammary Gland, Lactating, II; H&E
stain; 10 μm paraffin section; human.

There are no higher magnification images.

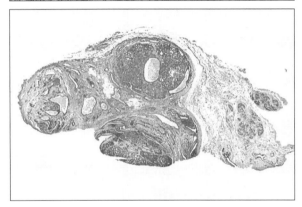

MAMMARY GLAND: LOBES
Slide #90: Mammary Gland, lobes; H&E stain; 10
μm paraffin section; human.

Higher magnification images:
  • (medium) lobules

becomes increasing infiltrated with lymphocytes, plasma cells, and eosinophils. In the later months of pregnancy the parenchymal cells enlarge and the alveoli and ducts become distended with colostrum, the first secretion of the mammary gland.

In the active mammary gland, most of the gland is represented by alveoli, with only narrow septa of connective tissue separating the large lobules. Not all alveoli may be in the same functional state at the same time. In some areas the alveoli are dilated with the milk and the glandular epithelium is thin, whereas in other areas the lumen is narrow and the alveolar epithelium is thick. Observe the sacculated alveoli that are closely packed within the well-demarcated lobules. Those saccules dilated by milk or colostrum have a low cuboidal epithelium, whereas those not so filled have a columnar one. The cell boundaries are indistinct, the nuclei round to oval and centrally located. Occasionally, myoepithelial cells can be seen between the glandular cells and the basement membrane. The intralobular ducts are lined with cuboidal cells and have longitudinally disposed myoepithelial cells.

21. THE EYE

The eyes are special sensory receptors that are specifically designed to detect visual stimuli and transmit meaningful signals regarding the external world to the brain. They are highly organized spherical bodies that permit light to enter within, focusing it onto a complex layer of photosensitive tissue.

The architecture of the eyeball corresponds to a fusion of segments of two spheres, each segment with an interior cavity. The anterior chambers of the eye are filled with aqueous humor (*aqua*, water; *umor*, liquid) whereas the posterior chamber is filled with the relatively solid, transparent vitreous body (*vitreous*, glass).

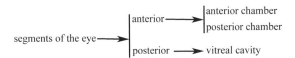

The wall of the entire eye consists of three concentric layers, with the innermost layer being a developmental outgrowth of the brain. Recognizing the structures that are part of each of the layers, or tunics, facilitates your understanding of the structural organization of the eye. The diagrammatic overview below of the principal component structures of the eye is based, in part, on the layers.

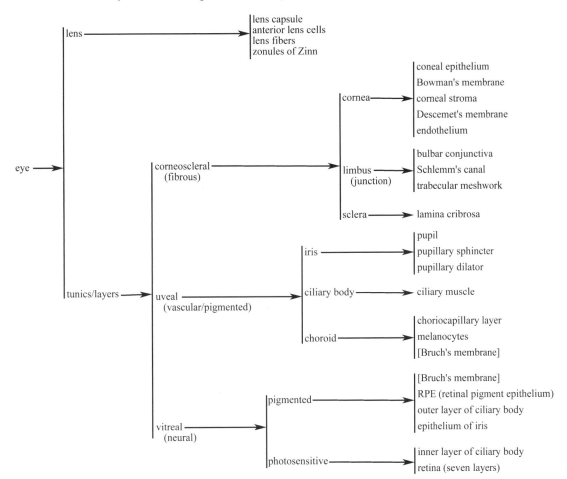

215

The eyeball is a difficult structure to preserve for histology without artifact because it is large and contains tissues with very different biochemical consistencies and physical properties, and these respond differently to standard preparative procedures. Thus, it is not unusual for the eyeball in tissue sections to be distorted in shape, or the retina to be separated artifactually from the interior of the eyeball. Quite frequently, as in the present tissue section, the lens is cracked and chipped. Look beyond these common artifacts of preparation as you examine this tissue section.

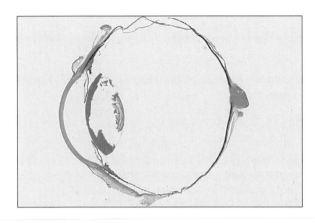

EYE

Slide #80: Eye; H&E; 10 μm paraffin section; human.

Higher magnification images:
- (medium) lens and pupil
- (medium) cornea
- (high) corneal epithelium
- (high) Descemet's membrane and endothelium
- (medium) limbus
- (high) Schlemm's canal
- (high) trabecular meshwork and Schlemm's canal
- (medium) sclera
- (medium lamina cribrosa
- (medium) sphincter pupillae
- (high) ciliary processes

The low–power view of this tissue section provides a general orientation to the eyeball. This eyeball has been sectioned in a horizontal plane in terms of the head and body, i.e., parallel to the floor. The transparent cornea is at its anterior pole and the optic nerve exits from the posterior pole toward the midline of the body or nasal side of the eyeball. The eyeball has two segments, an anterior and posterior segment. These segments differ in the radius of their curvature and in the nature of the material within the interior space, or chambers. The anterior segment is incompletely subdivided into an anterior and posterior chamber and is filled with the continuously circulating aqueous humor. The posterior segment has one chamber, the vitreal cavity, and it is occupied by the vitreal body. The vitreal body is a highly hydrated transparent gel composed of a stroma enclosing a watery fluid called the vitreous humor.

The three chambers of the eye are clearly identified by their boundaries. The anterior chamber, with a depth at its center of approximately 3 mm, is bounded by the cornea, the iris and the lens. The posterior chamber is a smaller area bordered anteriorly by the iris, posteriorly by the lens and its zonules, and laterally by the ciliary body. The large vitreal chamber or cavity corresponds to the posterior segment of the eye; it lies between the lens and the retina.

LENS

Examine the lens of the eye, which in this tissue section has been poorly preserved resulting in an artifactual chipping and distortion of its interior. In life, the lens can be quite elastic, but that elasticity decreases with increasing age. The lens is encapsulated by a homogeneous, transparent, highly refractile capsule composed of type IV collagen and proteoglycans. This extracellular capsule is a basement membrane and its position is explained by the embryonic development of the lens. Basically, the lens forms from embryonic ectoderm, the outermost tissue layer of the embryo. In the developing embryo, a plaque of ectoderm overlying the forming eyeball invaginates and pinches off a sphere of epithelium with its basement membrane on its outside surface. This sphere subsequently flattens and becomes the lens. The lens, therefore, is composed of modified epithelial cells. In the mature lens a single layer of cuboidal cells on the anterior surface (toward the cornea) is the subcapsular epithelium. Toward the lateral margin of the lens these epithelial cells undergo a process of maturation in which they become columnar in shape and hexagonal in cross-section. This morphological differentiation is accompanied by the loss of the cells' nuclei and cytoplasmic organelles, which are replaced by lens proteins termed crystallins. These crystallin-filled differentiated epithelial cells are termed lens fibers and they make up the bulk of the lens. The original lumen of the embryonic evagination from which the lens develops is obliterated in the mature lens, and the apical surfaces of the anterior lens cells (subcapsular epithelial cells) interdigitate with the lens fibers.

Suspensory ligaments (zonular fibers or zonules of Zinn) extend from the lens capsule, at the equator of the lens, to the inner surface of the ciliary body (described below) and hold the lens in place. These fibers are inelastic polymers of fine fibrils. It should be noted that with regard to designation of the position of the various structures of the eye and their parts, the side adjacent to the inside of the eye is called the inner side. Thus, the inner surface of the ciliary body is the surface facing the inside of the eye.

Consider the three tunics of the eye: (*1*) the outermost protective corneoscleral coat, (*2*) the middle uveal coat of vascularized connective tissue, and (*3*) the innermost layer, derived as an evagination of the embryonic brain. Each tunic has functionally and morphologically distinct component parts.

CORNEOSCLERA

The cornea (*corneus*, horny) is the transparent anterior portion of the corneoscleral layer, forming a dome-shaped elevation upon the eyeball. It is the principal site of refraction of light entering the eye. The cornea is avascular and highly innervated, and microscopically has five identifiable layers. These layers and the histological nature of these layers are listed in the following table, beginning with the outside.

layer of cornea	composition
corneal epithelium	stratified squamous epithelium that is normally kept moist by the tear film
Bowman's membrane	12 μ–thick dense mass of collagen fibrils
coneal stroma	composed of 200–250 highly ordered lamellae of mainly type I collagen fibril sheets, with scattered fibroblasts
Descemet's membrane	homogeneous basement membrane
corneal endothelium	single layer of flattened polygonal cells

The sclera (*skleros*, hard) is continuous with the cornea and encloses the rest of the eyeball. It is a dense irregular connective tissue that appears white and opaque in its fresh state. Like the cornea, it is avascular except for a few superficial blood vessels and, unlike the cornea, it is only sparsely innervated. Where it is exposed on the anterior portion of the eye, the sclera is covered by the bulbar conjunctiva, which is a transparent mucous membrane with a nonkeratinized stratified squamous epithelium that is continuous with the corneal epithelium. The bulbar conjunctiva is thin and transparent and sparsely vascularized. Laterally, the conjunctiva is continuous with the inside surfaces of the eyelids. Posteriorly, the sclera is covered by the fascial sheath of the eyeball. The sclera provides attachments for the extraocular eye muscles, which rotate the eye within the orbit.

There are two specialized regions of the corneoscleral coat: the lamina cribrosa and the limbus. The lamina cribrosa (*lamina*, thin plate; *cribrum*, a sieve) is the perforated disc in the sclera at the posterior pole where the axons of the optic nerve exit the interior of the eye. Most of the holes in the lamina cribrosa are small, allowing fascicles of fibers to exit, but a larger central hole is traversed by the central retinal artery and vein. Not surprisingly, this small lattice is the weakest part of the encasing corneoscleral coat and can bulge outward when intraocular pressure is elevated.

The limbus (*limbus*, a border), or sclerocorneal junction, marks the transition between the transparent cornea and the opaque sclera, and corresponds to the point where the segments of the two spheres of different radii conjoin to form the eyeball. Just deep to its inner surface, in the angle where the iris is attached, a circumferential space, called Schlemm's canal, is located. The endothelium-lined Schlemm's canal drains aqueous humor from the anterior chamber into veins of the circulatory system. A band of the stroma between Schlemm's canal and the anterior chamber is made up of strands of connective tissue covered by endothelium. The endothelium is continuous with the corneal endothelium. This region of the stroma, which the aqueous humor traverses en route to Schlemm's canal, is termed the trabecular meshwork.

UVEA

The middle tunic of the eye is the vascular tunic, called the uvea (*uva*, grape; presumably because it looks like a peeled grape when exposed). The anterior division of the uvea is the iris. The iris is a disc-shaped diaphragm with a hole at its center, termed the pupil. It is anchored peripherally in the ciliary body and separates the anterior and posterior chambers of the eye. The interior of the iris is a loose connective tissue containing the melanocytes that determine the color of the iris. The anterior surface of the iris is a discontinuous layer of fibroblasts and melanocytes. The posterior surface is covered by a heavily pigmented epithelium that is a continuation of the innermost (unpigmented) covering of the ciliary body. There are two sets of muscles located within the stroma of the iris and these control the diameter of the pupil. The sphincter muscle (sphincter pupillae) is a circumferentially oriented flat ring of smooth muscle cells at the inner margin of the pupil; it constricts of the pupil. The dilator muscle (dilator pupillae) is a thin, radially oriented layer of myoepithelial cells that is located anterior to the pigmented epithelial layer of the iris. It is diffusely organized and less conspicuous in tissue sections than the sphincter muscle. These muscles are innervated by fibers of the autonomic nervous system.

The ciliary body is the second principal component of the uveal layer. It is a circumferential thickened region of the uvea lying between the iris and the choroid. Bundles of smooth muscle in the base of the ciliary body make up its bulk. Several short projections, called ciliary projections extend from its surface toward the interior of the eye. The zonule fibers that extend from the capsule of the lens attach to the ciliary processes, holding the lens in place. The action of the ciliary muscles alters the shape and position of the lens to bring light into focus on the retina. Two epithelial layers, which are in fact parts of the vireal layer of the eye, cover the ciliary body. The outer layer, away from the lumen of the posterior chamber, is pigmented and the inner layer, adjacent to posterior chamber, is not. The nonpigmented inner layer is primarily responsible for the production of aqueous humor. An irregular region termed the ora serrata (*os*, pl. *ora*, mouth; *serra*, a saw) marks the junction of the ciliary body with the retina. The ora serrata is an anterior circumferential zone lining the vitreous chamber marking the transition where the thick multilayered retina becomes a thin layer containing no photoreceptor cells.

The choroid (from *choio-*, a membrane) is the third principal component of the vascular uvea. It is a thin, highly vascularized layer lying immediately interior to the sclera. It contains pigmented melanocytes that give it a brown color. The inner portion of the choroid, called the choriocapillaris, contains a dense bed of fenestrated capillaries that provides for the nutritional needs of the outer half of the retina. The choroid is well illustrated in the following tissue section. At the interface between the choroid and the pigmented epithelial cells of the retina is the refractile Bruch's membrane.

Bruch's membrane is a tripartite structure, consisting of a middle layer of elastic tissue bordered by the basement membrane of the retinal pigment epithelium and the basement membranes of the capillaires in the choriocapillaris.

VITREA

The innermost layer of the eye is the vitreal layer (*vitreo-*, glassy). The larger posterior component of this tunic is the photosensitive tissue of the eye and the nonphotosensitive anterior component forms the epithelial lining of the ciliary body and the iris. Embryology again provides a key to understanding the structure of this part of the eye: the entire vitreal layer originates as an evagination of the brain, one evagination on each side of the brain. What begins as a spheroid evaginated outgrowth of diencephalon subsequently invaginates into itself to form a two-layered cup-shaped extension of the brain. The outer wall of this cup gives rise to the thin retinal pigment epithelium (RPE), the inner layer of this cup gives rise to the neural retina, and the stalk of this evagination becomes the optic nerve.

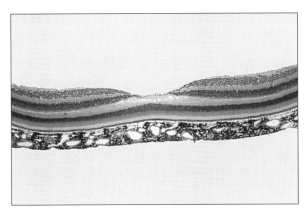

RETINA
Slide #79: Fovea; H&E stain; 3 μm methacrylate section; nonhuman primate.

Higher magnification images:
- (high) retina
- (higher) outer retina and RPE
- (medium) fovea

This tissue section, Slide # 79, provides cellular details of the retina that cannot be seen in the previous tissue section. The prominent depression in this tissue section is the fovea, described below.

The retinal pigment epithelium, or RPE, is single layer of cuboidal cells having a basal surface that rests on Bruch's membrane. The apical surfaces of these cells have long microvilli that project between the outer ends of the rods and cones, the photoreceptor cells of the neural retina. Tips of the outer segments of the rods deeply insert into the apical cytoplasm of these RPE cells although the two cell types are not physically bound to each other. The apical cytoplasm of these pigmented epithelial cells is filled with melanin granules that serve to absorb light and the phagocytosed ends of rods and cones that are undergoing lysosomal digestion within the RPE cells. Tight junctions between the cells of the RPE are responsible for the blood–retina barrier that protects the sensitive microenvironment of the retina.

RETINA

The sensory retina is a complex multilaminar structure that includes sensory and neural cells. These cells form a synaptically connected chain to relay signals from the retina to the brain. Basically, the photoreceptors (the rod and the cone cells) connect to first order neurons (bipolar cells) that connect to second order neurons (ganglion cells) that have axons that collect on the inner surface of the retina and exit the eyeball as the optic nerve. Additional cells include special interneurons (amacrine and horizontal cells) and neuroglial elements. The retina is best viewed as a special area of the brain and as such is a network of interconnected neurons and interneurons. As is the case with light microscope tissue sections of central nervous tissue, neuronal and neuroglial nuclei and cell bodies are identifiable but their attenuated processes become tangled in a feltwork of neuropil.

The neuroglial supporting cells of the retina are called Müller cells. Expanded endfeet of these supporting cells form the inner limiting membrane of the retina. This glial membrane is covered with a basement membrane that marks the boundary between the retina and the gel-like vitreous body in the vitreous chamber. On the other side of the retina, these supporting cells form intercellular junctions with the photoreceptors and these junctions comprise the outer limiting membrane of the retina. The nuclei of the Müller cells are located in the inner nuclear layer, but their cytoplasm is distributed throughout the thickness of the retina. Müller cells cannot be recognized in this material without special stains. Astrocytes, one of the main neuroglial cells of the central nervous system, are present in the ganglion and nerve fiber layers.

The layers of the retina represent zones where specific cellular components are clustered. These layers extend uninterrupted throughout the retina except at two areas: the optic disc where the nerve fibers (axons of the ganglion cells) exit and at the fovea where photoreceptors predominate and visual acuity is greatest. The names of the layers of the retina reflect both the main components within them as well as their position within the thickness of the retina. Note again, the convention is that structures near the vitreous cavity are designated inner, and those nearer the choroid are designated outer.

The receptors and neurons of the retina are arranged in seven alternating nuclear and plexiform (*plexus*, a braid + *forma*, form) layers. The layer of rods and cones is closest to the RPE; the nerve fiber layer is closest to the vitreous body. The layers and the principal components of each are as follows:

layer of retina (from inside of eye)	principal components
nerve fiber layer	unmyelinated axons of retinal ganglion cells that terminate in the brain
layer of ganglion cells	cell bodies and nuclei of retinal ganglion cells
inner plexiform layer	complex synaptic connections among the processes of neurons in the adjacent layers
inner nuclear layer	nuclei of horizontal cells, bipolar cells, Muller, and amacrine cell
outer plexiform layer	complex synaptic connections among the processes of cells in the adjacent layers
outer nuclear layer	several tiers of rod and cone nuclei and their cell bodies
layer of rods and cones	inner and outer segments of the rod and cone cellular processes

The fovea (*fovea*, a pit) is a small oval depression of the inner retina, approximately 1.5 mm in diameter. It is the area of highest visual acuity. It is located temporal to the optic disc, in the direct visual axis of the eye. This modified area of the retina contains only tightly packed cones. At its center all the other layers of the retina are pushed aside. Light rays can pass directly to the outer segment of the cones without passing through the normally intervening inner six layers.

The optic disc is the exit point for the optic nerve fibers as well as the entry and exit point for the central retinal artery and vein. The sensory retina does not extend into this region and because of this, this small area is called the blindspot of the retina. The optic disc is usually somewhat elevated and is also termed the optic papilla (*papilla*, a nipple).

The retina receives blood from two sets of arteries and veins. The inner half of the retina contains and is supported by branches of the central retinal vein and artery, which enter the eye through the optic nerve. The outer half of the retina depends on the vascular choroid for its metabolic requirements.

22. ULTRASTRUCTURE OF THE CELL

The purpose of this chapter is to illustrate common organelles, inclusions, and other cellular details visible in an electron micrograph. However, it should be appreciated that the ability to recognize these elements is only the first step in the knowledge to be acquired regarding them. It is important to comprehend the following:

- the basic function of each organelle, inclusion, and surface specialization,
- the functional significance of structural variability,
- the functional significance of numerical frequency, and
- the relationship between a cell's ultrastructural image and its light microscope image.

This chapter summarizes these interpretive issues, many of which have been addressed in previous chapters with respect to specific cells and tissues. Providing details of the molecular biology of the organelles, inclusions, and surface specializations is not the purpose of this chapter and a comprehensive textbook should be consulted for in-depth elaboration of the functional aspects.

MICROSCOPY IN HISTOLOGY

Histology is a visual discipline that is based on the study of structures that require optical aids in order to be seen. The principal optical instrument available to most people in the biomedical sciences is the light microscope, not the electron microscope. However, the light microscope has its limitations, for it does not permit detailed analysis of histology's fundamental unit of structure — the cell. The limit of resolution for a light microscope is approximately 200 nanometers (nm), whereas that of an electron microscope is approximately 0.2 nm. For the histologist, it is important to relate a cell's light microscope image to its fine structure, and vice versa. A student should understand what can and cannot be seen in the light microscope, and why, and appreciate that much of what we understand about the structure and function of cells is based on ultrastructural images. In the present chapter, a light microscope slide is referenced as a source of an example of the cell or tissue used to illustrate some ultrastructural feature. Locate the light microscope slide in the section of the CD-ROM in which the images are indexed by slide number.

STANDARD PREPARATIVE PROCEDURES IN ELECTRON MICROSCOPY

To prepare biological material for standard transmission electron microscopy, the tissue must be processed and embedded in a relatively hard plastic medium. The tissue sections are typically very thin (less than 0.08 µm, or 80 nm) and illuminated in the electron microscope by a beam of electrons traveling in a vacuum. The tissue is stained with heavy metals: osmium is incorporated into the cell membranes as part of the preparative techniques, and uranium and lead salts are used as stains after the thin section has been cut and mounted on a small copper grid that is inserted into the electron microscope for viewing. The images are recorded on photographic film exposed by the electrons that are able to pass through the tissue section. There is no color in an electron micrograph, just shades of black that are described as levels of electron density that range from electron dense to electron lucent.

CELLULAR ULTRASTRUCTURE

The flow chart on the following page diagrammatically lists the principal ultrastructural components of a generic cell, grouped into categories and subcategories for easier understanding of the relationships among them. These items represent a standard vocabulary of the fine structural composition of a cell.

This chapter will focus on the interpretative aspect of cellular ultrastructure — what a cell's ultrastructure can reveal of its function. It begins with a discussion of cell membranes, then progress to protoplasm and the nucleus and other cellular organelles. A discussion of cytoskeletal elements completes the overview.

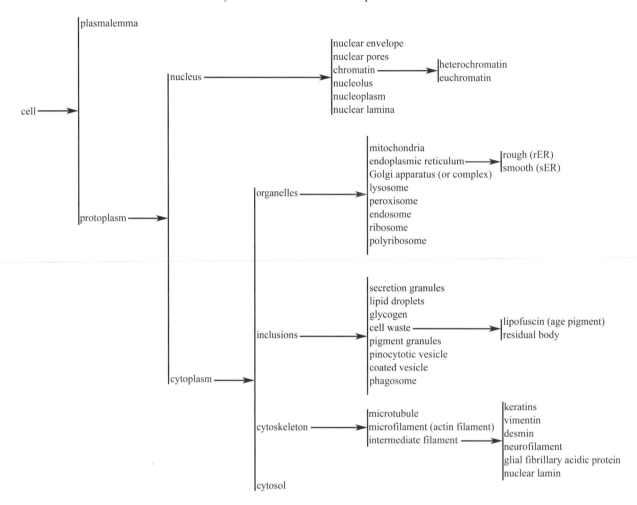

CELL MEMBRANES

Cell membranes are lipid bilayers within which are incorporated a great variety of proteins that are responsible for many of the properties that enable cells to interact with each other and their microenvironment. The ultrastructure of the membrane is visible principally because the electron dense osmium cross-links membrane lipid molecules, stabilizing the membranes and rendering them electron dense. The transmembrane proteins are not indentifiable in standard electron microscope thin sections without the use of specific immunocytochemical or ligand-binding markers. In electron micrographs, with the appropriate magnification and plane of section like that illustrated in Electron Micrograph #28, the cell membrane appears as a three-layered structure: two electron dense layers and an intervening electron lucent layer. This trilaminar structure is termed the unit membrane. It is approximately 7.5 nm thick and not visible in the light microscope. In low magnification electron micrographs, like most of the ones in this exercise, the membranes are visible as single electron dense lines.

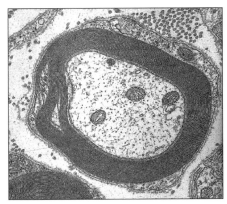

UNIT MEMBRANE
Electron Micrograph #28: Peripheral Myelin; rat.
(EM negative provided by Dr. Alan Peters)

Higher magnification image:
  • myelin lamellae (trilaminar membrane)

A cell membrane envelops the entire cell. It forms the interface between the cell's protoplasm and its external environment and controls the interaction of that cell with its environment. This enveloping membrane is specifically termed the plasmalemma or plasma membrane. Most of the intracellular organelles and inclusions are surrounded by a cell membrane of similar basic lipid bilayer composition that facilitates the function of the organelle or inclusion within the cytosol. These internal membranes are simply known as cell membranes.

PROTOPLASM

Protoplasm refers to the nucleus and the cytoplasm of the cell. The following series of electron micrographs illustrate a variety of cells in which the nuclear morphology, and the morphology and numerical density of the organelles, can be used to interpret the cell's function.

NUCLEUS

Electron Micrograph #1 illustrates a collection of cells and a range of nuclear morphologies. The characteristic appearance of a cell's nucleus is usually noted in its description. The shape of the nucleus — round, oval, or indented — is not particularly significant unless the observed shape varies from what normally characterizes the cell. The nucleus contains the cell's genomic DNA, which together with histones is termed chromatin. The nucleus is the site of DNA replication and of RNA synthesis. The electron dense chromatin is known as heterochromatin and it is transcriptionally inactive. The electron lucent chromatin is known as euchromatin and it is transcriptionally active. Thus, the relative amount of heterochromatin and euchromatin in a nucleus is a functionally significant feature; if cell's nucleus contains mostly euchromatin it is considered to be transcriptionally active and therefore to be metabolically active as well.

The following electron micrograph (#2) illustrates a hepatocyte, the parenchymal cell of the liver. A large round euchromatic nucleus and prominent nucleolus are characteristic of this cell. This image illustrates details of the structural organization of

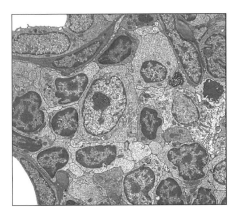

NUCLEUS
Electron Micrograph #1: Nuclear Morphologies; lymph node; rat.
Light microscopic view: Slide #71: Lymph Node (cortex)

Higher magnification images:
  • nuclei and cytoplasm
  • heterochromatin euchromatin and nucleolus

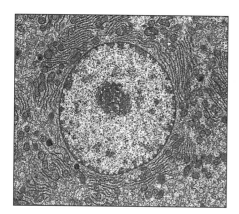

PROTOPLASM
Electron Micrograph #2: Nucleus and Cytoplasm; rat.

Higher magnification images:
• smooth and rough endoplasmic reticulum
• nucleoplasm and cytoplasm

the electron dense nucleolus, which differs in texture from the heterochromatin. The nucleolus is the site where ribosome particles are produced. A cell that is actively generating ribosomes will have one or more prominent nucleoli. Nucleoli are usually clearly visible in light microscope preparations. They are especially visible in the large euchromatic nuclei of neurons, like those in Slide #41, and the nuclei of hemopoietic precursor cells, like the myeloblsts in Slide #18.

CYTOPLASM

The volume of cytoplasm is another functionally significant morphological characteristic of cells. Cytoplasm contains three basic categories of formed elements: organelles, inclusions, and cytoskeleton. Organelles are specialized for carrying out some particular metabolic or synthetic function in the cell, and inclusions are metabolically inert. The cytoskeleton provides order and structure to the cytoplasm, which is approximately 70% water and contains dissolved organic and inorganic substances. The cell's cytosol is its cytoplasm minus the formed elements; it is the site of many metabolic events. Generally, the more metabolically active a cell, the more cytoplasm and organelles it has. Most of the cells depicted in the earlier micrograph (#1) are small lymphocytes in the cortex of the lymph node and have scant cytoplasm and few organelles. The high packing density of the nuclei, visible in the light microscope, reflects the small volume of cytoplasm that characterizes most lymphocytes in a lymph node. Upon antigenic stimulation, the lymphocyte nucleus becomes more euchromatic and the volume of cytoplasm increases as the cells become active.

Unlike the lymphocytes in the previous micrograph, the hepatocyte is a cell with ample cytoplasm containing a variety of membrane bound organelles. One of the most prominent organelles in this cell is the endoplasmic reticulum, a continuous membranous system of interconnected sacs and tubules. The lumen of the sacs and tubules is termed the cistern. The endoplasmic reticulum is subcategorized according to whether ribosomes are attached to its cytoplasmic surface. The endoplasmic reticulum to which ribosomes are attached is known as the rough endoplasmic reticulum (rER); it is the site of synthesis for proteins that are to be exported from the cell or to become integral membrane proteins. The attached ribosomes generate proteins that collect within the cisterns. The cytoplasm of a cell with substantial amounts of rER is basophilic in a standard light microscope preparation on account of the ribosomes. It should be noted that in the light microscope it is not possible to differentiate between basophilia that is attributed to free ribosomes or to ribosomes bound to endoplasmic reticulum, as in in the case of a basophilic erythroblast (Slide #18) vs. a plasma cell (Slide #33).

The smooth endoplasmic reticulum (sER) is a membranous system with no attached ribosomes. The three dimensional shape of the sER is that of anastomosing tubules, in contrast to the rER's arrangement of interconnected flattened plates. The sER has a variety of functions in various cells. In the hepatocyte, the smooth endoplasmic reticulum is involved in the detoxification of substances like barbiturates that are transported to the liver in the blood. In skeletal muscle, the sER sequesters calcium and is specifically known as the sarcoplasmic reticulum. In cells of the adrenal gland and ovary, the sER is well developed and involved in the synthesis of steroid hormones. In most cells, however, the sER is not especially abundant. Abundant or not, sER is not visible in the light microscope.

Mitochondria are ubiquitous organelles. They generate adenosine triphosphate (ATP) via oxidative phosphorylation. Therefore, cell with a high level of aerobic metabolism, like a cardiac muscle cell, has a high numerical density of mitochondria. In the hepatocyte of Electron Micrograph #3, the mitochondria are small and uniform and dispersed throughout the cytoplasm where they reside in proximity to the organelles that use the ATP they generate. A mitochondrion has a complex shape: a smooth outer membrane encloses an inner membrane that has multiple folds, termed cristae, extending plate-like into an internal matrix space. The inner membrane contains the ATP synthase and respiratory chains, so the greater the internal surface area, the greater the ability to generate ATP. Mitochondria are typically not visible in standard light microscope preparations.

Peroxisomes are small membrane bound vesicles involved in the catabolism of long-chain fatty acids. Peroxisomes generate hydrogen peroxide, which detoxifies various noxious agents in the cell. These organelles, like lysosomes, can only be identified with certainty using histochemical techniques that can localize any of their many oxidative enzymes.

The hepatocyte cytoplasm also contains glycogen, which is the common storage form of glucose. Glycogen appears as electron dense particles slightly larger in diameter than the ribosomes and it usually clusters around the smooth endoplasmic reticulum. Hepatocytes and white (glycolytic) skeletal muscle fibers typically have abundant glycogen. In the light microscope, glycogen is best visualized with the PAS stain, as in the glycolytic skeletal muscle fibers illustrated in Slide # 37.

The following electron micrograph (#3) provides additional details of the nuclear envelope. The nuclear envelope is an enveloping structure consisting of two cell membranes enclosing a narrow lumen termed the perinuclear cistern. The outer nuclear membrane is continuous with the rough endoplasmic reticulum and ribosomes on the cytoplasmic surface of the nuclear envelope function in a manner similar to those of the rER. The nuclear envelope has apertures known as nuclear pores that provide a means for material to pass between the nucleoplasm and the cytoplasm. Each pore is surrounded by an intricate nuclear pore complex that regulates the material that passes into and out of the nucleus. The number of nuclear pores in a nucleus is related to the metabolic activity of a cell: the greater the metabolic activity, the greater the number of pores. Nuclear pores are not visible in light microscope preparations.

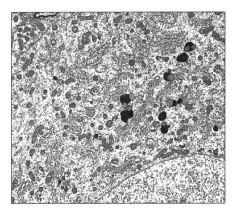

CYTOPLASMIC ORGANELLES AND INCLUSIONS
Electron Micrograph #3: Perikaryal Cytoplasm; neuron; nonhuman primate.

Higher magnification images:
• nuclear envelope
• Golgi apparatus
• rough endoplasmic reticulum and polysomes

The numerous small mitochondria scattered throughout the cytoplasm of this neuron (Electron Micrograph #3) reflect its high level of metabolic activity. The rER in this cytoplasm assembles into stacks surrounded by additional cytoplasmic ribosomes and polyribosomes. Polyribosomes are ribosomes that are actively synthesizing cytosolic proteins; several ribosomes are linked together upon the common strand of mRNA that is being translated. The neuronal cell body can be viewed in light microscope Slide #41. In the light microscope, these stacks of rER and ribosomes are visible and known as Nissl bodies.

Multiple complexes of the Golgi apparatus encircle the neuron's nucleus. These are not evident in the light microscope without the use of special stains. This membranous organelle is involved in the modification, packaging, and sorting of proteins and lipids within the cell. Its compound morphology of curved membranous cisterna and associated transport and transitional vesicles reflect its functional polarization. Products are delivered to the cisternae on the convex side of this organelle, processed through the series of stacked membranous cisternae, and released on the concave side. The packaged products may be delivered to another organelle or secreted from the cell.

Lipofuscin is the membrane bound residual debris that accumulates with advancing age in neurons like this one, and cardiac muscle cells. In these two cell types lipofuscin is also called age pigment and it serves as a biomarker of advancing age. In cells other than neurons and cardiac myocytes, similar membrane bound packages of undigested debris represent the final stage of lysosomal intracellular digestion and are termed residual bodies. Lipofuscin and residual bodies, when abundant, are visible in light microscope preparations.

The characteristic basophilia of the plasma cell, illustrated below in Electron Micrograph #10 is attributed to ribosomes upon the surface of the rough endoplasmic reticulum that dominates the cytoplasm of this connective tissue cell. The plasma cell generates antibodies that are synthesized in the rER. Polyribosomes cluster on the surface of the rER and clusters are visible in regions where surfaces of the rER have been sectioned tangentially. Another characteristic feature of the plasma cell, which also can be viewed in light microscope images of Slide #33, is its pale cytocentrum. Although the Golgi apparatus is only barely within the plane of this electron micrograph, its location in the center of the cell and its lack of ribosomes account for the characteristic pale cytocentrum of the plasma cell. The absence of secretion granules in this cell's cytoplasm indicates that the synthesized product is released continuously.

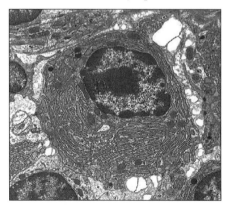

PROTEIN SYNTHESIS
Electron Micrograph #10: Plasma Cell; rat.

Higher magnification images:
- nucleus and rough endoplasmic reticulum
- cytocentrum
- rough endoplasmic reticulum

Electron Micrograph #4 illustrates two morphologically and functionally distinct cell types, one that is involved in exocytosis of a stored product and the other involved in absorption from the lumen it borders. The goblet cell, which has been viewed in a number of light microscope images, such as Slide #117, synthesizes mucinogen and stores it in apical secretion granules until it is to be released into the lumen of the gut. Organelles associated with this exocrine function appear in the apical perinuclear cytoplasm of the goblet cell: rER and a small Golgi apparatus. The nascent mucinogen granules in the perinuclear area are to be added to the coalesced apical droplet.

The principal function of the absorptive cell is reflected in the regular array of microvilli on its apical surface; microvilli increase the amount of membrane exposed to the luminal contents thereby increasing the cell's ability to absorb materials. The

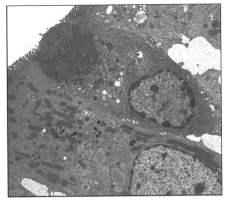

SECRETION AND ABSORPTION
Electron Micrograph #4: Simple Columnar Epithelium; gut; rat.

Higher magnification images:
* intercellular interdigitation (plasmalemma)
* mucinogen inclusions (secretory granules)

cytoplasm of the absorptive cell includes mitochondria that are necessary to provide energy to fuel the absorptive and processing activities. Lysosomes in the cytoplasm digest endocytosed material. Irregular bodies of amorphous material in the deep perinuclear cytoplasm of this cell are lipid droplets, which coalesce in the aqueous environment of the cytosol. Generally, the columnar absorptive cell is recognized in the light microscope by its striated border.

The fibroblast in Electron Micrograph #8 is the connective tissue cell responsible for synthesizing and secreting the principal constituents of the extracellular matrix. Typically this cell has relatively sparse cytoplasm, as observed in light microscope Slide #33. Inspection of its ultrastructure reveals cytoplasmic organelles associated with the fibroblast's role in the constant turnover of the matrix: profiles of rER, a Golgi apparatus for packaging the matrix material for export, and numerous transport vesicles. Pinocytotic vesicles opening onto the surface of the fibroblast may be involved in export or import functions. In a static image such as this, it is not possible to determine whether the vesicles are filling, emptying, or simply returning membrane to the plasmalemma.

The nuclear lamina is illustrated in this image of the fibroblast. This nuclear structure is a 100 nm wide feltwork of nuclear lamin that lines the nucleoplasm side of the inner membrane of the nuclear envelope and provides structure to the nucleus. Nuclear lamin is one of several types of intermediate filaments.

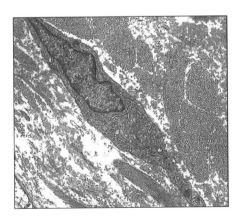

NUCLEAR LAMINA AND SYNTHETIC ACTIVITIES
Electron Micrograph #8: Fibroblast; rat.

Higher magnification images:
* rough ER and pinocytotic vesicles
* transport and secretory vesicles

Continuing on the topic of intracellular inclusions, Electron Micrograph #9 illustrates how electron microscope images may provide less information than light microscope images. The macrophage and the eosinophil in this micrograph both contain electron dense inclusions in their cytoplasm. The eosinophil is the granulocyte observed in slides #33 and #17 that contains characteristic eosinophilic granules and azurophilic lysosomal granules. Since an electron micrograph depicts images in shades of grey and black, the cytoplasmic granules of the eosinophil must be recognized by characteristics other than color. Because these cell-specific granules do have a characteristic fine

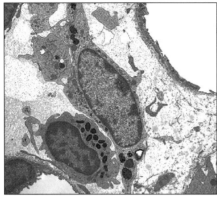

CELLULAR INCLUSIONS
Electron Micrograph #9: Macrophage and Eosinophil; rat.

Higher magnification images:
- macrophage cytoplasm (lysosomes)
- secretory granules and residual bodies
- fenestrated capillary

structure—an electron dense core, the internum, surrounded by a less dense externum—the eosinophil is easily recognized in the electron microscope. The dense core of the eosinophil's cell-specific granule is responsible for the characteristic refractile nature of these granules when viewed in the light microscope.

Compare the fine structure of the macrophage with that of the eosinophil. The phagocytic and digestive activity of the macrophage is reflected in its cytoplasmic organelles: rER, Golgi apparatus, and mitochondria share perinuclear cytoplasm with numerous small vesicles that are likely to be lysosomes. It is not possible to identify lysosomes for certain without using a histochemical technique to demonstrate the presence of acid hydrolases within them. The cytoplasm of the macrophage contains several secondary lysosomes and residual bodies. A secondary lysosome is a membrane bound vacuole containing phagocytosed substrate and lysosomal enzymes; the residual body is a membrane bound body containing the undigested remnants of enzymatic digestion. The heterogeneous content of these various inclusions indicates they are part of the macrophage's lysosomal digestion system. In the light microscope, the macrophage is frequently recognized by its characteristic empty appearing phagocytic vacuoles (emptied of their contents by the standard preparative procedures) as in slide #33, or by specific phagocytosed material, as in slide #7.

Finally, with regard to the functional significance of nuclear morphology: the nucleus of the macrophage is more euchromatic than that of the eosinophil, reflecting the greater transcriptional activity of this cell compared to the terminally differentiated eosinophil. The fact that the nucleus of the eosinophil does not appear lobed is not unusual given the thinness of the tissue section.

Electron Micrograph #19 illustrates morphological features of cells actively engaged in transepithelial transport. The transport process clearly requires high levels of energy as reflected in the number of mitochondria concentrated in the basal compartment of these cells. The mitochondria are aligned with the basally infolded plasmalemma, a location that brings the ATP they produce into proximity with the energy-dependent transmembrane proteins that pump ions out of the cells against a concentration gradient. The elaboration of the plasmalemma in the base of these cells provides

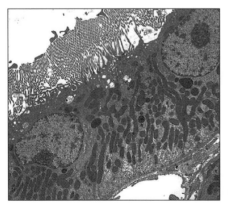

TRANSCELLULAR TRANSPORT
Electron Micrograph #19: Microvilli and Basal Enfoldings; rat.

Higher magnification images:
- basal infoldings (mitochondria)
- endocytotic vesicles and vacuoles

increased surface area across which to pump ions. These infolded membranes and aligned mitochondria may be light microscopically visible in the basal compartment of striated ducts, as illustrated in the ducts of Slide #102.

The luminal surface of the cells in Electron Micrograph #19 is also involved in transport across a membrane, in this case, absorption into the cell. The microvilli amplify the luminal surface area and thereby provide the increased means for trans-membrane transport into the cell. At the base of the microvilli tubular invaginations and vesicles and vacuoles, collectively termed endosomes, transport larger materials into the cell by endocytosis. In the light microscope this microvillous border is the brush border of the proximal tubules in the kidney, Slide #160.

CYTOSKELETON

The final two electron micrographs illustrate cytoskeletal elements. A cell's cytoskeleton is a network of intracellular filaments and tubules that functions to maintain cell shape and to provide intracellular pathways. They are bolow the resolution of the light microscope, and therefore not individually visible light microscopically. Microtubules and neurofilaments are visible in the axoplasm of the transversely sectioned myelinated axon illustrated in Electron Micrograph #13. Microtubules are hollow cylindrical polymers of tubulin dimers, approximately 25 nm in diameter; in this micrograph the microtubules appear as uniform circular profiles. Microtubules are frequently closely associated with organelles, like mitochondria, which they transport within the cell with the aid of microtubule-associated molecular motors. The small solid dots in the axoplasm are transversely sectioned neurofilaments, the intermediate filaments of neurons. Intermediate filaments are approximately 10 nm in diameter and provide the cell with the ability to withstand tensile forces. Microtubules and intermediate filaments are also present in the cytoplasm of the associated Schwann cell that surrounds the axon. The intermediate filament in the supporting cell is glial fibrillary acidic protein, abbreviated GFAP. Morphologically the intermediate filaments are not distinguishable from each other (except by location), but they can be easily identified using immuno-cytochemical methods because they are protein polymers.

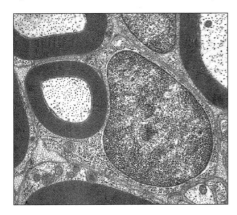

MICROTUBULES AND INTERMEDIATE FILAMENTS
Electron Micrograph #13 Myelinated Axon.
(EM negative providd by Dr. Alan Peters.)

Higher magnification image:
 • myelinated axon (neurofilaments and microtubules)

Extracellular collagenous fibers of the endoneurium surround the Schwann cells in this peripheral nerve fiber. Do not confuse the intracellular cytoskeletal elements with the extracellular fibers. These extracellular collagen fibrils constitute the endoneurium of peripheral nerves, like the one illustrated in light microscope Slide #52

The final electron micrograph is an oblique section through the apical portion of absorptive enterocytes in which there reside several cytoskeletal elements. Polymerized actin comprises the cell's population of microfilaments. These microfilaments are approximately 6 nm in diameter and difficult to visualize unless they are bundled together or uniformly oriented. The core of the microvillus is formed of a bundle of stable actin filaments whose purpose is to provide structural support. Individual actin filaments are visible in the I–band of skeletal muscle, as in Electron Micrograph #16.

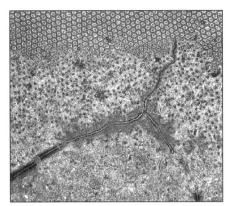

Microfilaments and Intermediate Filaments
Electron Micrograph #6: Junctional Complex; rat.

Higher magnification images:
- microvilli (actin core)
- tight junction (plasmalemma)
- desmosome and zonula adherens

A dense meshwork of actin filaments and unpolymerized actin is typically concentrated in the cytoplasm just beneath the plasma membrane of most cells, in a region referred to as the cell cortex. In such a location the actin provides support to the cell surface and mediates changes in the shape of the cell, as for the purpose of phagocytosis or ameboid movement through the matrix. The cell cortex is particularly well developed in the area of the terminal web illustrated in this plate.

The electron density associated with the zonula adherens in this micrograph is attributed to the concentrated presence of actin and actin binding proteins. Extracellularly linked transmembrane proteins in the zonula adherens link intracellularly to actin binding proteins that in turn link to the actin of the terminal web. In this way, the zonula adherens links the terminal web of one cell to the terminal webs of the adjacent cells. The terminal web is illustrated in Slide #117.

The desmosomes in this micrograph are associated with a third class of intermediate filament, keratin, the intermediate filament of epithelial cells. Bundles of keratin form the tonofilaments that loop into the desmosomes and provide the linked cells with strong resistance to tensile forces. Desmosomes are not visible in the light microscope although they do account for the intercellular bridges visible in the statum spinosum of the epidermis, viewed in Slide # 84.

INDEX

SYSTEM REQUIREMENTS:

PC MSWindows 95/98/NT, 586 133 Mhz
Macintosh System 7.1, 68030 processor

Requires also:
256 color, 680 x 480 pixel monitor,
CD-ROM drive (double speed or faster),
World Wide Web Browser